SLEEP-RELATED BREATHING DISORDERS

LUNG BIOLOGY IN HEALTH AND DISEASE

Executive Editor

Claude Lenfant
Director, National Heart, Lung and Blood Institute
National Institutes of Health
Bethesda, Maryland

The opinions expressed in these volumes do not necessarily represent the views of the National Institutes of Health.

SLEEP-RELATED BREATHING DISORDERS

EXPERIMENTAL MODELS AND THERAPEUTIC POTENTIAL

Edited by

David W. Carley
Miodrag Radulovacki

University of Illinois
Chicago, Illinois, U.S.A.

MARCEL DEKKER, INC.　　　　　NEW YORK · BASEL

Library of Congress Cataloging-in-Publication Data
A catalog record for this book is available from the Library of Congress.

ISBN: 0-8247-0877-6

This book is printed on acid-free paper.

Headquarters
Marcel Dekker, Inc.
270 Madison Avenue, New York, NY 10016
tel: 212-696-9000; fax: 212-685-4540

Eastern Hemisphere Distribution
Marcel Dekker AG
Hutgasse 4, Postfach 812, CH-4001 Basel, Switzerland
tel: 41-61-260-6300; fax: 41-61-260-6333

World Wide Web
http://www.dekker.com

The publisher offers discounts on this book when ordered in bulk quantities. For more information, write to Special Sales/Professional Marketing at the headquarters address above.

Current printing (last digit):
10 9 8 7 6 5 4 3 2 1

PRINTED IN THE UNITED STATES OF AMERICA

INTRODUCTION

*The gods confound the man who first found out how to distinguish hours.
Confound him, too, who in this place set up a sundial, to cut and hack my
day so wretchedly into small portions!*

Titus Maccius Plautus, 250–184 BC

Nowadays, the portions may not be so small, as one is for sleep and the
other is for wakefulness. The balance between these two phases of our life
has become an important issue for modern medicine and human behavior.
To put it simply, this balance controls the rhythm of our life, at least up to a
point. As is often the case in human biology, it is because of disruptions in
the equilibrium between sleep and wakefulness that clinicians and medical
researchers have focused on learning about the mechanisms controlling the
rhythmicity of our life.

Over the past decades, a good deal of work has been done to
understand sleep and its disorders. Although much more needs to be done,
much is already known. For example, we know that many of the
manifestations of sleep disorders are circulatory (such as hypertension) or

iii

respiratory (apnea) or even a combination of both. But, many other functions, such as behavior, are also affected by sleep disorders.

This Lung Biology in Health and Disease series recognized very early the importance of research on sleep, its mechanisms, and its disorders. Since 1981, the series has presented 12 volumes discussing sleep, including six exclusively devoted to this function. All along, however, one approach to the study of sleep has been missing: the development and study of well-characterized animal models. This is an obvious deficiency that contrasts with what has been done almost systematically in the study of most other known biological functions and their disorders. Furthermore, it is well known that what is viewed as "abnormal" in humans is often "normal" in other species. Thus, the study of animal models is a powerful tool for understanding human biology.

This volume, edited by Drs. David Carley and Miodrag Radulovacki, fills an important gap in this series of monographs, and in the field itself. Those who work in the field will benefit from the knowledge presented in this volume, and so eventually will all the patients who can only dream of a good night's sleep!

Drs. Carley and Radulovacki and their authors are making an important contribution. As the editor of this series, I thank them for giving me the opportunity to present this volume to the readership.

Claude Lenfant, M.D.
Bethesda, Maryland

PREFACE

Sleep-related breathing disorders have been recognized and described by astute clinicians for millennia. The past several decades have witnessed intensive and accelerating investigation into the epidemiology, genetics, pathophysiology, and clinical as well as behavioral consequences of sleep-related breathing disorders. The Lung Biology in Health and Disease series has played an important role in consolidating the accumulating knowledge in this area and in providing a focused view of the state of the art. The recent volume *Sleep Apnea*, edited by Allan Pack, highlights the public health significance of sleep-related breathing disorders in terms of their high prevalence and significant morbidity, as well as our lack of fully adequate treatment options. Despite these advances, progress toward defining the exact pathogenic mechanisms of sleep-related breathing disorders and their consequences has been slow. Elucidation of these mechanisms will undoubtedly yield new insights to improve both diagnosis and treatment of these disorders.

A lack of well-defined animal model systems for sleep-related breathing disorders has been an important factor limiting progress in this area of knowledge. Over the past decade, several approaches have been developed based on spontaneously occurring and experimentally induced apnea and hypoxia in sleeping rodents, cats, dogs, sheep, and pigs. In parallel with these efforts, tools of modern molecular biology and functional neuroanatomy have increasingly been applied to investigate the neurobiology of sleep and respiration. The synthesis of these two approaches has led to significant recent advances in understanding the pathogenesis of sleep-related breathing disorders and their consequences at the molecular, cellular, and integrative systems levels.

Our goal in this volume is to provide a synthesis of the current knowledge. To this end, we present a series of comprehensive reviews of experimental approaches to the pathogenesis and consequences of sleep-related breathing disorders based on a solid foundation of basic science. Accordingly, we have divided the volume into four sections. First, we provide an introduction to the subject. The second part illustrates the application of fundamental methods of modern neuroscience to important questions regarding brainstem control of sleep and breathing. The third provides comprehensive reviews of experimental methods utilizing experimentally induced breathing disorders in sleeping animals. These methods represent a valuable new approach to define the pathogenic mechanisms leading to the clinical *consequences* associated with sleep-related breathing disorders such as sleep apnea. Part Four highlights the complementary strengths of several methods based on spontaneously occurring apnea in animals to further our understanding of the *causes* of sleep-related breathing disorders. Parts Three and Four also emphasize the potential opportunities for developing improved diagnostic and therapeutic strategies using these experimental approaches.

Sleep-Related Breathing Disorders: Experimental Models and Therapeutic Potential is intended to serve the needs and interests of clinician investigators and basic scientists alike. It is our hope that clinicians will broaden the scope of these experimental approaches, using evolving knowledge of the epidemiology, genetics, risk factors, and pathobiology of sleep-related breathing disorders, and that basic scientists, stimulated to see the clinical relevance of their work, will continue to expand the armamentarium of methods used to examine the control of sleep and breathing in health and disease.

We thank all the contributors to this volume for their thoughtful, thorough, and trenchant reviews. We are especially grateful to Dr. Claude Lenfant for his encouragement, support, and assistance in producing this volume.

David W. Carley
Miodrag Radulovacki

CONTRIBUTORS

Julie Arsenault, M.Sc. Physiology and Respiratory Research Unit, University of Sherbrooke, Sherbrooke, Quebec, Canada

Helen A. Baghdoyan, Ph.D. Professor of Anesthesiology and Pharmacology, Department of Anesthesiology, University of Michigan, Ann Arbor, Michigan, U.S.A.

David W. Carley, Ph.D. Professor of Medicine, Bioengineering, and Pharmacology, Department of Medicine, College of Medicine, University of Illinois, Chicago, Illinois, U.S.A.

Michael A. Castellini, Ph.D. Professor and Director, Institute of Marine Sciences, University of Alaska Fairbanks, Fairbanks, Alaska, U.S.A.

Nancy L. Chamberlin, Ph.D. Assistant Professor, Department of Neurology, Harvard Medical School, and Beth Israel Deaconess Medical Center, Boston, Massachusetts, U.S.A.

Maria F. Czyżyk-Krzeska, M.D., Ph.D. Associate Professor, Department of Molecular and Cellular Physiology, University of Cincinnati, Cincinnati, Ohio, U.S.A.

Eugene C. Fletcher, M.D. Professor and Director, Division of Pulmonary and Critical Care Medicine, Department of Medicine, University of Louisville School of Medicine, Louisville, Kentucky, U.S.A.

David Gozal, M.D. Professor, Vice Chair for Research, and Director, Department of Pediatrics, Kosair Children's Hospital Research Institute, University of Louisville School of Medicine, Louisville, Kentucky, U.S.A.

Joan C. Hendricks, V.M.D., Ph.D. Professor, Department of Clinical Studies, School of Veterinary Medicine, University of Pennsylvania, Philadelphia, Pennsylvania, U.S.A.

Richard L. Horner, Ph.D. Assistant Professor, Departments of Medicine and Physiology, University of Toronto, Toronto, Ontario, Canada

R. John Kimoff, M.D., F.R.C.P.(C) Director, Sleep Disorders Center, Respiratory Division, McGill University Health Centre, Montreal, Quebec, Canada

Leszek Kubin, Ph.D. Research Associate Professor, Department of Animal Biology, University of Pennsylvania, Philadelphia, Pennsylvania, U.S.A.

Ralph Lydic, Ph.D. Bert La Du Professor, Department of Anesthesiology; Professor, Department of Physiology; and Associate Chair, Anesthesiology Research, University of Michigan, Ann Arbor, Michigan, U.S.A.

Christopher Paul O'Donnell, Ph.D. Associate Professor, Department of Medicine, Johns Hopkins School of Medicine, Baltimore, Maryland, U.S.A.

Jean-Paul Praud, M.D., Ph.D. Professor, Department of Pediatrics and Department of Physiology and Surgery, University of Sherbrooke, Sherbrooke, Quebec, Canada

Miodrag Radulovacki, M.D., Ph.D. Professor of Pharmacology and Medicine, Department of Pharmacology, University of Illinois, Chicago, Illinois, U.S.A.

Sylvain Renolleau, M.D. Pediatric and Neonatal Intensive Care Unit, Armand-Trousseau Children's Hospital, Paris, France

Clifford B. Saper, M.D., Ph.D. James Jackson Putnam Professor and Chairman, Department of Neurology, Harvard Medical School, and Beth Israel Deaconess Medical Center, Boston, Massachusetts, U.S.A.

Richard Stephenson, Ph.D. Associate Professor, Departments of Physiology and Zoology, University of Toronto, Toronto, Ontario, Canada

Kingman P. Strohl, M.D. Professor, Department of Medicine, Case Western Reserve University, and Louis Stokes Cleveland VA Medical Center, Cleveland, Ohio, U.S.A.

Sigrid Carlen Veasey, M.D. Assistant Professor, Department of Medicine, University of Pennsylvania, Philadelphia, Pennsylvania, U.S.A.

CONTENTS

SLEEP-RELATED
BREATHING DISORDERS

Part One

OVERVIEW

1

Pathophysiology of Sleep-Related Breathing Disorders
Unanswered Questions

DAVID W. CARLEY and MIODRAG RADULOVACKI

University of Illinois
Chicago, Illinois, U.S.A.

The last two decades have witnessed an exponential increase in knowledge regarding sleep-related breathing disorders (SRBD). Significant strides have been made in our understanding of these disorders with respect to epidemiology and risk factors, pathogenesis, clinical and behavioral consequences, and appropriate diagnostic and treatment strategies. Still, work to understand these factors in terms of the underlying cellular and molecular processes is in its infancy. As detailed in the subsequent chapters of this volume, fundamental tools and approaches of molecular biology and quantitative neuroscience are now being employed to study SRBDs. The next decade should mark important advances in this area, with significant progress in therapies directed at the specific pathophysiology of these disorders.

Patients with SRBD can exhibit a spectrum of respiratory disturbances during sleep, including: central apneas, operationally defined as cessation of respiratory effort for more than 10 sec; obstructive apneas, characterized by continued inspiratory efforts against an occluded upper airway; mixed apneas, which present with an initial central component followed immediately by an obstructive component; hypopneas, associated with partial collapse of the upper airway and an attendant drop in pulmonary ventilation; and respiratory event-related arousals, characterized by increased inspiratory force generation leading to arousal from sleep but not impaired gas exchange (1). Disordered breathing events may be a normal phenomenon during transitions from wakefulness to sleep and during rapid eye movement (REM) sleep in man (2,3). However, when the frequency of disordered breathing events becomes high, daytime symptoms and clinical sequelae can result. A generalized respiratory disturbance index (RDI) is most often used clinically to assess the overall frequency of disordered breathing events of any type during sleep. Although early studies suggested that healthy subjects rarely exhibited an RDI > 5 (2–5), it has thus far proven impossible to identify a threshold RDI above which behavioral or clinical morbidity results.

I. Public Health Significance

Sleep-related breathing disorders are a significant public health concern, with a prevalence in the U.S. general population of at least 2–5% (6,7). Accumulating evidence suggests that morbid consequences of untreated SRBD include hypertension, coronary artery disease, myocardial infarction, arrhythmia, stroke, dementia, depression, cognitive dysfunction, sexual dysfunction, and injury due to accidents. Partinen and Guilleminault (8) demonstrated that sleep apnea patients to have three times the prevalence of heart disease and four times the prevalence of cerebrovascular disease compared to the general population. This may reflect the fact that the risk of developing hypertension, a major risk factor for cardiovascular and cerebrovascular disease, is elevated in patients with sleep apnea, irrespective of age, gender, or body mass index (9,10). In a group of elderly nursing home residents, Ancoli-Israel et al. (11) demonstrated a strong correlation between apnea and dementia and between the severity of apnea and severity of dementia. Untreated sleep apnea has also been associated with increased mortality (12,13).

Chapters 6 and 7 detail recent experimental approaches to the systematic study of the pathophysiological consequences of SRBD in animal model systems. These methods may help to define the causative pathways responsible for the consistent associations of SRBD with both cardiovascular and cerebrovascular morbidity and mortality (8–10,12,13).

Significant neurocognitive changes are also commonly associated with SRBD. Excessive daytime sleepiness is reported by almost every patient with sleep apnea and related syndromes (14). This symptom is often presumed to result from the disruption of sleep continuity attendant to repetitive disordered breathing events during sleep. However, strong associations between quantitative measures of sleepiness and sleep fragmentation have rarely been demonstrated. Still, some correlation has been found consistently between SRBD severity and both subjective (15) and objective (16,17) assessments of sleepiness. Impairment of mood, memory, problem-solving ability, vigilance, reaction time, and motor coordination have been associated with SRBD (18,19). Each of these impairments can negatively impact perceived quality of life, and can return toward normal, but often not to normal, with institution of therapy (20). Considerable work remains to define the constellation of factors that contribute neurocognitive deficits associated with SRBD, and to the recovery of these functions with treatment. This understanding may yield strategies for better diagnostic and treatment procedures.

II. Pathogenic Mechanisms

No general agreement exists regarding mechanisms underlying the generation or termination of apneas during sleep. It is now clear, however, that in general, patients with primarily obstructive apnea have redundant pharyngeal tissue with relatively narrow and collapsible upper airways (for recent reviews, see Refs. (21–24). These anatomical defects can predispose to upper airway collapse during sleep, launching the vicious cycle of sleep apnea–arousal–ventilation that is a hallmark of the syndrome. Still, the change in behavioral state from wakefulness to sleep is necessary for airway collapse even in the most severe presentations of sleep apnea. Numerous investigations of state-dependent activation of upper airway muscles demonstrate the importance of active and coordinated control of motor outputs to the upper airway in avoiding airway collapse or flow limitation (23–27; for a review, see Ref. 28).

It now appears that in most patients, total (apnea) or partial (hypopnea) collapse of the pharyngeal airway during sleep arises from both deficient airway anatomy and state-related influences on airway muscle function. Changes in airway geometry and collapsibility are associated with transitions among behavioral states in everyone. These changes primarily result from state-dependent alteration in reflex control of the intrinsic upper airway muscles (29). Activation of pharyngeal dilator muscles, such as the genioglossus, can widen and stiffen the extrathoracic airways. Some evidence suggests that augmented reflex activation of pharyngeal dilators, possibly by phasic negative intraluminal pressure, is an important compensatory mechanism during wakefulness in patients with obstructive sleep apnea (30). The ability to sense and respond to changes in inspiratory resistence and negative pressure is attenuated during sleep even in healthy individuals (31,32). Thus, a patient with an anatomically narrow airway who relies on reflex activation of dilator muscles to maintain airway patency during wakefulness will be vulnerable to airway collapse during sleep.

This viewpoint suggests that interventions intended to specifically maintain upper airway reflexes at their waking levels throughout sleep might provide an effective treatment strategy for obstructive SRBD. Many of the intrinsic pharyngeal dilator muscles are directly innervated by neurons residing in the hypoglossal nucleus of the medulla (33,34). Unfortunately, the anatomy, connectivity, neuropharmacology, electrophysiology, and molecular biology of this nucleus cannot be readily explored in man. Chapters 2–5 present approaches to these and related questions using quantitative investigational methods applied in several animal systems.

Factors independent of upper airway anatomy and physiology have also been suggested to contribute to the pathophysiology of SRBD. It has been argued that general instability of ventilatory control produces fluctuating drive to the diaphragm and to the pharyngeal muscles in SRBD (35,36). Such fluctuations cause attendant alterations in upper airway resistance and collapsibility even in normal individuals (35,37). In fact, Önal and Lopata (38) showed that tracheostomized SRBD patients exhibit obstructive apnea when breathing through their anatomical upper airways, but exhibit central apneas when these airways are bypassed by the tracheostomy. One study also demonstrated a desynchronization between diaphragmatic and pharyngeal muscle activation during sleep in patients with obstructive apnea (39). Delayed activation of upper airway muscles with respect to the diaphragm may allow negative pressure to develop in the upper airway at a time when it is vulnerable to collapse. To date, this hypothesis has been neither confirmed nor rejected by subsequent investigation.

These findings suggest that unstable or desynchronized respiratory drive is an important factor contributing to SRBD. In circumstances where the upper airway is predisposed to collapse by anatomical or neuromuscular factors, mixed and obstructive events may predominate. In conditions where the upper airway is mechanically stable, central events may predominate. This view is in accord with the observation that most patients with SRBD exhibit a combination of central, mixed, and obstructive events within a single sleep period. Furthermore, a detailed understanding of central apnea pathogenesis may provide important insights into the mechanisms of obstructive events, and vice versa.

These observations highlight an additional important gap in our knowledge: little is known about the brainstem and forebrain mechanisms mediating state-dependent changes in respiratory control. Virtually nothing is known about the effects of aging on these central processes and nothing at all is known regarding possible defects in these mechanisms associated with sleep apnea syndrome. This lack of knowledge stems in part from a paucity of animal models to study naturally occurring apnea across all behavioral states. Chapters 8–12 describe recent work using animal models of spontaneously occurring central and obstructive apnea and hypopnea. These model systems hold great promise to move us toward a detailed mechanistic understanding of SRBD from the level of the molecule to the whole organism.

III. Age-Related Influences
A. Developmental Aspects

Sleep-related breathing disorders can be expressed in all life stages. Because the average child spends almost half of each day sleeping, SRBD can be of particular importance during childhood. The breathing pattern becomes erratic during REM sleep, with variable tidal volume and respiratory rate, including central apneas, even in healthy children and adults (40–42). Thus, REM sleep is a state that can be provocative of SRBD. This can be especially important in children, because they sleep more than adults and spend a greater fraction of their sleep period in REM sleep than adults. In neonates, active sleep (an REM-like state) can occupy up to two-thirds of total sleep time (43), as compared to about one-fifth of sleep time in adults (44).

Central apneas, especially during REM sleep, are common in infants and children (44). Central apneas in children have often been considered significant if they are very frequent, are longer than 20 sec in duration, or are associated with severe oxygen desaturation, arrhythmia, or arousal (45). However, in view of recent observations in normal infants, the clinical significance of these events remains unclear (45). In contrast, obstructive apneas in normal children are rare (46).

Sleep-related breathing disorders, particularly obstructive sleep apnea syndrome, are common in childhood. Studies in the United States and Britain have shown similar prevalence rates of approximately 2% (47,48). The peak prevalence of childhood SRBD occurs at age 2–8 years (45). Although the data remain preliminary, it appears that SRBD occurs with equal frequency in children of each gender (48).

Obstructive SRBD in children is most often associated with adenotonsillar hypertrophy, and clinical improvement is usually observed after adenotonsillectomy (49). Still, the pathogenesis of airway obstruction in children, as in adults, appears to reflect a combination of anatomical and neuromuscular factors. As in adults, children with obstructive SRBD have no difficulty maintaining airway patency during wakefulness, suggesting that structural factors cannot be the sole causative factor. In addition, no clear correlation has been demonstrated between airway or adenotonsillar dimensions and SRBD incidence or severity in children (50,51). Moreover, some children with adenotonsillar hypertrophy as the sole recognizable risk factor are not cured by adenotonsillectomy (49). Finally, one study reported a group of children initially "cured" of obstructive SRBD by adenotonsillectomy who experienced a recurrence of the disorder during adolescence (52).

It is now feasible to investigate developmental aspects of SRBD pathogenesis and associated morbidity. Spontaneous sleep-related central and obstructive apneas have been described in preterm lambs as well as in newborn and infant rats. These model systems already are proving valuable for exploring maturational aspects of cardiorespiratory control as they may contribute to SRBD. For example, the importance of sleep continuity in the neonate for appropriate autonomic regulation in the adult is illustrated by the observation that disruption of sleep continuity in newborn rats caused significant SRBD that persisted into adulthood (53). Applications of this basic investigational approach are detailed in Chapters 8 and 9.

B.   Sleep-Related Breathing Disorders in the Elderly

The high prevalence of SRBDs in the elderly is well established (7,54–61). Although sleep apnea syndrome is most commonly diagnosed among patients in the fifth to seventh decades of life, studies of more general populations reveal a clear age-related increase in sleep apnea that extends to at least the eighth decade (54,61). Prevalence rates for apnea index greater than 5/hr are wide ranging: 28–67% for elderly males and 20–54% for elderly females (61).

Several studies of elderly subjects reported correlations between apnea and dysfunctions including heart failure (62), sleep fragmentation (63,64), hypersomnolence (65), daytime sleepiness (66), neuropsychiatric deficits (67,68) and mortality (57) in heterogeneous groups that included patients. Elucidating the mechanisms underlying disordered breathing events will help to identify circumstances under which they represent a clinical risk factor, and may suggest improved therapeutic modalities.

Basic experimental approaches in animals have not yet been applied systematically to study age-related changes in the causes and consequences of SRBD. There is little doubt that the pace of such investigations will soon increase. Animal model systems play a valuable role in studies of age-related aspects of many disease processes. Initial observations of age-related changes in state-dependent respiratory function in animals are noted in Chapters 10–12.

IV. Other Risk Factors

A. Behavioral

Although not a risk factor in the traditional sense, transitions from wakefulness to sleep are clearly a necessary "permissive" factor for expression of SRBDs, as used in this volume. In normal subjects and patients, disordered breathing events of all sorts are most especially associated with the transitional state of "sleep onset" and with REM sleep (2,3,69). A significant gap in our current understanding of SRBD is a detailed knowledge of the anatomical connectivity and molecular basis of action for the brainstem and forebrain networks that govern sleep and arousal, and the means by which they influence respiratory function. Basic approaches and current work in this area are presented in Chapters 2–5.

B. Biometric

Numerous studies have confirmed strong and consistent correlations between obesity and obstructive SRBD (70–72). Estimates for the relative risk of SRBD due to obesity can be greater than 10 (70–72). The mechanism underlying this effect, however, remains uncertain. It has been suggested that excess fat deposition in the pharynx may be a direct contributor to SRBD pathogenesis, and overall obesity may be an indirect marker for such upper airway changes. In accord with this possibility, upper body or trunk obesity (73) and neck circumference (71) may be better predictors for SRBD than overall body mass index. Indeed, these may also prove to be useful SRBD predictors in thin subjects.

The basic impact of pharyngeal anatomy, tissue mechanics, and neuromuscular control on expression of SRBD is also being investigated in animal model systems. Obstructive and central apnea is spontaneously expressed in both preterm lambs and neonatal rats, a setting in which the bony and cartilaginous support of the upper airways in not fully developed. In contrast, mature adult sheep and rats with fully developed and anatomically normal pharyngeal airways do not exhibit obstructive SRBD, but rats demonstrate impressive respiratory pattern instability, including central apnea. Ongoing work in this area is described in Chapters 8–10.

English bulldogs uniformly demonstrate significant whole-body obesity, including anatomically narrow pharyngeal airways with excess and redundant soft tissues marked by fat deposition. These animals snore and experience obstructive hypopneas during nonrapid eye movement (NREM) sleep, as well as frequent obstructive apnea and arterial oxygen desaturation during REM sleep. Thus, this model system is well suited to explore the whole-body and pharyngeal obesity in airway collapse during sleep, although breeding and clinical management of these animals can be difficult. Work using bulldogs to investigate the pathophysiology of SRBD and to identify improved therapeutic strategies is presented in Chapter 11. The connection between obesity and SRBD is also being explored in obese rodents. Genetically obese homozygous Zucker rats express SRBD in the form of central apnea with a frequency similar to that of phenotypically lean heterozygous rats. However, obese rats may also experience transient obstructive events during sleep, whereas lean rats do not. More recently, obese Zucker rats were demonstrated to have blunted reflex activation of upper airway dilator muscles (74). It has even been suggested that both obesity and SRBD may be due to leptin resistance. These preliminary findings are discussed in Chapters 2 and 10.

Another important risk factor for SRBD is male gender. Estimates for the ratio of males to females with SRBD depend on the population and sampling methods employed, but range from about 3:1 to as high as 10:1 (75). The reasons for the risk of male gender remain poorly defined. Gender difference in pharyngeal anatomy, neuromuscular control, respiratory control, and body fat distribution have been suggested as potential contributors to the male-associated risk for SRBD. The gender difference in SRBD prevalence appears to narrow with age (60), suggesting that hormonal status may also play a role in predisposition to SRBD. These questions have not yet been systematically approached using the experimental methods and experimental model systems detailed in this volume. However, all of the approaches presented are suitable for investigations of gender-related mechanisms.

Congenital or acquired abnormalities of craniofacial structure can also contribute to SRBD risk, but appear to account for only a small fraction of the total prevalence. For example, retrognathia, micrognathia, macroglossia, palatal abnormalities, and nasal septal abnormalities can contribute to the development of SRBD.

C. Genetic

Genetic factors exert a strong influence. Sleep-related breathing disorders cluster in families, with the relative risk being 2–4 times higher in first-degree relatives of diagnosed patients (76). A significant fraction of the population variance in RDI may depend on genetic factors that may persist after the influences of obesity and craniofacial structure are removed (76). In accordance, even thin relatives of patients with obstructive sleep apnea are at increased risk for SRBD (77). Risk for SRBD is almost certainly polygenic and complex; these facts have hindered human investigation in this area. The existence of rodent models of SRBD will provide an important opportunity to examine the genetics of respiratory control and of SRBD risk from a complimentary direction. Preliminary work of this type is noted in Chapters 2, 5, and 10.

D. Vascular

Only about 5% of adult patients with SRBD express purely central apneas (78). However, nearly 50% of patients with stable congestive heart failure (CHF) may exhibit SRBD characterized by central apneas (79). Moreover, Ancoli-Israel et al. (62) demonstrated that increasing severity of central SRBD was predictive of increasingly poor prognosis in patients with CHF.

Central SRBD has also been reported in the context of acquired brain lesions of both vascular and nonvascular origin. Anatomical lesions ranging from the cerebral cortex to the pons have been associated with a diathesis of SRBD characterized by central apnea (80). A failure of experimental medullary lesions to elicit periodic breathing with central apnea led to the hypothesis that SRBD following brain injury resulted from a loss of supramedullary inhibition to an intrinsic brainstem oscillator (81).

These findings again emphasize the importance of understanding the interactions between the brainstem respiratory control systems and the homeostatic systems that regulate sleep and wakefulness (80). It is now feasible to approach such questions using modern tools of molecular biology, neuropharmacology, neuroanatomy, and electrophysiology. The state of the art in this field of inquiry is presented throughout the remaining chapters of this volume.

References

1. Sleep-related breathing disorders in adults: recommendations for syndrome definition and measurement techniques in clinical research. The Report of an American Academy of Sleep Medicine Task Force. Sleep 1999; 22:667–689.
2. Bulow, K. Respiration and wakefulness in man. Acta Physiol Scand 1963; 59:1–110.
3. Webb, P. Periodic breathing during sleep. J Appl Physiol 1974; 37:899–903.
4. Block, A. J., Boysen, P. G., Wynne, J. W., and Hunt, L. A. Sleep apnea, hypopnea and oxygen desaturation in normal subjects. A strong male predominance. N Engl J Med 1979; 300:513–517.

5. Lavie, P. Incidence of sleep apnea in a presumably healthy working population: a significant relationship with excessive daytime sleepiness. Sleep 1983; 6:312–318.
6. Redline, S., Tishler, P. V., Hans, M. G., Tosteson, T. D., Strohl, K. P., and Spry, K. Racial differences in sleep-disordered breathing in African-Americans and Caucasians. Am J Respir Crit Care Med 1997; 155:186–192.
7. Young, T., Palta, M., Dempsey, J., Skatrud, J., Weber, S., and Badr, S. The occurrence of sleep-disordered breathing among middle-aged adults [see comments]. N Engl J Med 1993; 328:1230–1235.
8. Partinen, M. and Guilleminault, C. Daytime sleepiness and vascular morbidity at seven-year follow-up in obstructive sleep apnea patients. Chest 1990; 97:27–32.
9. Millman, R. P., Redline, S., Carlisle, C. C., Assaf, A. R., and Levinson, P. D. Daytime hypertension in obstructive sleep apnea. Prevalence and contributing risk factors. Chest 1991; 99:861–866.
10. Peppard, P. E., Young, T., Palta, M., and Skatrud, J. Prospective study of the association between sleep-disordered breathing and hypertension. N Engl J Med 2000; 342:1378–1384.
11. Ancoli, I. S., Kripke, D. F., Klauber, M. R., Mason, W. J., Fell, R., and Kaplan, O. Sleep-disordered breathing in community-dwelling elderly. Sleep 1991; 14:486–495.
12. He, J., Kryger, M., Zorick, F., Conway, W., and Roth, T. Mortality and apnea index in obstructive sleep apnea: experience in 385 patients. Chest 1988; 94:9–14.
13. Partinen, M., Jamieson, A., and Guilleminault, C. Long-term outcome for obstructive sleep apnea syndrome patients: mortality. Chest 1988; 94:1200–1204.
14. Roth, T., Roehrs, T., and Rosenthal, L. Hypersomnolence and neurocognitive performance in sleep apnea. Curr Opin Pulm Med 1995; 1:488–490.
15. Johns, M. W. A new method for measuring daytime sleepiness: the Epworth sleepiness scale. Sleep 1991; 14:540–545.
16. Engleman, H. M., Cheshire, K. E., Deary, I. J., and Douglas, N. J. Daytime sleepiness, cognitive performance and mood after continuous positive airway pressure for the sleep apnoea/hypopnoea syndrome. Thorax 1993; 48:911–914.
17. Lamphere, J., Roehrs, T., Wittig, R., Zorick, F., Conway, W. A., and Roth, T. Recovery of alertness after CPAP in apnea. Chest 1989; 96:1364–1367.
18. Greenberg, G. D., Watson, R. K., and Deptula, D. Neuropsychological dysfunction in sleep apnea. Sleep 1987; 10:254–262.
19. Mitler, M. M. Daytime sleepiness and cognitive functioning in sleep apnea. Sleep 1993; 16:S68–S70.
20. Flemons, W. W. and Tsai, W. Quality of life consequences of sleep-disordered breathing. J Allergy Clin Immunol 1997; 99:S750–S756.
21. Badr, M. S. Pathogenesis of obstructive sleep apnea. Prog Cardiovasc Dis 1999; 41:323–330.

22. Pepin, J. L., Levy, P., Veale, D., and Ferretti, G. Evaluation of the upper airway in sleep apnea syndrome. Sleep 1992; 15:S50–S55.

23. Schwab, R. J. Properties of tissues surrounding the upper airway. Sleep 1996; 19:S170–S174.

24. Shepard, J. W. Jr, Gefter, W. B., Guilleminault, C., Hoffman, E. A., Hoffstein, V., Hudgel, D. W., Suratt, P. M., and White, D. P. Evaluation of the upper airway in patients with obstructive sleep apnea. Sleep 1991; 14:361–371.

25. Kuna, S. T. and Smickley, J. S. Superior pharyngeal constrictor activation in obstructive sleep apnea. Am J Respir Crit Care Med 1997; 156:874–880.

26. Marcus, C. L., McColley, S. A., Carroll, J. L., Loughlin, G. M., Smith, P. L., and Schwartz, A. R. Upper airway collapsibility in children with obstructive sleep apnea syndrome. J Appl Physiol 1994; 77:918–924.

27. Schwartz, A. R., Eisele, D. W., Hari, A., Testerman, R., Erickson, D., and Smith, P. L. Electrical stimulation of the lingual musculature in obstructive sleep apnea. J Appl Physiol 1996; 81:643–652.

28. Kuna, S. T. and Sant'Ambrogio, G. Pathophysiology of upper airway closure during sleep. JAMA 1991; 266:1384–1389.

29. Tangel, D. J., Mezzanotte, W. S., Sandberg, E. J., and White, D. P. Influences of NREM sleep on the activity of tonic vs. inspiratory phasic muscles in normal men. J Appl Physiol 1992; 73:1058–1066.

30. Mezzanotte, W. S., Tangel, D. J., and White, D. P. Waking genioglossal electromyogram in sleep apnea patients versus normal controls (a neuromuscular compensatory mechanism). J Clin Invest 1992; 89:1571–1579.

31. Wheatley, J. R., Tangel, D. J., Mezzanotte, W. S., and White, D. P. Influence of sleep on response to negative airway pressure of tensor palatini muscle and retropalatal airway. J Appl Physiol 1993; 75:2117–2124.

32. Wiegand, L., Zwillich, C. W., and White, D. P. Sleep and the ventilatory response to resistive loading in normal men. J Appl Physiol 1988; 64:1186–1195.

33. Berger, A. J. Determinants of respiratory motoneuron output. Respir Physiol 2000; 122:259–269.

34. Sawczuk, A. and Mosier, K. M. Neural control of tongue movement with respect to respiration and swallowing. Crit Rev Oral Biol Med 2001; 12:18–1237.

35. Onal, E., Burrows, D. L., Hart, R. H., and Lopata, M. Induction of periodic breathing during sleep causes upper airway obstruction in humans. J Appl Physiol 1986; 61:1438–1443.

36. Skatrud, J. B. and Dempsey, J. A. Interaction of sleep state and chemical stimuli in sustaining rhythmic ventilation. J Appl Physiol 1983; 55:813–822.

37. Warner, G., Skatrud, J. B., and Dempsey, J. A. Effect of hypoxia-induced periodic breathing on upper airway obstruction during sleep. J Appl Physiol 1987; 62:2201–2211.

38. Önal, E. and Lopata, M. Periodic breathing and the pathogenesis of occlusive sleep apneas. Am Rev Respir Dis 1982; 126:676–680.

39. Hudgel, D. W. and Harasick, T. Fluctuation in timing of upper airway and chest wall inspiratory muscle activity in obstructive sleep apnea. J Appl Physiol 1990; 69:443–450.

40. Carskadon, M. A., Harvey, K., Dement, W. C., Guilleminault, C., Simmons, F. B., and Anders, T. F. Respiration during sleep in children. West J Med 1978; 128:477–481.

41. Marcus, C. L., Omlin, K. J., Basinki, D. J., Baily, S. L., Rachal, A. B., Von Pechmann, W. S., Keers, T. G., and Ward, S. L. Normal polysomnographic values for children and adolescents. Am Rev Respir Dis 1992; 146:1235–1239.

42. Millman, R. P., Knight, H., Kline, L. R., Shore, E. T., Chung, D. C., and Pack, A. I. Changes in compartmental ventilation in association with eye movements during REM sleep. J Appl Physiol 1988; 65:1196–1202.

43. Curzi-Dascalova, L., Peirano, P., and Morel-Kahn, F. Development of sleep states in normal premature and full-term newborns. Dev Psychobiol 1988; 21:431–444.

44. Carskadon, M. and Dement, W. Normal human sleep: an overview. In: Kryger, M., ed. Principles and Practice of Sleep Medicine. Philadelphia: Saunders, 1994:16–25.

45. Marcus, C. L. Sleep-disordered breathing in children. Curr Opin Pediatr 2001; 12:208–212.

46. Kahn, A., Franco, P., Kelmanson, I., Kato, I., Dan, B., and Scaillet, S. Breathing during sleep in infancy. In: Loughlin, G. M., Carroll, J. L., and Marcus, C. L. eds. Sleep and Breathing in Children—A Developmental Approach. New York: Marcel Dekker, 2000:405–422.

47. Ali, N. J., Pitson, D. J., and Stradling, J. R. Snoring, sleep disturbance, and behaviour in 4–5 year olds. Arch Dis Child 1993; 68:360–366.

48. Redline, S., Tishler, P. V., Schluchter, M., Aylor, J., Clark, K., and Graham, G. Risk factors for sleep-disordered breathing in children. Associations with obesity, race, and respiratory problems. Am J Respir Crit Care Med 1999; 159:1527–1532.

49. Suen, J. S., Arnold, J. E., and Brooks, L. J. Adenotonsillectomy for treatment of obstructive sleep apnea in children. Arch Otolaryngol Head Neck Surg 1995; 121:525–530.

50. Fernbach, S. K., Brouillette, R. T., Riggs, T. W., and Hunt, C. E. Radiologic evaluation of adenoids and tonsils in children with obstructive sleep apnea: plain films and fluoroscopy. Pediatr Radiol 1983; 13:258–265.

51. Laurikainen, E., Erkinjuntti, M., Alihanka, J., Rikalainen, H., and Suonpaa. Radiological parameters of the bony nasopharynx and the adenotonsillar size compared with sleep apnea episodes in children. Int J Pediatr Otorhinolaryngol 1987; 12:303–310.

52. Guilleminault, C., Partinen, M., Praud, J. P., Quera-Salva, M. A., Powell, N., and Riley, R. Morphometric facial changes and obstructive sleep apnea in adolescents. J Pediatr 1989; 114:997–999.

53. Thomas, A., Austin, W., Friedman, L., and Strohl, K. A model of ventilatory instability induced in the unrestrained rat. J Appl Physiol 1992; 73:1530–1536.
54. Ancoli, I. S. Epidemiology of sleep disorders. Clin Geriatr Med 1989; 5:347–362.
55. Ancoli, I. S. and Kripke, D. F. Prevalent sleep problems in the aged. Biofeedback Self Regul 1991; 16:349–359.
56. Berry, D. T., Phillips, B. A., Cook, Y. R., Schmitt, F. A., Gilmore, R. L., Patel, R., Keener, T. M., and Tyre, E. Sleep-disordered breathing in healthy aged persons: possible daytime sequellae. J Gerontol 1987; 42:62062–62066.
57. Bliwise, D. L., Bliwise, N. G., Partinen, M., Pursley, A. M., and Dement, W. C. Sleep apnea and mortality in an aged cohort. Am J Public Health 1988; 78:544–547.
58. Dickel, M. J. and Mosko, S. S. Morbidity cut-offs for sleep apnea and periodic leg movements in predicting subjective complaints in seniors. Sleep 1990; 13:155–166.
59. Knight, H., Millman, R. P., Gur, R. C., Saykin, A. J., Doherty, J. U., and Pack, A. I. Clinical significance of sleep apnea in the elderly. Am Rev Respir Dis 1987; 136:845–850.
60. Redline, S. Generalizability of findings in older populations. In: Kuna, S., ed. Sleep and Respiration in Aging Adults. New York: Elsevier, 1991:189–193.
61. Redline, S. and Young, T. Epidemiology and natural history of obstructive sleep apnea. Ear Nose Throat J 1993; 72:20–21.
62. Ancoli-Israel, S., Engler, R. L., Friedman, P. J., Klauber, M. R., Ross, P. A., and Kripke, D. F. Comparison of patients with central sleep apnea. With and without Cheyne-Stokes respiration. Chest 1994; 106:780–786.
63. Carskadon, M. A., van den Hoed, J., and Dement, W. C. Sleep and daytime sleepiness in the elderly. J Geriatr Psychiatry 1980; 13:135–151.
64. Carskadon, M. A., Brown, E. D. and Dement, W. C. Sleep fragmentation in the elderly: relationship to daytime sleep tendency. Neurobiol Aging 1982; 3:321–327.
65. Carskadon, M. A. and Dement, W. C. Respiration during sleep in the aged human. J Gerontol 1981; 36:420–423.
66. Morewitz, J. H. Evaluation of excessive daytime sleepiness in the elderly. J Am Geriatr Soc 1988; 36:324–330.
67. Bliwise, D. L., Yesavage, J. A., Sink, J., Widrow, L., and Dement, W. C. Depressive symptoms and impaired respiration in sleep. J Consult Clin Psychol 1986; 54:734–735.
68. Yesavage, J., Bliwise, D., Guilleminault, C., Carskadon, M., and Dement, W. Preliminary communication: intellectual deficit and sleep-related respiratory disturbance in the elderly. Sleep 1985; 8:30–33.
69. Remmers, J. E., deGroot, W. J., Sauerland, E. K., and Anch, A. M. Pathogenesis of upper airway occlusion during sleep. J Appl Physiol 1978; 44:931–938.

70. Dealberto, M. J., Ferber, C., Garma, L., Lemoine, P., and Alperovitch A. Factors related to sleep apnea syndrome in sleep clinic patients. Chest 1994; 105:1753–1758.
71. Grunstein, R., Wilcox, I., Yang, T. S., Gould, Y., and Hedner, J. Snoring and sleep apnoea in men: association with central obesity and hypertension. Int J Obes Relat Metab Disord 1993; 17:533–540.
72. Rajala, R., Partinen, M., Sane, T., Pelkonen, R., Huikuri, K., and Seppalainen, A. M. Obstructive sleep apnoea syndrome in morbidly obese patients. J Intern Med 1991; 230:125–129.
73. Mortimore, I. L., Marshall, I., Wraith, P. K., Sellar, R. J., and Douglas, N. J. Neck and total body fat deposition in nonobese and obese patients with sleep apnea compared with that in control subjects. Am J Respir Crit Care Med 1998; 157:280–283.
74. Nakano, H., Magalang, U. J., Lee, S. D., Krasney, J. A., and Farkas, G. A. Serotonergic modulation of ventilation and upper airway stability in obese Zucker rats. Am J Respir Crit Care Med 2001; 163:1191–1197.
75. Fogel, R. and White, D. Obstructive sleep apnea. Adv Intern Med 2000; 45:351–389.
76. Redline, S., Tishler, P. V., Tosteson, T. D., Williamson, J., Kump, K., Browner, I., Ferrette, V., and Krejci, P. The familial aggregation of obstructive sleep apnea. Am J Respir Crit Care Med 1995; 151:682–687.
77. Mathur, R. and Douglas, N. J. Family studies in patients with the sleep apnea-hypopnea syndrome. Ann Intern Med 1995; 122:174–178.
78. DeBacker, W. A., Verbraecken, J., Willemen, M., Wittesaele, W., DeCock, W., and Van deHeyning, P. Central apnea index decreases after prolonged treatment with acetazolamide. Am J Respir Crit Care Med 1995; 151:87–91.
79. Javaheri, S., Parker, T. J., Wexler, L., Michaels, S. E., Stanberry, E., Nishyama, H., and Roselle, G. Occult sleep-disordered breathing in stable congestive heart failure. Ann Intern Med 1995; 122:487–492.
80. Khoo, M. Periodic breathing. In: Crystal, R., West, J., Barnes, P., and Weibel, E. eds. The Lung: Scientific Foundations. Vol. 2. New York: Raven, 1997:1851–1863.
81. Wuyam, B., Pepin, J. L., Tremel, F., and Levy, P. Pathophysiology of central sleep apnea syndrome. Sleep 2000; 23(suppl 4):S213–S219.

Part Two

GENERAL TECHNIQUES

2

Instrumentation and Methods for Chronic Studies of Sleep and Breathing in Rodents

RICHARD L. HORNER and RICHARD STEPHENSON

University of Toronto
Toronto, Ontario, Canada

CHRISTOPHER PAUL O'DONNELL

Johns Hopkins School of Medicine
Baltimore, Maryland, U.S.A.

I. Overview: Research on Sleep and Breathing in Rodents

Disorders of sleep and breathing constitute a major public health problem (1,2). Obstructive sleep apnea, for example, affects approximately 4% of adults (3) and causes recurrent asphyxia, arousals from sleep, and cardiovascular changes. The clinical consequences associated with obstructive apneas include excessive daytime sleepiness; impaired driving and work performance (4,5); hypertension (6); increased risk for stroke, angina, and myocardial infarction (7); and suppressed ventilatory and arousal responses to altered blood gases and airway occlusions (8,9).

Given this clinical relevance, there is major interest in determining the role of stimuli involved with sleep-disordered breathing (e.g., intermittent hypoxia or arousals from sleep) and the mechanisms underlying the adverse physiological consequences (10–12). Because rats tolerate well the implantation of chronic electrodes for long-term studies, this species is well suited for investigations of the control of breathing and cardiovascular activity in sleep. As discussed in Chapter 3, rats are also particularly well suited for experiments aimed at determining the brain mechanisms controlling cardiorespiratory activity awake and asleep because stereotaxic brain maps are well established for rats (13) as are brainstem pathways involved in sleep–wake regulation (14). Moreover, automated analysis and sleep staging from the electroencephalogram (EEG) and neck electromyogram (EMG) signal allow rapid and accurate assessment of large quantities of data, and the ability to apply experimental stimuli in sleep, or particular stages of sleep, in long-term experiments. Such studies will contribute to determining mechanisms underlying the physiological consequences of stimuli associated with sleep-disordered breathing and be relevant to human clinical disorders.

Typically, however, many previous studies investigating the effects of intermittent stimuli relevant to sleep-disordered breathing in rats as an animal model have not measured sleep–wake states. For example, the effects on blood pressure and cardiovascular responses of repetitive intermittent hypoxia or arousal stimuli applied for several hours during the day have been reported (15–20). For such studies to have more direct relevance to understanding the adverse physiological consequences of sleep-related breathing disorders, however, the intermittent stimuli should be timed to sleep episodes and terminated by arousal. Indeed, the robust ultradian rhythm of the sleep–wake cycle in rodents (21) ensures that there are prolonged periods of wakefulness even during the resting phase (22). Therefore, it can not be assumed that simply applying stimuli for several hours in the rest phase of the animal will result in those stimuli being applied in sleep, especially because the rats will likely shift their sleep to the dark phase when the stimuli are not applied. Moreover, even if the intermittent stimuli happen to be applied coincidentally in sleep in such a protocol, it would be highly unlikely that the offset of hypoxia would be coincident with arousal, as occurs in clinical disorders. These observations suggest that application of stimuli in sleep, and removal of stimuli at arousal, should be prerequisites to study the effects of respiratory-related stimuli on sleep mechanisms and other physiological processes in a way that most effectively models the clinical sleep-related breathing problems.

Despite the prominence of studies of sleep and breathing in rats, an increasing number of studies are also being performed in mice. Such studies are important because the mouse allows use of new advances in molecular biology and genetic manipulations of neurotransmitter systems to address questions that are unfeasible in other preparations. However, the small size of the mouse poses technical difficulties in measurements of sleep and breathing, and in miniaturization of the techniques used in rats. This chapter summarizes techniques currently used to measure sleep and breathing in rats and mice, and also describes methods that can be used to apply respiratory-related stimuli in sleep. This chapter is not meant to review the range of different techniques applied in different laboratories and to compare their validity. Rather, this chapter intends to assist those who do not currently make chronic recordings of sleep and breathing in rodents in their own laboratory, and provides practical details of methods that can be used to implement these techniques.

II. Sleep Recordings in Rats
A. Implantation of EEG and Neck EMG Electrodes

A variety of approaches have been used for the implantation of electrodes for chronic recording of sleep–wake states in rats. Sterile surgery needs to be performed under general anesthesia, and intraperitoneal ketamine (85 mg/ kg) and xylazine (15 mg/kg) is a commonly used and well-tolerated anesthetic (23). Among other anesthetics, intraperitoneal pentobarbital sodium (60 mg/kg) is also commonly used (21). Before surgery, the rats should also be given premedication to control potential postoperative pain (e.g., buprenorphine, 0.03 mg/kg), atropine (1 mg/kg) to reduce airway secretions, and sterile saline (3 mL, 0.9%) for fluid loading. To fix body position during surgery, the rats can be placed in a stereotaxic apparatus with blunt ear bars. The corneas should be coated with ophthalmic ointment to prevent drying. A mask (24) placed over the snout for the administration of a volatile anesthetic (e.g., halothane or isoflurane in air) is an excellent way to maintain tight control over levels of anesthesia for long surgeries. This is preferable to, for example, applying periodic bolus doses of injected anesthetic for which it is more difficult to effectively titrate anesthetic depth. The additional advantage of an anesthetic mask is that supplemental O_2 (e.g., 50% in air) can also be delivered during surgery. Body temperature can also be measured with a rectal probe and maintained at normal levels (36 to 38°C) with a heating pad. In this way animals are well maintained during surgery and recover well postoperatively.

Implantation of Wire Electrodes

Electroencephalogram recordings can simply be made by implanting two stainless steel screws (0–80, 1.5 mm diameter, Plastics One Inc., Roanoke, VA) attached to ~5 cm of insulated wire (30 gauge, R30R0100, Wire Wrapping Wire, O.K. Industries) onto the skull over the frontal–parietal cortex. For example, our laboratory uses one electrode placed approximately 2 mm anterior and 2 mm to the right of the bregma skull reference, and the other approximately 3 mm posterior and 2 mm to the left of the bregma (23). A second pair of electrodes can be implanted in case one of the original placements becomes dysfunctional at some point in the chronic experiments. A reference electrode placed approximately 5 mm anterior and 3 mm to the left of the bregma acts as a suitable ground. Recordings of neck

EMG can be obtained from two ~8-cm-long insulated, multistranded stainless steel wires (AS636, Cooner Wire, Chatsworth, CA) bared at the tips and sutured onto the dorsal cervical neck muscles. The EEG and neck EMG electrodes are connected to pins inserted into an appropriate miniature plug (e.g., STC-89PI-220ABS, Carleton University, Ottawa). The wires are coiled and the plug is then affixed to the skull with dental acrylic and anchor screws. The skull can be cleaned with 3% H_2O_2 to facilitate in the bonding of the dental acrylic to the skull. In this way, chronic EEG and neck EMG electrodes can be maintained for several weeks in adult animals. Figure 1 shows examples of the types of EEG and EMG wire electrodes that are suitable for chronic recordings in rats.

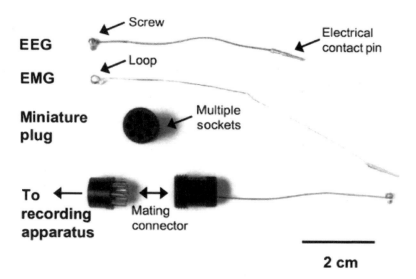

Figure 1 Examples of EEG and EMG wire electrodes and connectors suitable for chronic recordings in rats. The EEG electrode consists of single-stranded wire wrapped around a small screw with the other end soldered to an electrical contact pin. The EMG electrode is looped and knotted at one end for suturing directly onto the neck muscles. The electrical contact pins are connected to the underside of a miniature plug (the top of a nine-pin plug is shown in the picture). The plug is later attached to a mating connector that transfers the signals from the EEG and neck EMG electrodes to the recording apparatus via a shielded cable (not shown).

Telemetry

Recording of EEG and neck EMG signals by telemetry is an excellent way of avoiding the physical connection of the rat to the recording apparatus, i.e., without the use of a cable and swivel system (described below). Telemetry also permits experiments in which measurements of sleep are made in a sealed chamber, such as with whole-body plethysmography (see Sec. IV).

Rats undergo surgical implantation of a telemetry transmitter for recording EEG and neck EMG. Other signals such as body temperature or arterial blood pressure (see Sec. II.E) can also be recorded. Suitable telemetry transmitters are available from companies such as Data Sciences International (St. Paul, MN) and Mini Mitter Inc. (Bend, OR). To implant such transmitters, midline incisions are made in the scalp and abdomen to expose the skull and peritoneal cavity. The radiotransmitter is then inserted into the peritoneal cavity and loosely sutured to the rectus abdominus muscle. The electrode leads from the implant are tunneled from the peritoneal cavity and led subcutaneously to the head. The muscle and skin of the abdomen are then sutured closed. The rats are placed in a stereotaxic apparatus to fix body position and the EEG and neck EMG electrodes are attached to the skull and dorsal neck muscles as described above for wire electrodes. Figure 2 shows a telemetry transmitter for chronic recording of EEG, EMG, and body temperature in rats.

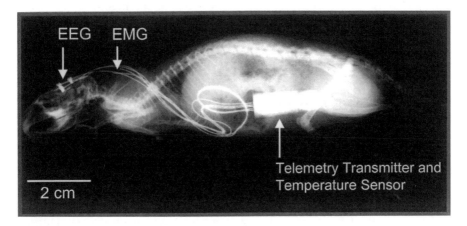

Figure 2 X-ray of a rat implanted with EEG and neck EMG electrodes attached to a telemetry unit in the peritoneal cavity. A temperature sensor is also located in the peritoneal cavity.

B.   Chronic EEG and EMG Recordings in Rats

The animals should be allowed to recover fully prior to the onset of the experiments, e.g., at least 7 days. Normal eating, drinking, and grooming are signs of good health. After surgery the rats should be handled regularly and habituated to the recording apparatus and experimental chamber for the experiments.

When wire electrodes are used to record the EEG and neck EMG signals, a lightweight shielded cable is connected to the plug on the rat's head and this is attached to a commutator and counterbalanced swivel. The commutator/swivel connection is necessary to allow unrestricted movement of the rats while the electrical signals are recorded. The commutator allows 360° rotation of the lower half of the unit while the upper half remains fixed. The commutator is placed directly above the center of the cage. When telemetry is used, the EEG and neck EMG signals are sent by radio signal to an appropriate receiver placed under the rats' cage. Sources of AM radio noise, such as computer monitors, should be kept well away from the telemetry receivers. Sources of interference can be checked using a hand-held radio tuned to the low end of the AM dial. Passing a battery close to the animal's abdomen turns on the transmitter, and the unit is turned off between experiments.

The EEG and EMG signals from the commutator, or telemetered system, are amplified and filtered and sent to chart and/or a computerized data acquisition system. Typical filters used are 1–50 Hz for EEG and 10–100 Hz for neck EMG. The sampling frequency of the computerized data acquisition system should be at least twice that of the highest frequencies expected in the raw signal. If the sampling frequency is not fast enough then high frequencies are aliased to lower frequencies. However, sampling at inappropriately high frequencies leads to a full data storage disk in a short time.

C.   Analysis of EEG and EMG Signals in Rats
Visual Analyses

Wakefulness, nonrapid eye movement (NREM), and REM sleep can be simply determined by visual analyses from chart records using standard EEG and EMG criteria (Fig. 3). Chart speeds of 5 mm · sec^{-1} are sufficient. Periodic observations of the animal should also be performed via camera or one-way mirror as an aid to determination of sleep–wake states. In wakefulness, the EEG displays low-voltage, high-frequency activity. During NREM sleep, the EEG shows high-voltage, low-frequency activity and during REM sleep, the EEG is dominated by low-voltage, high-frequency activity and neck muscle is silent, except for occasional muscle twitches.

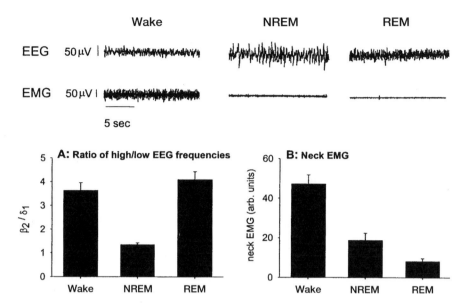

Figure 3 Example of the raw EEG and neck EMG activities recorded in wakefulness, NREM sleep, and REM sleep in chronically instrumented rats. Also shown are the group ($\pm$SEM) data for changes in (A) β_2/δ_1 EEG frequencies and (B) neck EMG amplitude across sleep–wake states. The data show that in NREM sleep, compared to wakefulness and REM sleep, there were significant decreases in β_2/δ_1 EEG frequencies and decreases in neck EMG. Despite the similarity in EEG activities between wakefulness and REM, note the major suppression of neck EMG amplitude in REM sleep. (Data modified from Ref. 22.)

Transitions to REM sleep can also be determined by visual inspection using a modification of the criteria of Benington et al., (25). Transitions to REM sleep can be determined from epochs containing low delta activity, high-amplitude spindles, and greater than 50% theta rhythm (23). Brief arousals from sleep can also be identified from the EEG and neck EMG using the same criteria as in humans (26).

Computer Analyses

Continuous visual scoring of sleep–wake states from polygraphic records and manual application of stimuli in sleep is obviously not practical for chronic animal experiments that can last many hours or days. A variety of techniques have been described for computerized analysis of sleep–wake states from EEG and EMG recordings in rats. Such techniques include spectral and interval histogram frequency analyses, auto-regressive modeling, fuzzy logic, neural network approaches, and detection of EEG and EMG amplitudes following integration (see Refs. 27–31). Detailed reviews of these various techniques and sleep-detection algorithms have appeared elsewhere (see Refs. 27,28) and are outside the scope of this chapter. Nevertheless, for studies aimed at determining the effects of specific respiratory-related stimuli on sleep mechanisms and other physiological processes in a way that most effectively models the clinical sleep-related breathing problems, computerized sleep-detection systems need to fulfill two basic criteria: (1) they must able to analyze sleep–wake states *on line*, and (2) they must be able to deliver stimuli in sleep and remove stimuli at arousal.

Bergmann et al. (31,32) pioneered a computer algorithm for on-line detection of sleep–wake states in freely behaving rats from chronic EEG and neck EMG recordings in order to apply stimuli exclusively in sleep. This algorithm has been used extensively in rats in studies of full or partial sleep deprivation (31,33–35). The original algorithm uses the amplitudes of the integrated EEG and neck EMG signals to separate sleep–wake states with two EEG signals filtered between 5 and 15 Hz and 0.5 and 15 Hz (31,32). However, the original validation of this algorithm was restricted to the light phase of the light–dark cycle and was performed in few rats (32). Validation data were presented only in the light phase in that study, probably because constant illumination is routinely used in sleep deprivation experiments to dampen or eliminate circadian rhythms (31,34). However, such criteria for detection of sleep-wake states in constant illumination may not be readily applicable to studies using the normal light–dark cycle. In addition, restricting analysis of EEG frequencies to below 15 Hz precludes analysis of a significant portion of EEG frequencies that change across sleep–wake states in rats. For this reason, a recent study re-evaluated the effects of sleep–wake states on EEG frequencies and EMG values across sleep–wake states in rats in the light–dark cycles with the purposes of: (1) developing and validating an on-line sleep-detection algorithm in rats (22), and (2) determining the consequences of sleep-related intermittent hypoxia on sleep regulation (36).

In the former study (22), 12 rats were studied with implanted EEG and neck EMG electrodes in the light–dark phases. Although there were general shifts in the distribution of EEG frequencies in NREM sleep compared to wakefulness and REM, those frequencies in the high (β_2, 20–30 Hz) and low (δ_1, 2–4 Hz) ranges showed the greatest magnitude of change. The increase in slow EEG frequencies in NREM sleep and decrease in fast frequencies were better reflected in the β_2/δ_1 ratio, which showed a larger percentage change in NREM sleep compared to when the other frequency bands were considered alone with less variance (22). Notably, the β_2/δ_1 ratio also varied consistently with sleep–wake states, but not light–dark cycle, making it a robust parameter to distinguish NREM sleep (Fig. 3). Although EEG frequencies were generally similar between wakefulness and REM sleep, the low neck EMG distinguished REM sleep (Fig. 3). Unlike EEG frequencies, however, EEG amplitudes in NREM sleep were affected by light–dark cycle. This observation fits with the demonstrated time-of-day dependence of homeostatic sleep regulation that produces high-intensity NREM sleep at the beginning of the sleep phase after prolonged wakefulness, which then diminishes over time (21,37). This observation meant, however, that EEG amplitude would not be a reliable criterion to distinguish sleep–wake states in experiments in rats that cover several hours because the ability to detect a difference between NREM sleep and the other states would vary with time of day and the light–dark cycle.

Given these observations, the β_2/δ_1 ratio and neck EMG were incorporated into a simple two-step computer algorithm for detection of sleep–wake states, as shown in Figure 4. After appropriate threshold values were set in a preliminary experiment in each rat, this algorithm produced detection accuracies of 94.5 ± 1.0% (standard error of the mean [SEM]) for wakefulness, 96.2 ± 0.8% for NREM sleep, and 92.3 ± 1.6% for REM sleep compared with blinded human scorers. This degree of accuracy, especially for REM sleep, is similar to or better than that for other computerized systems typically employed in rodents (25,28,32,38,39). The advantage of this newly developed algorithm is that it is derived from extensive analysis of EEG and EMG signals in a relatively large number of rats studied in both the light and dark phases. This degree of validation was also more stringent than that described in most previous studies (28,32). Notably, this algorithm was similar to that developed and validated in dogs (40,41), and has recently been validated for mice (see below). Applicability across species may also extend to humans, although this has not yet been tested.

D. Application to Trigger Respiratory Stimuli Exclusively in Sleep

Frequency and amplitude analysis of EEG and neck EMG signals is readily performed using a variety of commercially available data acquisition and analysis systems, which are also capable of producing voltage outputs based on threshold criteria. Incorporation of algorithms, for example as described by Bergmann et al. (31,32), Bennington et al. (25), Hamrahi et al. (22,36), or others (28), into such computerized systems can then simply be used to trigger stimuli exclusively in sleep. The feasibility of this approach has been shown recently where hypoxic stimuli were applied during natural sleep in freely behaving rats (Fig. 5) and produced significant modulation of sleep–

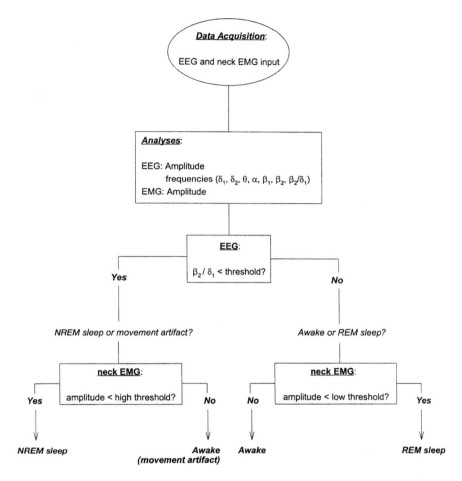

Figure 4 Flow chart to show algorithm for computerized judgment of sleep–wake states. Neck EMG amplitude and EEG frequencies in each of six bandwidths are analyzed: δ_2 (0.5–2 Hz), δ_1 (2–4 Hz), θ (4–7.5 Hz), α (7.5–13.5 Hz), β_1 (13.5–20 Hz), and β_2 (20–30 Hz). If the EEG signal shows predominantly slow frequencies relative to high frequencies (i.e., low β_2/δ_1), and the neck EMG is below a high-amplitude threshold, then the rat is judged to be in NREM sleep. If the EEG is dominated by slow frequencies, but the EMG is above the high-amplitude threshold, then the rat is judged to be in active wakefulness (i.e., EEG movement artifact associated with grooming). In contrast, if the EEG shows predominantly high frequencies relative to low frequencies (i.e., high β_2/δ_1) and the neck EMG is below a low-amplitude threshold, then the rat is judged to be in REM sleep. If the EEG is dominated by fast frequencies, but the EMG is above the low-amplitude threshold, then the rat is awake. (Modified from Ref. 22.)

wake regulation both during and after application of the stimuli (36). Of particular relevance, sleep-related hypoxia produced profound decreases in REM sleep and rebound increases after removal of the hypoxic stimuli (36). These changes in REM sleep mimic those observed in obstructive sleep apnea (OSA) patients after treatment (42) and are important given the suggested role of REM sleep in functions related to memory and cognitive processes (43,44). Application of progressively increasing arousal stimuli, and hypercapnic and/or hypoxic stimuli only in sleep in future studies will lead to determination of mechanisms underlying the independent effects of stimuli associated with sleep-related breathing disorders in a fashion that more effectively approximates OSA.

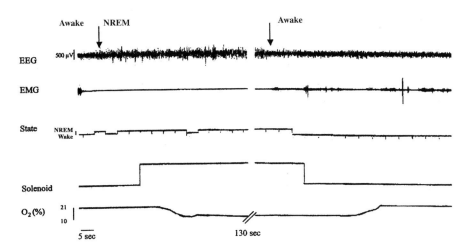

Figure 5 Example of the application of hypoxia during natural sleep in a freely behaving rat. The first arrow shows the onset of continuous NREM sleep detected by a computer, and following two consecutive sleep epochs, a voltage pulse switches a solenoid to deliver the hypoxic stimuli. The second arrow shows the point of arousal from sleep detected by the computer, and following two consecutive epochs of wakefulness, a switch back to room air is triggered by the solenoid. Sleep–wake states are shown as a hypnogram with demarcations separating each computer epoch. (From Ref. 22.)

E. Combining Measurements of the Sleep–Wake State with Other Physiological Parameters in Rats

Respiratory Muscle Activities

Electromyogram electrodes of the type shown in Figure 1 can also be used to record other muscles of interest, for example the genioglossus or diaphragm (23,45). Direct suturing of such electrodes onto muscle can lead to longer and more stable recordings than simply using wire hook electrodes (46). For chronic experiments, the genioglossus muscle is exposed following a small (~ 2 cm) midline submental incision with the rat supine and surgically anesthetized. The ventral surface of genioglossus is accessed after careful dissection of the overlying geniohyoid and mylohyoid muscles. The genioglossus electrodes are ~ 11 cm long and placed bilaterally under direct vision into the body of the tongue. Responses to electrical stimulation of the genioglossus wires can be used to ascertain correct placement (47). To record diaphragm activity, two electrodes ~ 18 cm long can be sutured onto the costal diaphragm via an abdominal approach. The wires from the diaphragm and genioglossal electrodes are tunneled subcutaneously to the neck incision and subsequently attached to the miniature plug along with the EEG and neck EMG electrodes. In this way, chronic measurements of respiratory pump and pharyngeal muscle activities can be made across sleep–wake states in freely behaving rats (45). The electrocardiogram can be removed from the diaphragm signal using an electronic blanker (e.g., model SB-1, CWE Inc., Ardmore, PA) prior to obtaining the moving-time average (23).

Blood Pressure

Sleep-related breathing disorders are a cause of hypertension (6) and are associated with other adverse cardiovascular sequelae (7). Several studies have been performed in rats to determine underlying mechanisms. For example, the long-term effects of intermittent hypoxia applied for several hours during the day on blood pressure and cardiovascular responses have been studied (15–19), as have the effects of arousal stimuli (20). Although there is the caveat that the stimuli were applied without reference to sleep–wake states (Sec. I), these studies have led to much-improved knowledge of the effects of certain stimuli associated with sleep-disordered breathing on heart rate and blood pressure (48). The following is a brief summary of the options available to record blood pressure in conscious rats; some advantages and disadvantages are highlighted.

The tail cuff method is one of the most convenient methods to record blood pressure noninvasively in rodents. Although noninvasive tail cuff measurements correlate with direct measurements of arterial blood pressure, inconsistent differences between the two methods lead to uncertainties of the exact pressure with tail cuff measurements (49,50). However, in naturally sleeping and freely behaving animals, the tail cuff method has major disadvantages compared to the other methods described below. These disadvantages include physical restraint, cuff inflation arousing the animal, and errors of measurement increasing with progressive alterations in blood pressure, such as in hypertension (49,51–53).

Unlike noninvasive measurements, chronic implantation of cannulae into blood vessels has the advantage of providing direct measurements of arterial blood pressure on a beat-by-beat basis. Catheters can be implanted into the abdominal aorta or femoral artery (54) and are typically exteriorized at the nape of the neck and exit the recording chamber alongside the EEG and neck EMG electrodes. A major advantage of such a system is that periodic calibration of the pressure transducers can be performed to ensure the validity of the measurements. However, there is the potential for exit site infection with chronic implantation of arterial catheters, and repeated flushing of the catheter with an antithrombogenic solution may be required to maintain patency. Indeed, catheter clotting and maintenance is the major limiting factor in long-term experiments.

For these reasons, in the last several years increasing numbers of studies have used telemetry for the long-term continuous measurements of arterial blood pressure (6,55–60). Implantation of commercially available telemetry units into the peritoneal cavity, with the tip of the blood pressure catheter placed in the abdominal aorta, is readily performed in rats (60,61). The major advantages of telemetry include no physical connection between the sensor and the animal, and hence no restraint or movement artifact occur, and less risk of exit site infection exists. Moreover, the antithrombogenic tips of currently available catheters remove the need for antithrombogenic therapy. Indeed, implanted catheters in dogs have been maintained for years (6). In such cases, the time limit for telemetered blood pressure measurements is typically related to the life of the battery in the transmitter. To prolong battery life, the transmitter is turned off between experiments using a magnet.

The one disadvantage of telemetry units for measurement of blood pressure is the inability to calibrate and validate the pressure sensor during the experiment. Although the sensors can be calibrated before implantation and after removal from the animal, calibration is not easily performed in rodents during the experiments once the unit is implanted. In larger animals, e.g., dogs, periodic comparisons of the telemetered blood pressure signal with pressure recorded from a catheter transiently inserted into the femoral artery can be performed to check for accuracy (62). Periodic comparisons of the telemetered blood pressure signal are necessary for accurate blood pressure measurements in chronic experiments lasting several weeks (62). Indeed, although telemetry systems can accurately measure absolute blood pressures and acute changes, the stability of the signal can only be properly judged if the system is periodically validated to protect against inherent drift (62). Moreover, the telemetry pressure sensors measure absolute pressures and hence need to be referenced to atmosphere to provide accurate measurements of arterial blood pressure fluctuations. Although this compensation for ambient pressure can be performed with additional software and hardware components from the telemetry suppliers, failure to compensate for fluctuations in atmospheric pressure over time can lead to artifactual changes in pressure measured from the arterial catheter. For example, changes in atmospheric pressure can lead to shifts in arterial pressure that have nothing to do with the status of the animal.

F. Summary

Because the rat is well suited for implantation of chronic electrodes for long-term studies, it has been well utilized for studies of the control of breathing and cardiovascular activity in sleep. Moreover, automated analysis and sleep staging from EEG and neck EMG signals allow rapid and accurate assessment of large quantities of data, and offer the ability to apply experimental stimuli in sleep or particular stages of sleep. Such studies, if performed with knowledge of sleep–wake states, will be a major benefit in determining mechanisms underlying the physiological consequences of stimuli associated with sleep-disordered breathing and will be more relevant to human clinical disorders.

III. Sleep Recordings in Mice

Implanting electrodes for chronic recording of EEG and neck EMG in an animal the size and weight of the mouse poses several unique technical problems. Nevertheless, a small number of studies measuring sleep in mice began appearing in the literature from the late 1960s (63–68). In the 1990s, however, a large number of laboratories around the world routinely made sleep recordings in mice. The rise in popularity of polysomnography in mice paralleled the sequencing of the human and mouse genomes and the rapid development of transgenic mice as a new tool for biologists to explore basic mechanisms of sleep homeostasis and cardiorespiratory regulation. The benefits of using transgenic mice to uncover potential causes of sleep disorders was illustrated dramatically in recent studies of hypocretin/orexin knockout mice, which developed behavioral arrest akin to narcolepsy (69), and in prion protein-deficient mice, which exhibited features of fatal familial insomnia (70). Studies of sleep in mice have also identified important roles for other genes such as interleukin-1 beta (71) and 5-HTI$_B$ receptors (72). Thus, despite the small size of the mouse, recent advances in genome sequencing and transgenic technology make it an important animal for biological studies of sleep.

A. Implantation of EEG and Neck EMG Electrodes

A variety of approaches have been utilized for the implantation of electrodes for chronic recording of sleep–wake states in mice. The mouse needs to be anesthetized throughout the surgical procedure, and inhaled anesthetics such as halothane or isoflurane are preferable to precisely control the depth of anesthesia (73). Because of the very small size of the skull, most investigators have described the positioning of electrodes only qualitatively over the frontal and parietal lobes. Generally, electrodes are positioned bilaterally approximately 1–2 mm lateral to the midline and 1–2 mm anterior and posterior to the bregma (74,75). Suitable positioning of electrodes in mice can be routinely accomplished without the use of stereotaxic equipment (73). A minimum of two electrodes, plus a separate ground, is required to record EEG activity, but many investigators implant extra electrodes and use the combination of the three electrodes, which provides the best tracing for discriminating sleep–wake states (76). For short-term use (0–10 days), fine wire electrodes can be inserted through small drilled holes in the skull and fixed with dental acrylic (77,78).

To implant the EEG and neck EMG electrodes, a midline incision is made to expose the skull and the muscles immediately posterior to the skull (73). The underlying fascia is gently cleared from the skull surface and two bilateral pairs of holes (0.015 cm; drill bit E-HSD-97, Small Parts Inc., Miami Lakes, FL) are drilled through the skull in the frontal and parietal regions. Four 40-cm EEG electrodes are fashioned from Teflon-coated stainless steel wire (outside diameter 0.018 cm Teflon coated and 0.013 cm bare; A-M Systems, Inc., Everett, WA). The end 0.15 cm of each electrode is stripped of the Teflon coating, bent at 90°, and inserted into the skull through each of the predrilled holes. The four electrodes are bonded to the dorsal surface of the skull with dental acrylic. Two 45-cm nuchal EMG electrodes are made from the identical Teflon-coated stainless steel wires used for the EEG electrodes. The end of each of the EMG electrodes is fashioned into a small loop (approximately 0.15 cm diameter) from which the Teflon coating is removed with a bunsen burner. The two EMG electrodes are stitched (6-0 silk) flat onto the surface of the muscle immediately posterior to the dorsal area of the mouse skull. The skin overlying the skull and posterior muscles are sutured together and the six electrodes exit the skin dorsally approximately 1.25 cm posterior to the point of EMG attachment. We have obtained high quality, short-term recordings of EEG and neck EMG activities using such an approach with fine wire electrodes (73,77).

For longer-term use (weeks to months) a detachable electrode system provides more reliable measurements. Electrodes are connected to small screws implanted in the skull, which in turn are attached to a connector/ pedestal system cemented to the skull (74–76). The surgical preparation and electrode positioning are identical to those described above for placement of fine wire electrodes. The components necessary for implanting a detachable electrode system in mice are commercially available; for example, Plastics One Inc., provides a full range of anchoring screws (0-80 × 1/16), EEG electrodes (E363/1), EMG electrodes (E363/76), pedestals (MS363), and connector cables (363-SL/6 6TCS). An advantage of the connector/pedestal approach is that animals need only be tethered to recording apparatus during experiments, and can be housed in normal cages at other times, such as during recovery from surgery or between experimental manipulations.

Because of the extremely small size of the mouse, it is necessary for the commutator to turn with a minimum of torque application to allow the mice to behave freely, i.e., while grooming, feeding, and drinking. Mercury swivels operate with extremely low torque properties, and as such are preferable for use in mice (79,80), compared to the more standard slip-ring commutators used routinely for larger animals (described above for rats).

B. Recording and Analysis of EEG and EMG Signals in Mice

The electrical signals from the commutator are amplified and filtered and normally sent to a computerized data acquisition system. The filters used should encompass the range of interest and are similar to those used in rats (Sec. II.B). The combination of low-torque commutators and computer technology, therefore, allows EEG and EMG signals to be recorded continuously for days or weeks at a time in mice.

The amount of digitized polysomnographic data acquired in a single 24-hr period in one mouse is substantial. As with rats, therefore, it is impractical to attempt to score such a large amount of data manually. Accordingly, some researchers have developed computer programs to automate the sleep-scoring process in mice (38,74). Most commonly, spectral analysis of the EEG frequency is used to determine differences between wakefulness, NREM sleep, and REM sleep using an appropriate algorithm. Because sleep cycles are short in mice compared to those in larger animals (81), automated sleep detection programs routinely score data in epochs of 10 sec or less (38,74). In mice, as in other species, NREM sleep tends to be dominated by EEG frequencies in the delta (<4 Hz) and theta (6–9 Hz) range, and the amplitude of the EEG tends to be high, whereas the amplitude of the EMG is low. In contrast, REM sleep is characterized by regular low-amplitude EEG waves in the theta range and a low-amplitude EMG. Wakefulness is characterized by low amplitude EEG of variable frequency and a high EMG (38,74). One approach to scoring large amounts of polysomnography data in mice is to use automated off-line analyses (74). Analyzing polysomnographic data off-line allows the investigator to establish accurate estimates of key threshold values for parameters such as EMG amplitude, delta frequency, and theta frequency to separate wakefulness, NREM sleep, and REM sleep. Off-line analyses, however, do not permit continual monitoring of sleep–wake states with the purpose of acting upon those judgments; for example, for application of certain stimuli in chosen sleep–wake states (22,36).

If an on line automated sleep detection system is required, however, the threshold values need to be set prior to starting the experiment after several hours of analysis across all sleep–wake states. In our laboratory, we have successfully adapted an on-line automated sleep detection program previously used and validated in dogs (40,41) and rats (22,36) for use in a mouse model of sleep-disordered breathing. This on-line system was described in detail above for rats (see Fig. 4). Thus, the extensive generation of data in murine sleep studies can be successfully scored and analyzed either off line or on line using automated sleep detection programs.

C. Potential Problems of Sleep Recordings in Mice

Polysomnography in mice presents some caveats associated with accurate sleep detection. One potential complication of sleep assessment is that the rapid breathing frequency of mice is in the frequency range that characterizes NREM sleep (i.e., the delta range). Consequently, when an electrode connection or lead deteriorates, a breathing artifact may be observed that resembles NREM sleep. One other caveat for scoring sleep in mice is that the amplitude of the EMG does not always decrease in the transition from NREM sleep to REM sleep. However, the amplitude of the EMG in REM sleep is always below wakefulness levels, allowing accurate separation of these two sleep states.

The environmental status of the mouse is also important in any accurate assessment of sleep–wake states. Sufficient time is required for the mouse to recover from the surgical stress related to implantation of chronic recording electrodes, as it is with rats. Recovery time is best assessed by resumption of normal eating and weight gain. After surgical recovery, the animal must next adjust to being tethered while performing the normal daily routines of eating, drinking, grooming, foraging, etc. One study proposed that up to 15 days is necessary for REM cycling to stabilize in tethered mice (82). Other environmental considerations include maintaining the external temperature in the thermoneutral zone of the mouse (83), and determining an intensity of light that is appropriate for sleeping during the light phase. Thus, attention to environmental factors such as tethering, temperature, and lighting will likely maximize the quality of polysomnographic data in mice.

D. Combining Measurements of Sleep–Wake State with Other Physiological Parameters in Mice

Apart from the study of the sleep architecture per se of mice, note that sleep has important influences on other physiologic parameters. A pertinent example is the application of whole-body barometric plethysmography in mice (73,84), a technique to noninvasively quantify the frequency and depth of respiration (see Sec. IV). The accurate recording of tidal breathing from barometric plethysmography requires an animal that is stationary, and mice that are not moving are usually either asleep or transitioning into sleep. Sleep, however, is a powerful modifier of the respiratory control system (73) and understanding the sleep–wake state of the mouse could markedly alter interpretation of any respiratory data. We have developed techniques for simultaneously performing polysomnography and barometric plethysmography in mice while also challenging their ventilation with a range of hypercapnic gases from 0–8% CO_2 (73). In male C57BL/6J mice, we found that the slope of the relationship between ventilation and inspired CO_2 varied from $16.8 \pm 1.1\,mL/min/\%CO_2$ during wakefulness, to $6.1 \pm 0.5\,mL/min/\%CO_2$ during NREM sleep, to $1.3 \pm 0.5\,mL/min/\%CO_2$ during REM sleep (73). Clearly, without knowledge of the sleep–wake states of the mouse, it is extremely difficult to interpret findings related to respiratory control. Similarly, we have shown that systemic arterial blood pressure can vary on average by 15–20 mmHg across the range of wakefulness to REM sleep in C57BL/6J mice (77). Furthermore, given the rapid sleep cycling of mice, no particular state is held for any significant period of time (81). Consequently, the measurement of polysomnography in mice can enhance the interpretive value of other physiological experiments.

E. Summary

The measurement of polysomnography in mice is routinely performed in many laboratories. Commercially available or custom-made tethering systems and commutators enable long-term electrical recordings of EEG and EMG activity in mice with chronically implanted electrodes. As with rats, automated analysis of sleep staging from the frequency distribution of the EEG and the amplitude of the neck EMG signal allow rapid and accurate assessment of large quantities of data both off line and on line. Although polysomnography in mice is technically difficult, there is clearly a mounting interest in the area of the genetic basis of sleep homeostasis and sleep disorders, resulting in the continued growth of sleep-related research in mice (75,85–88).

IV. Application of Plethysmography to Research in Sleep and Breathing in Rodents

Whole-body plethysmography has proven to be a very useful technique in the study of breathing and metabolism in sleeping rodents. The main advantage of the technique is that it is noninvasive and therefore enables long-term recordings from unanesthetized and unrestrained animals. This section presents an overview of the basic theory underlying the technique and suggests practical approaches to implementation of the method in studies using rodents.

A. Basic Principles
Measurement of Lung Ventilation

When an animal is placed inside a closed chamber, pressure of the gas inside the chamber increases and decreases during inspiration and expiration, respectively (89,90). The respiratory pressure deflection (ΔP_{resp}) arises for two basic reasons: (1) the combined effect of changes in tidal gas temperature and water vapor pressure due to differences between chamber conditions and alveolar conditions (this is generally considered the primary cause of ΔP_{resp}) (90–92); and (2) mechanical expansion and compression of the gas as a result of muscular contractions, or elastic and gravitational forces. This is a source of artifact and, perhaps more importantly in the present context, may be relevant under conditions when airway resistance (R_{aw}) is elevated. The latter can occur in several sleep-related breathing disorders, and this potential source of error will be considered later.

The following description is not intended to be an exhaustive account of the thermodynamic basis of the method. The reader is referred to the original paper by Drorbaugh and Fenn (90), a theoretical analysis by Chaui-Berlinck and Bicudo (93), and a recent review (92) for further discussion. Basically, during inspiration a tidal volume of air (V_T) at chamber temperature (T_c, K) and chamber water vapor pressure (P_{wc}, mmHg) is drawn into the lungs. During inspiration V_T is warmed to body (alveolar) temperature (T_b) and becomes saturated with water vapor (P_{wb}) at T_b.

Heating and humidification of the air increases its volume and because the animal is sealed within a fixed-wall (i.e., noncompliant) chamber, this in turn results in an increase in pressure within the entire chamber. Therefore, the magnitude of the pressure deflection depends mainly upon the differences between the lung and the chamber in terms of their temperatures, water vapor pressures, and volumes.

Calculation of V_T requires a knowledge of barometric pressure (P_B), relative humidity of the air in the chamber (RH, %), T_c, T_b, and ΔP_{resp}. According to the Drorbaugh and Fenn method (90), ΔP_{resp} is taken as the average of the trough-to-peak pressure difference during inspiration and the peak-to-trough pressure difference during the subsequent expiration (Fig. 6). Fortunately, by use of a simple calibration technique, it is not necessary to know the volumes of the chamber and the respiratory system, nor is it necessary to calibrate the pressure transducer in absolute units. This calibration involves injection of a known volume of air at T_c (V_{cal}, typically 0.5 or 1 mL in rat studies) while the resulting pressure deflection (ΔP_{cal}) is recorded. This should be done during each experiment with the animal in the chamber because the animal's body occupies a significant volume. The ratio $V_{cal}/\Delta P_{cal}$ represents the relationship between effective volume and pressure change (according to the ideal gas law) for a specific animal in a given chamber.

Multiplication of ΔP_{resp} by this ratio yields the relative change in volume of the inhaled gas resulting from heating and humidification. Thus, V_T (mL, at body temperature and ambient pressure, and saturated with water vapor [BTPS]) can be derived from ΔP_{resp} using a proportionality constant that expresses the ratio of V_T to volume expansion. The proportionality derives from differences in temperature and pressure, and is therefore calculated from these variables (90):

$$V_T = \Delta P_{resp}(V_{cal}/\Delta P_{cal})[T_b(P_B - P_{wc})]/\{[T_b(P_B - P_{wc})] - [T_c(P_B - P_{wb})]\} \tag{1}$$

Inspiratory time (t_I, sec) and expiratory time (t_E, sec) are measured as the interval between minimum and maximum, and maximum and minimum, respectively, of the respiratory pressure waveform (Fig. 6). Total breath time (t_{TOT}, sec) is the sum of t_I and t_E, and respiratory frequency (f_R, breaths $\cdot$ min^{-1}) is $60/t_{TOT}$. For each breath, inspired ventilation V_I (mL $\cdot$ min^{-1} BTPS) $= V_T f_R$.

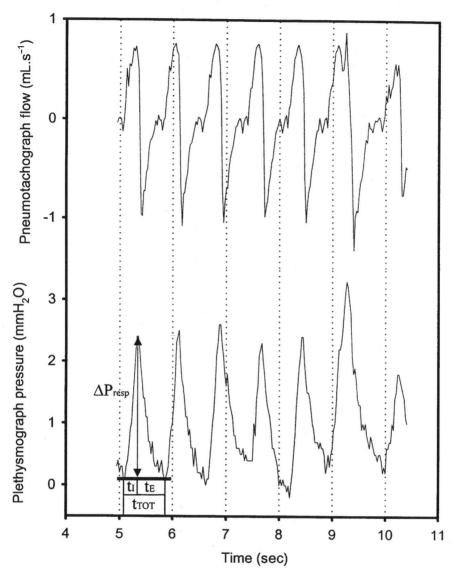

Figure 6 Representative recording of respiration by whole-body plethysmography and pneumotachography in an anesthetised Wistar rat. The magnitude of the respiratory pressure wave (ΔP_{resp}) is illustrated by the double-headed arrow on one breath. Note that according to the method of Drorbaugh and Fenn (90), ΔP_{resp} represents the mean of the maximum–minimum difference for both inspiration and expiration. Inspiratory time (t_I, sec) expiratory time (t_E, sec), and total breath duration (t_{TOT}) are measured as shown.

Measurement of Metabolic Rate

For a full interpretation of ventilatory changes, it is often advantageous to measure metabolic rate (94,95). Fortunately, the plethysmographic technique enables this by indirect calorimetry (i.e., respiratory gas exchange). The rates of oxygen consumption ($\dot{V}_{O_2}$, $mL \cdot min^{-1}$ a volume of gas at standard temperature and pressure that contains no water vapor [STPD]) and carbon dioxide production ($\dot{V}_{CO_2}$, $mL \cdot min^{-1}$ STPD) can be estimated in several ways, depending upon the specific design of the plethysmograph. A plethysmograph can be operated as an open-flow or a closed system, or as a combination of both (intermittent flow) (Fig. 7).

In open-flow systems oxygen uptake and carbon dioxide production are calculated as follows (96,97):

$$V_{o_2} = \dot{V}_i(F_i o_2 - F_e o_2)/[1 - (1 - R)F_e o_2] \tag{2}$$

$$V_{co_2} = \dot{V}_i(F_e co_2 - F_i co_2)/[1 - (1 - 1/R)F_e co_2] \tag{3}$$

The respiratory exchange ratio (R) can be estimated with negligible error as follows:

$$R = (F_e co_2 - F_i co_2)/(F_i o_2 - F_e o_2) \tag{4}$$

If only one gas analyzer is available, R can be assumed to be 0.85 with a maximum relative error of only 3%.

When the chamber is closed, air can be sampled from the chamber and recirculated rapidly via the gas analyzers back to the chamber. During experiments, the rates of changes in $F_e O_2$ and $F_E\ CO_2$ can be used to calculate metabolic rate (98):

$$\dot{V}_{o_2} = [F_e o_{2,1} \cdot V_c - (\{F_e o_{2,2} \cdot V_c[1 - (F_e o_{2,1} + F_e co_{2,1})]\}$$
$$/[1 - (F_e o_{2,2} + F_e co_{2,2})])]/t_2 - t_1 \tag{5}$$

$$\dot{V}_{co_2} = [(\{F_e co_{2,2} \cdot V_c[1 - (F_e o_{2,1} + F_e co_{2,1})]\}$$
$$/[1 - (F_e o_{2,2} + F_e co_{2,2})]) - F_e co_{2,1} \cdot V_c]/t_2 - t_1 \tag{6}$$

where the subscripts 1 and 2 refer to measurements at the start (t_1) and end (t_2) of the measurement interval, respectively. This calculation takes into account the effect of $R < 1$. The measurement interval should be as short as the resolution of the gas analyzers will allow. The volume of the air in the chamber (V_c, mL) must be known, and can be measured by gas dilution using a known volume (V_{CO_2}) of pure CO_2:

$$V_c = V_{co_2}/\Delta F_{co_2}, \tag{7}$$

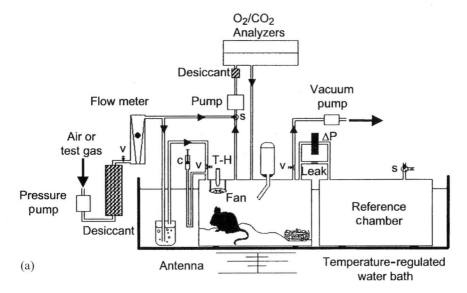

(a)

Figure 7 Schematic diagram of the essential features of two types of whole-body plethysmographs for measurement of lung ventilation and metabolic rate. For clarity, the electrical connections between sensors and a recording device are not shown. ΔP, differential pressure transducer; PnT, pneumotachograph; T-H, thermohygrometer; s, solenoid value or stopcock; v, needle value. Arrowheads indicate direction of airflow. High-resistance apertures are indicated as short, thick-walled segments. The antenna is placed beneath the animal chamber to receive radio transmitter signals. In long-term experiments, animals are provided with food, water, and bedding materials. (a) Open-flow design. The figure illustrates Pappenheimer's (95) design for use in continuous flow mode. Dry air or test gas is supplied under pressure (left) via a calibrated flow meter. It enters the animal chamber via a high-resistance aperture after humidification at chamber temperature. A vacuum pump withdraws air from the animal chamber via a high-resistance aperture, regulated by a needle valve to maintain atmospheric pressure within the chamber. This can also be operated in intermittent flow mode if the high-resistance inlet and outlet valves are replaced by low-resistance stopcocks or solenoid valves. In both operating modes, the respiratory pressure deflection is calibrated by injection of a known volume of air (c). (b) Closed design (98). Air is recirculated via a canister of CO_2 absorbent at a rate sufficient to maintain CO_2 concentrations below 0.5%. O_2 consumed by the animal is replaced from a gas cylinder. Infusions of O_2 can be regulated by a solenoid valve under feedback control from the O_2 analyzer. The pneumotachograph measures the quantity of O_2 infused, which serves to measure steady state $\dot{V}O_2$ and also to calibrate the respiratory pressure deflection. The CO_2 by-pass enables stimulation of the animal by progressive asphyxia, and feedback control of the CO_2 scrub/by-pass solenoid valves using the output of the CO_2 analyzer can hold CO_2 concentration at any desired level. Note that the leak between chambers is used only for pressure equilibration and is occluded during experiments.

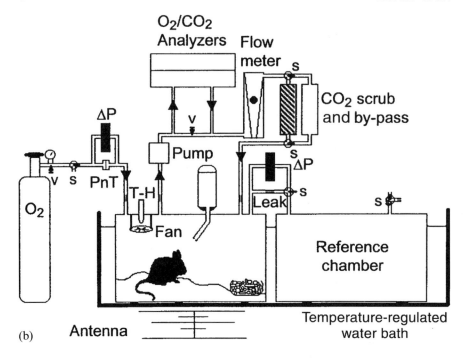

Figure 7 Continued

where ΔFCO_2 is the increase in the fractional concentration of CO_2 following injection. If the above measurement of V_c is done without an animal in the chamber, the measured V_c must be corrected (V_c') to subtract the volume of the animal during an experiment:

$$V_c' = V_c - M_b/\rho \tag{8}$$

where M_b is body mass (g) and ρ is body density, which can be assumed to be equal to $1.03 \, g \cdot mL^{-1}$ (99).

Because $\dot{V}_{o_2}$ and $\dot{V}_{co_2}$ are reported as standardized quantities (i.e., corrected to STPD), barometric pressure and temperature of the air in the flow meter (which should be the same as chamber temperature) should be recorded for both open-flow and closed systems.

B. Potential Sources of Error

Measurement of Lung Ventilation

Since the formal introduction of the technique nearly 50 years ago, several potential sources of error have been identified, and the means by which to eliminate those errors have been proposed (93,100–102). The following discussion of these issues will be brief, and the reader is referred to the original articles for more detail. Here we emphasize that numerous validation studies, comparing whole-body plethysmography with other "standard" methods such as pneumotachography, have confirmed the accuracy of the method (89–91,103–108).

A single-chamber, whole-body plethysmograph (89,90) is subject to significant baseline drift and other noise originating from external factors such as changes in temperature and mechanical vibrations. These problems are substantially reduced by the use of a second (reference) chamber (103). A differential pressure transducer is used to measure differences in pressure between the animal chamber and the reference chamber so that external disturbances (which affect both chambers equally) are canceled. Furthermore, surrounding the plethysmograph by a water bath, even if experiments are to be done at room temperature, attenuates temperature fluctuations that originate both externally and from the experimental animal. The lid of the plethysmograph should be shielded from direct radiant heat (i.e., incandescent light bulbs).

Errors in the computation of V_T can arise from inaccuracies in the measurement of any of the variables contributing to the calculation: pressure, relative humidity, temperature, or calibration. Errors in barometric pressure (P_B, mmHg) and water vapor pressures (P_{wc} and P_{wb}) give rise to small relative errors in V_T (e.g., ± 5 mmHg introduces an error of $<2\%$ in V_T).

In general, the greater the difference between T_b and T_c, the smaller is the effect on V_T of inaccuracy in the measurement of these temperatures. Under most circumstances, however, this will be unimportant, because for euthermic rodents in a chamber at room temperature ($T_b - T_c \sim 15°C$), a $0.5°C$ error in one of the temperature readings yields a relative error in V_T of ~ 2–3%. However, in studies where $T_b - T_c$ is low, the errors are greater. For example, if $T_b - T_c$ is $4°C$, an inaccuracy of $0.5°C$ would yield a relative error in V_T of $\sim 35\%$.

T_c can be measured accurately provided that the air in the chamber is adequately mixed. However, T_b is more susceptible to error. It is technically difficult to measure alveolar temperature directly, so core body temperature, usually abdominal or rectal temperature, is measured and assumed to be the same as alveolar temperature. This is likely to be a reasonable assumption, except under conditions of very low ambient temperature combined with high ventilation (109). The optimum method is to use surgically implanted telemetry transmitters (110). Care must be taken in the calibration of the transmitter, not only with respect to the accuracy and resolution of the signal, but also the time constant of response. The latter determines the temporal resolution of the temperature recording, which for example, determines the minimum time after a change in sleep–wake state before a recording accurately reflects that of the new state.

The differential pressure signal is calibrated by single injections or repetitive injection–withdrawal cycles of a known volume of air (V_{cal}) into the animal chamber during the course of experiments. In practice, V_{cal} is chosen to produce a ΔP_{cal} that is about three or more times the magnitude of ΔP_{resp}. This is sufficient to reduce the effect of ΔP_{resp}, which contaminates the calibration recording. In a closed system, ΔP_{cal} will attain a peak value (overshoot) and then decay to a steady asymptote after a few seconds. The steady level provides an accurate calibration; the overshoot results from nonisothermal conditions in the plethysmograph during the first few seconds following injection. Note that any slow leak connecting the animal and reference chambers must be closed during the calibration procedure. In open-flow systems or "leaky" closed systems (i.e., incorporating either physical leaks or electronic coupling), ΔP_{cal} is dissipated over time so a steady-state value cannot be obtained. Thus, the closed system is superior with respect to accuracy of calibration.

A source of potential error that has generated much debate since it was first recognized in 1978 (100) challenges the assumption that inspiration and expiration are symmetrical with respect to changes in temperature and water vapor pressure. Epstein and Epstein 100 assumed that cooling of expired air occurs more slowly than warming of inspired air. They suggested that expired air cools rapidly to nasal temperature (T_n) and then further cooling to T_c occurs too slowly to contribute to the phasic respiratory pressure waveform. Jacky (102) developed a simplified computational method based on Epstein and Epstein's (100) theory.

To our knowledge, four studies have directly tested these ideas. Two studies by the authors of the modified theory were confirmatory (101,102), finding that neglecting to adjust for nasal temperature (T_n) underestimated V_T by between 11% and 37%. In contrast, two independent studies (104,108) found that adjusting for T_n resulted in slight overestimation of V_T.

The modified theory (100–102) requires knowledge of T_n, which is extremely difficult to measure in conscious rodents. Attempts have been made to estimate T_n based on separate recordings made on anesthetized animals (96,102,109), but this inevitably introduced an error of uncertain magnitude. In view of the additional experimental and analytical complexity that the modified theory introduces, and the repeated demonstrations that the traditional formula provides estimates of V_T that correspond well with other "standard" methods (89–91,103–108), we conclude that for most experimental situations there is little or no justification in adjusting for T_n.

Finally, we consider a potential source of error that has particular relevance to studies of sleep-disordered breathing: changes in airway resistance (R_{aw}). In healthy animals, the peak and trough of the respiratory pressure waveform are assumed to represent end inspiration and end expiration, respectively. Airflow is zero at these times in the respiratory cycle and alveolar pressure is assumed to be equivalent to chamber pressure. During inspiration and expiration, however, air flows because alveolar pressure is different from chamber pressure. Thus, during inspiration air in the alveolus expands as a result of work done by the respiratory pump muscles, in addition to the simultaneous effects of warming and humidification emphasized above. The latter effect will increase when R_{aw} is increased.

The pressure deflection measured in a plethysmograph due to mechanical compression and expansion of flowing alveolar air is a function of the ratio of lung volume to plethysmograph volume. In a relatively large whole-body plethysmograph used for long-term measurements of lung ventilation, this ratio is of the order of 0.0005–0.001. Therefore, a transthoracic pressure of $\pm 5 \, mmH_2O$ will generate a plethysmograph pressure deflection of only approximately 0.25–0.5% of ΔP_{resp}. When R_{aw} is increased, however, such as during upper airway obstructions (e.g., obstructive sleep apnea) or bronchoconstriction (e.g., nocturnal asthma), the quantitative relationship between mechanical and thermohygrometric factors is changed.

In total upper airway occlusion (as would occur in an animal model of obstructive sleep apnea), intrathoracic pressure deflections may decrease to $-10 \, cmH_2O$ or more, generating an apparent ΔP_{resp}. Clearly, ΔP_{resp} is no longer proportional to V_T, because airflow is zero under these conditions, and whole-body plethysmography is therefore not an appropriate method for studies of obstructive apnea. Apneas that do not involve active breathing attempts against a resistance are not subject to these methodological difficulties, and as such, whole-body plethysmography is a valid technique for the study of central apneas (111).

Measurement of Metabolic Rate

For open-flow systems, errors can arise because of inappropriate flow rates and inaccurate measurement of flow. Airflow must be low enough for a detectable signal ($F_iO_2 - F_eO_2$ and $F_iCO_2 - F_eCO_2$) to develop. This obviously depends upon the metabolic rate of the animal. However, it is also important to ensure sufficient flow to prevent excessive accumulation of CO_2 in the animal chamber and to allow rapid changes in gas composition if gaseous stimuli such as hypercapnia or hypoxia are to be applied. Clearly, the higher the resolution of the gas analyzers, and the higher the metabolic rate, the faster the airflow can be. Because this technique is limited to steady-state conditions, signal conditioning (zero suppression, amplification, and low pass filtering) can be employed to enhance the accuracy of the analyzers. A 10% error in the measurement of flow rate $(\dot{V}_i)$ will produce a commensurate error in the estimation of $\dot{V}_{o_2}$ and $\dot{V}_{co_2}$, so good quality flowmeters are essential.

C. Practical Implementation

Perhaps the most easily implemented plethysmograph is the original intermittent flow design (Fig. 7a) (89,90,103). However, when used in the traditional way, it has the disadvantage that ventilation and metabolic rate are measured sequentially, and recordings of each are therefore interrupted periodically (109). Furthermore, after measurement of ventilation, several minutes must pass for the system to regain steady-state conditions before another recording of metabolic rate can be made [using Eqs (2) and (3)]. This problem can be circumvented by raising airflow rates to effect rapid restoration of chamber gas concentrations, and measuring ventilation and metabolic rate simultaneously in the closed intervals [using Eqs. (5) and (6)]. Two additional practical difficulties are apparent with the intermittent flow approach. Changes in flow can be disturbing to the experimental animals and a conditioning period of several days may be needed to ensure that sleep–wake patterns are "normal." Second, it is necessary to ensure that the inlet gas is fully equilibrated to chamber temperature and saturated with water vapor to avoid baseline drift following closure of the system.

Pappenheimer (95) and Jacky (112) realized that it is not necessary to close the plethysmograph in order to make ventilatory measurements. The system will faithfully register the respiratory pressure waveform as long as the rate of dissipation of pressure through leaks in the system is significantly slower than the rate of pressure fluctuation due to respiration. Thus, continuous simultaneous recordings of ventilation and metabolic rate are possible in an open-flow plethysmograph. Pappenheimer's (95) design (Fig. 7A) uses a high-resistance orifice at both the inlet and outlet air tubes of the animal chamber. Sufficient airflow is ensured by high-pressure supply at the inlet. The barometric pressure inside the animal chamber is maintained at atmospheric levels by adjusting the outflow resistance (using a needle valve) and withdrawing the air from the chamber under vacuum. In practice, the outflow resistance must be monitored and adjusted occasionally to prevent pressure drift.

Jacky's (112) design differs from that of Pappenheimer (95) in that it features relatively low impedance inlet tubes. Air is drawn by vacuum through the plethysmograph and the low-impedance inlet ensures maintenance of near-ambient barometric pressure. The inlet tube is long (3–5 m), imparting high inertance to the inlet gas so that changes in gas flow rate due to pressure oscillations within the chamber are resisted. Thus, pressure changes are dissipated slowly and an undamped respiratory pressure waveform is observed. A practical difficulty with Jacky's (112) design is that both animal and reference chambers must be ventilated and the impedances of the two must be matched. This involves adjusting the length of the reference chamber inlet tube to achieve coarse matching, then using a needle valve for fine adjustments of reference chamber airflow. The system must be monitored and reference chamber flow adjusted occasionally to prevent drift of differential pressure.

For experiments lasting longer than a working day, the problems of pressure drift can be overcome through the use of a computer-mediated feedback control system, as was demonstrated recently for a Pappenheimer-type open-flow system (107).

A closed-system plethysmograph (Fig. 7b) avoids some of the problems discussed above in relation to the intermittent and continuous open-flow systems. It offers the advantages of continuous operation and good temporal resolution of metabolic rate measurements, enabling state-specific assessment in animals such as rats and mice that exhibit short sleep cycles. Although this system is simple in principle, in practice considerable effort is required during construction to eliminate leaks, dampen pressure fluctuations generated by the pump, and match impedances of the inlet and outlet orifices, in order to achieve a stable baseline. Another disadvantage of the closed design is the relative difficulty in exposing the experimental animals to steady-state test gases, such as hypoxia, hypercapnia, or aerosolized histamine. The closed system is ideally suited to experiments involving stimulation with progressive asphyxia (98). The animal chamber is ventilated with a recirculating airflow. Carbon dioxide produced by the animal is scrubbed using alkaline pellets or solution and the oxygen consumed by the animal is replenished from a pressurized O_2 cylinder. An efficient way to match O_2 consumption and supply is to use the output of the O_2 analyzer to trigger a solenoid valve that regulates O_2 flow. Placement of a calibrated pneumotachograph in the O_2 supply tube allows measurement of O_2 infusion over time, which under steady-state conditions is equal to $\dot{V}_{O_2}$ (113). These O_2 infusions also serve as repeated calibrations for V_T because each time a volume of O_2 is infused (V_{cal}), the pressure in the system is increased (ΔP_{cal}). Furthermore, under steady-state conditions, $\dot{V}_{CO_2}$ can be calculated from Eq. (3) by measuring FCO_2 both before (F_eCO_2) and after (F_iCO_2) the CO_2 scrubber.

D. Summary

Whole-body plethysmography is well suited to studies of respiration in sleeping rodents. Because it is a noninvasive method, it enables quantification of lung ventilation and metabolic rate in chronic undisturbed animals. However, there are limitations to the technique, and several variations in the basic design have been used. No single design is suitable for all experimental situations. We recommend an intermittent or continuous open-flow system for short-term or long-term experiments in which test gases are to be supplied to the animals. If sleep-state-specific measurements of metabolic rate are required, the intermittent flow system is optimized by measuring ventilation, $\dot{V}_{O_2}$ and $\dot{V}_{CO_2}$ simultaneously during the closed intervals [Eqs. (5) and (6)]. The continuous flow design is better when rapid gas exchange measurements are not needed. The closed system combines the advantages of sleep-state-specific measurements with uninterrupted recording, but initial implementation of the system and application of test gases during experiments is difficult. In experiments where R_{aw} is expected to change substantially, respiratory frequency and metabolic rate can be quantified, but whole-body plethysmography cannot measure V_T accurately, so only qualitative impressions of respiratory effort are provided.

Acknowledgments

The work of RLH is supported by the Canadian Institutes of Health Research (Operating Grant 15563), Canada Foundation for Innovation, and the Ontario Research and Development Challenge Fund. RLH is a recipient of a Canadian Institutes of Health Research Scholarship. The work of RS is supported by Natural Sciences and Engineering Research Council of Canada. RS thanks E. J. Gucciardi for permission to use unpublished Figure 6. The work of CPO is supported by grants HL51292, HL63767, HL66324 from the Heart, Blood, and Lung Institute of the National Institutes of Health.

References

1. National Commission on Sleep Disorders Research. Wake Up America: A National Sleep Alert. Washington, DC: Government Printing Office, 1993, 302 pp.
2. Phillipson, E. A. Sleep apnea. A major public health problem. N Engl J Med 1993; 328:1271–1273.
3. Young, T., Palta, M., Dempsey, J., Skatrud, J., and Badr, S. The occurrence of sleep-disordered breathing among middle-aged adults. N Engl J Med 1993; 328:1230–1235.
4. George, C. F. P., Nickerson, W., Hanley, P. J., Millar, T. W., and Kryger, M. H. Sleep apnoea patients have more automobile accidents. Lancet 1987; 2:447.
5. Findley, L. J., Levinson, M. P., and Bonnie, R. J. Driving performance and automobile accidents in patients with sleep apnea. Clin Chest Med 1992; 13:427–435.
6. Brooks, D., Horner, R. L., Kozar, L. F., Render-Teixeira, C. L., and Phillipson, E. A. Obstructive sleep apnea as a cause of systemic hypertension: evidence from a canine model. J Clin Invest 1997; 99:106–109.
7. Shepard, J. W., Jr. Hypertension cardiac arrhythmias myocardial infarction and stroke in relation to obstructive sleep apnea. Clin Chest Med 1992; 13:437–458.
8. Kimoff, R. J., Brooks, D., Horner, R. L., Kozar, L. F., Render-Teixeira, C. L., Champagne, V., Mayer, P., and Phillipson, E. A. Ventilatory and arousal responses to hypoxia and hypercapnia in a canine model of obstructive sleep apnea. Am J Respir Crit Care Med 1997; 156:886–894.
9. Brooks, D., Horner, R. L., Kimoff, R. J., Kozar, L. F., Render-Teixeira, C. L., and Phillipson, E. A. Effect of obstructive sleep apnea versus sleep fragmentation on acute responses to airway occlusion in the dog. Am J Respir Crit Care Med 1997; 155:1609–1617.
10. National Institutes of Health. National Heart, Lung, and Blood Institute. Oxygen sensing during intermittent hypoxia. Request for Applications: HL-00-004. http://grants.nih.gov/grants/guide/rfa-files/RFA-HL-00-004.html, 1999, Nov. 29.
11. Sieck, G. C. Physiological and genomic consequences of intermittent hypoxia. J Appl Physiol 2001; 90:1187–1188.
12. Neubauer, J. A. Physiological and pathological responses to intermittent hypoxia. J Appl Physiol 2001; 90:1593–1599.
13. Paxinos, G. and Watson, C. The Rat Brain in Stereotaxic Co-Ordinates. San Diego: Academic Press, 1986.
14. Paxinos, G. The Rat Nervous System. 2nd ed. San Diego: Academic Press, 1995.
15. Fletcher, E. C., Lesske, J., Qian, W., Miller, C. C. III, and Unger, T. Repetitive, episodic hypoxia causes diurnal elevation of blood pressure in rats. Hypertension 1992; 19:555–561.

16. Bakehe, M., Miramand, J. L., Chambille, B., Gaultier, C., and Escourrou, P. Cardiovascular changes during acute episodic repetitive hypoxic and hypercapnic breathing in rats. Eur Respir J 1995; 8:1675–1680.

17. Fletcher, E. C. and Bao, G. The rat as a model of chronic recurrent episodic hypoxia and effect upon systemic blood pressure. Sleep 1996; 19:S210–212.

18. Greenberg, H. E., Sica, A., Batson, D., and Scharf, S. M. Chronic intermittent hypoxia increases sympathetic responsiveness to hypoxia and hypercapnia. J Appl Physiol 1999; 86:298–305.

19. Kraiczi, H., Magga, J., Sun, X. Y., Ruskoaho, H., Zhao, X., and Hedner, J. Hypoxic pressor response, cardiac size, and natriuretic peptides are modified by long-term intermittent hypoxia. J Appl Physiol 1999; 87:2025–2031.

20. Bao, G., Metreveli, N., and Fletcher, E. C. Acute and chronic blood pressure response to recurrent acoustic arousal in rats. Am J Hypertens. 1999; 12:504–510.

21. Trachsel, L., Tobler, I., and Borbély, A. A. Electroencephalogram analysis of non-rapid-eye-movement sleep in rats. Am J Physiol 1988; 255:R27–R37.

22. Hamrahi, H., Chan, B., and Horner, R. L. On-line detection of sleep-wake states and application to produce intermittent hypoxia exclusively in sleep in rats. J Appl Physiol. In press.

23. Horner, R. L., Sanford, L. D., Annis, D., Pack, A. I., and Morrison, A. R. Serotonin at the laterodorsal tegmental nucleus suppresses rapid-eye-movement sleep in freely behaving rats. J Neurosci 1997; 17:7541–7552.

24. Freedman, N. L. A sliding gas-delivery system and ventilating chamber for small animals fixed in standard stereotaxic instruments. Behav Res Methods Instrum Comput 1992; 24:423–425.

25. Benington, J. H., Kodali, S. K., and Heller, H. C. Scoring transitions to REM sleep in rats based on the EEG phenomena of pre-REM sleep: an improved analysis of sleep structure. Sleep 1994; 17:28–36.

26. American Sleep Disorders Association. EEG arousals: scoring rules and examples. Sleep 1992; 15:173–184.

27. Robert, C., Guilpin, C., and Limoge, A. Review of neural network applications in sleep research. J Neurosci Methods 1998; 79:187–193.

28. Robert, C., Guilpin, C., and Limoge, A. Automated sleep staging systems in rats. J Neurosci Methods 1999; 88:111–122.

29. Pardey, J., Roberts, S., Tarassenko, L., and Stradling, J. A new approach to the analysis of the human sleep/wakefulness continuum. J Sleep Res 1996; 5:201–210.

30. Carley, D. W., Önal, E., and Lopata, M. Quantitative analyses of state of vigilance in periodic breathing. In: Kuna, S. T., Suratt, P. M., Remmers, J. E., ed. Sleep and Respiration in Aging Adults, New York: Elsevier, 1991:287–296.

31. Bergmann, B. M., Kushida, C. A., Everson, C. A., Gilliland, M. A., Obermeyer, W., and Rechtschaffen, A. Sleep deprivation in the rat: II. Methodology. Sleep 1989; 12:5–12.

32. Bergmann, B. M., Winter, J. B., Rosenberg, R. S., and Rechtschaffen, A. NREM sleep with low-voltage EEG in the rat. Sleep 1987; 10:1–11.

33. Rechtschaffen, A., Gilliland, M. A., Bergmann, B. M., and Winter, J. B. Physiological correlates of prolonged sleep deprivation in rats. Science 1983; 221:182–184.

34. Shaw, P. J., Bergmann, B. M., and Rechtschaffen, A. Effects of paradoxical sleep deprivation on thermoregulation in the rat. Sleep 1998; 21:7–17.

35. Feng, P., Vogel, G. W., Obermeyer, W., and Kinney, G. W. An instrumental method for long-term continuous REM sleep deprivation of neonatal rats. Sleep 2000; 23:175–183.

36. Hamrahi, H., Stephenson, R., Mahamed, S., Liao, K. S., and Horner, R. L. Regulation of sleep-wake states in response to intermittent hypoxic stimuli applied only in sleep J Appl Physiol 2001; 90:2490–2501.

37. Borbély, A. A. Sleep homeostasis and models of sleep regulation. In: Kryger, M. H., Roth, T., and Dement, W. C., eds. Principles and Practice of Sleep Medicine. 2nd ed. Philadelphia: W. B. Saunders, 1994: 309–320.

38. Van Gelder, R. N., Edgar, D. M., and Dement, W. C. Real-time automated sleep scoring: validation of a microcomputer-based system for mice. Sleep 1991; 14:48–55.

39. Feng, P. and Vogel, G. W. A new method for continuous long-term polysomnographic recording of neonatal rats. Sleep 2001; 23:9–14.

40. Kimoff, R. J., Makino, H., Horner, R. L., Kozar, L. F., Lue, F., Slutsky, A. S., and Phillipson, E. A. A canine model of obstructive sleep apnea: model description and preliminary application. J Appl Physiol 1994; 76:1810–1817.

41. Horner, R. L., Brooks, D., Kozar, L. F., Leung, E., Hamrahi, H., Render-Teixeira, C. L., Makino, H., Kimoff, R. J., and Phillipson, E. A. Sleep architecture in a canine model of obstructive sleep apnea. Sleep 1998; 21:847–858.

42. Issa, F. G. and Sullivan, C. E. The immediate effects of nasal continuous airway pressure treatment on sleep pattern in patients with obstructive sleep apnea syndrome. Electroenceph Clin Neurophysiol 1986; 63:10–17.

43. Karni, A., Tanne, D., Rubenstein, B. S., Askenasy, J. J. M., and Sagi, D. Dependence on REM sleep of overnight improvement of a perceptual skill. Science 1994; 265:679–682.

44. Smith, C. Sleep states, memory processes and synaptic plasticity. Behav Brain Res 1996; 78:49–56.

45. Jelev, A., Sood, S., Liu, H., and Horner, R. L. Microdialysis perfusion of 5-HT into the hypoglossal motor nucleus differentially modulates genioglossus activity across natural sleep-wake states in rats. J Physiol 2001; 532:467–481.

46. Megirian, D., Hinrichsen, C. F. L., and Sherrey, J. H. Respiratory roles of genioglossus, sternohyoid, and sternohyoid muscles during sleep. Exp Neurol 1985; 90:118–128.

47. Fuller, D., Mateika, J. H., and Fregosi, R. F. Co-activation of tongue protruder and retractor muscles during chemoreceptor stimulation in the rat. J Physiol 1998; 507:265–276.

48. Fletcher, E. C. Physiological consequences of intermittent hypoxia: systemic blood pressure. J Appl Physiol 2001; 90:1600–1605.

49. Bunag, R. D. Facts and fallacies about measuring blood pressure in rats. Clin Exp Hypertens 1983; A5(10):1659–1681.
50. Pettersen, J. C., Linartz, R. R., Hamlin, R. L., and Stoll, R. E. Noninvasive measurement of systemic arterial blood pressure in the conscious beagle dog. Fundam Appl Toxicol 1988; 10:89–97.
51. Hassler, C. R., Lutz, G. A., Linebaugh, R., and Cummings, K. D. Identification and evaluation of noninvasive blood pressure measuring techniques. Toxicol Appl Pharmacol 1979; 47:193–201.
52. Kvetnansky, R., Sun, C. L., Lake, C. R., Thoa, N., Torda, T., and Kopin, I. J. Effect of handling and forced immobilization on rat plasma levels of epinephrine, norepinephrine, and dopamine-β-hydroxylase. Endocrinology 1978; 103:1868–1874.
53. Chiueh, C. C. and Kopin, I. J. Hyperresponsivity of spontaneously hypertensive rat to indirect measurement of blood pressure. Am J Physiol 1978; 234:H690–H695.
54. Lestage, P., Vitte, P. A., Rolinat, J. P., Minot, R., Broussolle, E., and Bobillier, P. A chronic arterial and venous cannulation method for freely moving rats. J Neurosci Methods 1985; 13:213–222.
55. Armentano, R., Cabrera-Fischer, E., Breitbart, G., Pichel, R., Levenson, J., and Chau, N. P. Telemetry of aortic pressure in unrestrained animals: validation of the method over a wide range of blood pressure (from 40 to 200 mm Hg). Med Prog Technol 1990; 16:125–129.
56. DePasquale, M. J., Ringer, L. W., Winslow, R. L., Buchholz, R. A., and Fossa, A. A. Chronic monitoring of cardiovascular function in the conscious guinea pig using radio-telemetry. Clin Exp Hypertens 1994; 16:245–260.
57. Guiol, C., Ledoussal, C., and Surge, J. M. A radiotelemetry system for chronic measurement of blood pressure and heart rate in the unrestrained rat: validation of the method. J Pharmacol Toxicol Methods 1992; 28:99–105.
58. Sadoff, D. A., Fischel, R. J., Carroll, M. E., and Brockway, B. Chronic blood pressure radiotelemetry in rhesus macaques. Lab Anim Sci 1992; 42:78–80.
59. Schnell, C. R. and Wood, J. M. Measurement of blood pressure and heart rate by telemetry in conscious, unrestrained marmosets. Am J Physiol 1993; 264:H1509–1516.
60. Carley, D. W., Trbovic, S, M., Bozanich, A., and Radulovacki, M. Cardiopulmonary control in sleeping Sprague-Dawley rats treated with hydralazine. J Appl Physiol 1997; 83:1954–1961.
61. Brockway, B. P., Mills, P. A., and Azar, S. H. A new method for continuous chronic measurement and recording of blood pressure, heart rate and activity in the rat via radio-telemetry. Clin Exp Hypertens 1991; A13:885–895.
62. Brooks, D., Horner, R. L., Kozar, L. F., Waddell, T. K., Render, C. L., and Phillipson, E. A. Validation of a telemetry system for long-term measurement of blood pressure. J Appl Physiol 1996; 81:1012–1018.
63. Oliverio, A. Sleep and activity rhythms in mice. Waking Sleeping 1980; 4:155–166.

64. Valatx, J. L., Bugat, R., and Jouvet, M. Genetic studies of sleep in mice. Nature 1972; 238:226–227.

65. Eleftheriou, B. E., Zolovick, A. J., and Elias, M. F. Electroencephalographic changes with age in male mice. Gerontologia 1975; 21:21–30.

66. Valatx, J. L. Enregistrement chronique des activites electriques cerebrales, musculaires et oculaires chez la souris. Soc Biol (Paris) 1971; 112–115.

67. Fishbein, W., Kastaniotis, C., and Chattman, D. Paradoxical sleep: prolonged augmentation following learning. Brain Res 1974; 79:61–75.

68. Van Twyver. Sleep patterns of five rodent species. Physiol Behav 1969; 4:901–905.

69. Chemelli, R. M., Willie, J. T., Sinton, C. M., Elmquist, J. K., Scammell, T., Lee, C., Richardson, J. A., Williams, S. C., Xiong, Y., Kisanuki, Y., Fitch, T. E., Nakazato, M., Hammer, R. E., Saper, C. B., and Yanagisawa, M. Narcolepsy in orexin knockout mice: molecular genetics of sleep regulation. Cell 1999; 98:437–451.

70. Tobler, I., Gaus, S. E., Deboer, T., Achermann, P., Fischer, M., Rulicke, T., Moser, M., Oesch, B., McBride, P. A., and Manson, J. C. Altered circadian activity rhythms and sleep in mice devoid of prion protein. Nature 1996; 380:639–642.

71. Fang, J., Wang, Y., and Krueger, J. M. Effects of interleukin-1 beta on sleep are mediated by the type I receptor. Am J Physiol 1998; 274:R655–R660.

72. Boutrel, B., Franc, B., Hen, R., Hamon, M., and Adrien, J. Key role of 5-HT1$_B$ receptors in the regulation of paradoxical sleep as evidenced in 5-HT1B knock-out mice. J Neurosci 1999; 19:3204–3212.

73. O'Donnell, C. P., Schaub, C. D., Haines, A. S., Berkowitz, D. E., Tankersley, C. G., Schwartz, A. R., and Smith, P. L. Leptin prevents respiratory depression in obesity. Am J Respir Crit Care Med 1999; 159:1477–1484.

74. Veasey, S. C., Valladares, O., Fenik, P., Kapfhamer, D., Sanford, L., Benington, J., and Bucan, M. An automated system for recording and analysis of sleep in mice. Sleep 2000; 23:1025–1040.

75. Franken, P., Malafosse, A., and Tafti, M. Genetic determinants of sleep regulation in inbred mice. Sleep 1999; 22:155–169.

76. Welsh, D. K., Richardson, G. S., and Dement, W. C. A circadian rhythm of hippocampal theta activity in the mouse. Physiol Behav 1985; 35:533–538.

77. Schaub, C. D., Tankersley, C., Schwartz, A. R., Smith, P. L., Robotham, J. L., and O'Donnell, C. P. Effect of sleep/wake state on arterial blood pressure in genetically identical mice. J Appl Physiol 1998; 85:366–371.

78. Harris, D. V. and Walker, J. M. A semi-chronic electrode implant for very small animals. Brain Res Bull 1980; 5:479–480.

79. Ryan, L. J., Hall, F. L., and Young, S. J. An inexpensive, enclosed pool mercury commutator suitable for use with small animals. Physiol Behav 1982; 29:393–396.

80. Holley, J. R. and Powell, D. A. Mercury commutator arrangement for simultaneously stimulating or recording from two small animals in a social situation. Physiol Behav 1975; 15:741–743.

81. Weiss, T. and Rokdan, E. Comparative study of sleep cycles in rodents. Experientia 1964; 20:280–281.

82. Sinton, C. M. and Jouvet, M. Paradoxical sleep and coping with environmental change. Behav Brain Res 1983; 9:151–163.

83. Roussel, B., Turrillot, P., and Kitahama, K. Effect of ambient temperature on the sleep-walking cycle in two strains of mice. Brain Res 1984; 294:67–73.

84. Tankersley, C., Kleeberger, S., Russ, B., Schwartz, A., and Smith, P. Modified control of breathing in genetically obese (ob/ob) mice. J Appl Physiol 1996; 81:716–723.

85. Toth, L. A. and Williams, R. W. A quantitative genetic analysis of slow-wave sleep and rapid-eye movement sleep in CXB recombinant inbred mice. Behav Genet 1999; 29:329–337.

86. Franken, P., Malafosse, A., and Tafti, M. Genetic variation in EEG activity during sleep in inbred mice. Am J Physiol 1998; 275:R1127–R1137.

87. Tafti, M., Chollet, D., Valatx, J. L., and Franken, P. Quantitative trait loci approach to the genetics of sleep in recombinant inbred mice. J Sleep Res 1999; 8(suppl 1):37–43.

88. Naylor, E., Bergmann, B. M., Krauski, K., Zee, P. C., Takahashi, J. S., Vitaterna, M. H., and Trek, F. W. The circadian *Clock* mutation alters sleep homeostasis in the mouse. J Neurosci 2000; 20:8138–8143.

89. Chapin, J. L. Ventilatory response of the unrestrained and unanesthetized hamster to CO_2. Am J Physiol 1954; 179:146–148.

90. Drorbaugh, J. E. and Fenn, W. O. A barometric method for measuring ventilation in newborn infants. Pediatrics 1955; 16:81–89.

91. Malan, A. Ventilation measured by body plethysmography in hibernating mammals and in poikilotherms. Respir Physiol 1973; 17:32–44.

92. Mortola, J. P. and Frappell, P. B. On the barometric method for measurements of ventilation, and its use in small animals. Can J Physiol Pharmacol 1998; 76:937–944.

93. Chaui-Berlinck, J. G. and Bicudo, J. E. P. W. The signal in total-body plethysmography: errors due to adiabatic-isothermic difference. Respir Physiol 1998; 113:259–270.

94. Mortola, J. P. and Gautier, H. Interaction between metabolism and ventilation: Effects of respiratory gases and temperature. In: Dempsey, J. A., Pack, A. I., eds. Regulation of Breathing, New York: Marcel Dekker, 1995:1011–1064.

95. Pappenheimer, J. R. Sleep and respiration of rats during hypoxia. J Physiol Lond 1977; 266:191–207.

96. Peever, J. H. and Stephenson, R. Day-night differences in the respiratory response to hypercapnia in awake adult rats. Respir Physiol 1997; 109:241–248.

97. Withers, P. C. Measurement of V_{O_2}, V_{CO_2}, and evaporative water loss with a flow-through mask. J Appl Physiol 1977; 42:120–123.

98. Woodin, M. A. and Stephenson, R. Circadian rhythms in diving behavior and ventilatory response to asphyxia in canvasback ducks. Am J Physiol 1998; 274:R686–R693.

99. Stephenson, R. The contributions of body tissues, respiratory system, and plumage to buoyancy in waterfowl. Can J Zool 1993; 71:1521–1529.
100. Epstein, M. A. and Epstein, R. A. A theoretical analysis of the barometric method for measurement of tidal volume. Respir Physiol 1978; 32:105–120.
101. Epstein, R. A., Epstein, M. A. F., Haddad, G. G., and Mellins, R. B. Practical implementation of the barometric method for measurement of tidal volume. J Appl Physiol 1980; 49:1107–1115.
102. Jacky, J. P. Barometric measurement of tidal volume: effects of pattern and nasal temperature. J Appl Physiol 1980; 49:319–325.
103. Bartlett, D. Jr. and Tenney, S. M. Control of breathing in experimental anemia. Respir Physiol 1970; 10:384–395.
104. Fleming, P. J., Levine, M. R., Goncalves, A. L., and Woolard, S. Barometric plethysmograph: advantages and limitations in recording infant respiration. J Appl Physiol 1983; 55:1924–1931.
105. Onodera, M., Kuwaki, T., Kumada, M., and Masuda, Y. Determination of ventilatory volume in mice by whole-body plethysmography. Jap J Physiol 1997; 47:317–326.
106. Polgar, G. Comparison of methods for recording respiration in newborn infants. Pediatrics 1965; 36:861–868.
107. Seifert, E. L., Knowles, J., and Mortola, J. P. Continuous circadian measurements of ventilation in behaving adult rats. Respir Physiol 2000; 120:179–183.
108. Stahel, C. D. and Nicol, S. C. Comparison of barometric and pneumotachographic measurements of resting ventilation in the little penguin (*Eudyptula minor*). Comp Biochem Physiol 1988; 89A,387–390.
109. Mortola, J. P. and Maskrey, M. Ventilatory response to asphyxia in conscious rats: effect of ambient and body temperatures. Respir Physiol 1998; 111:233–246.
110. Nattie, E. and Li, A. Muscimol dialysis in the retrotrapezoid nucleus region inhibits breathing in the awake rat. J App Physiol 2000; 89:153–162.
111. Carley, D. W., Trbovic, S., and Radulovacki, M. Sleep apnea in normal and REM sleep-deprived normotensive Wistar-Kyoto and spontaneously hypertensive (SHR) rats. Physiol Behav 1996; 59:827–831.
112. Jacky, J. P. A plethysmograph for long-term measurements of ventilation in unrestrained animals. J Appl Physiol 1978; 45:644–647.
113. Stephenson, R. Diving energetics in lesser scaup (*Aythya fuligula*). J Exp Biol 1994; 190:155–178.

3

Neurochemical Evidence for the Cholinergic Modulation of Sleep and Breathing

RALPH LYDIC and HELEN A. BAGHDOYAN

University of Michigan
Ann Arbor, Michigan, U.S.A.

Sleep is the only naturally occurring behavioral state in which humans experience repeated airway obstructions. Many patients are unaware of these airway obstructions and their major complaint is excessive daytime sleepiness. Elucidating the neurochemical control of sleep is essential, therefore, for a complete understanding of the etiology, characteristics, and treatment of obstructive sleep apnea. The goal of this chapter is to describe how neurochemical studies of rapid eye movement (REM) sleep are providing novel insights into pontine acetylcholine (ACh) as a regulator of sleep and breathing. The chapter is organized around three themes, beginning with an overview of the cholinergic model of REM sleep. The second section shows how enhancing cholinergic neurotransmission in a nonrespiratory region of the pontine reticular formation significantly alters upper airway muscle control, ventilation, chemosensitivity, and neuronal excitability. The third section presents evidence that protein profiling can specify pre- and postsynaptic proteins contributing to the · cholinergic modulation of sleep and breathing. A diverse assortment of molecules influence sleep and breathing. The chapter concludes with unifying evidence that many of the molecules that alter REM sleep do so by modulating pontine cholinergic neurotransmission.

I. Experimental Models for Mechanistic Studies of REM Sleep and Breathing

Much of what we know about the cellular mechanisms generating sleep and breathing has been derived from studies of cat brain (1–4). Shortly after the 1953 identification of REM sleep in humans (5), a homologous sleep state with an "activated" electroencephalogram (EEG) was recorded from the cat (6). The sleep cycle in the cat is homologous to human sleep but it is not identical. There are significant species-specific features of REM sleep. In the cat, REM sleep occurs about every 25 min, whereas in the human REM sleep occurs about every 90 min. In normal social settings, human sleep is consolidated and occurs during the night. Feline sleep is expressed as a polycyclic rhythm of non-REM (NREM) and REM sleep throughout the 24-hr day. Humans spend about one-third of their life sleeping, whereas cats spend about half of their life asleep (7). A nihilistic focus on the differences between cat and human sleep might have retarded the development of sleep and respiratory neurobiology. Valuing the similarities—as well as differences—between feline and human REM sleep contributed to Jouvet's success in localizing REM sleep-generating neurons to the pontine brain stem (8,9). An inappropriate focus on the lack of identity between cat and human REM sleep would not have encouraged the first electrophysiological recordings of respiratory neuron discharge during sleep in the cat (10). All of the foregoing discoveries were made in the absence of evidence that cats experience obstructive sleep apnea.

Available data make clear that multiple animal models and experimental methods are providing the most productive approach for understanding sleep and breathing. For example, gene mapping studies in the dog led to the discovery that canine narcolepsy was caused by a mutation in the hypocretin/orexin receptor 2 gene (11). Whereas narcoleptic dogs lack the hypocretin/orexin receptor 2, mice with the hypocretin/orexin gene knocked out lack the peptide and have abnormal sleep (12). The postmortem finding that brains from narcolepsy patients have fewer than normal hypocretin/orexin neurons (13) is consistent with the view that loss or dysfunction of hypocretin/orexin-containing neurons causally contributes to human narcolepsy (14). These narcolepsy data illustrate how multiple animal models are needed for a molecular characterization of complex human disorders (15).

Advances in comparative genomics provide a new perspective on the cat as a model for studies of sleep and breathing. The first cat gene map was published in 1982 (16), and subsequent mapping studies show a high degree of conservation between cat and human genomes (17). Relative to the human, the cat displays the fewest number of chromosome changes of all nonprimate species examined to date (18). There are fewer chromosomes in the cat (18 pair plus sex chromosomes) than in the dog (39 pair plus sex chromosomes) (17). The cat also has fewer rearrangements of chromosomes than the dog or mouse, and the cat shows promise as a model for more than 200 genetic diseases (17). The extensive sleep and breathing phenotype data already obtained from the cat ultimately will enrich the cat as a genetic model.

II. The Cholinergic Model of REM Sleep Generation

About the same time that Dement discovered a sleep state in cat characterized by EEG activation (6), Longo in Rome reported that the EEG was activated by the acetylcholinesterase (AChE) inhibitor eserine (physostigmine) (19). In the early 1960s, cat experiments using intracranial drug delivery suggested that brain ACh was a sleep-modulating molecule (20,21). Administration of microgram quantities of cholinergic agonists into the pontine reticular formation of an intact, unanesthetized cat caused a state that was polygraphically and behaviorally similar to REM sleep (21–23). The pharmacological model of REM sleep provided pioneering evidence in support of the view that ACh contributes to REM sleep generation (24,25). Additional evidence for cholinergic generation of REM sleep came from data showing that blocking the degradation of endogenous ACh enhanced REM sleep. Domino and colleagues were the first to demonstrate that REM sleep in the cat was increased by intravenous administration of physostigmine, an inhibitor of the degradative enzyme AChE (26). Of particular relevance to this volume on experimental models for the study of sleep and breathing is evidence that intramuscular administration of a muscarinic antagonist increases REM sleep latency (27) and intravenous administration of an AChE inhibitor significantly decreases latency to REM sleep onset (28) in humans. Thus, there is good agreement between cat and human data that ACh contributes to the regulation of sleep. Detailed accounts of these pioneering discoveries on ACh as a modulator of neuronal excitability and REM sleep are available elsewhere (1,29,30). Evidence from many laboratories concurs that the cholinergic model of REM sleep is remarkably similar to natural REM sleep (31–34).

III. Koch's Postulates Are Satisfied by Cholinergic Modulation of REM Sleep

The 1905 Nobel Prize in Medicine was awarded to Robert Koch (1843–1910), who developed four criteria that must be satisfied for identifying the causal agent of an infectious disease (35). Koch's postulates illustrate the importance of conceptual as well as experimental models. By changing the focus from agents causing infectious disease to molecules causing REM sleep, one can apply Koch's postulates to the cholinergic control of sleep. Presently available data satisfy Koch's four postulates and confirm the cholinergic hypothesis of REM sleep generation (36).

First, for a molecule to be considered as causing a REM sleep state, the state must be reproduced when the putatively causal agent is administered. This first postulate has been addressed by many laboratories where experiments using intracranial drug delivery have significantly advanced sleep neurobiology (reviewed in Ref. 37). Pontine administration of cholinergic agonists (38) and AChE inhibitors (39) significantly enhances REM sleep. Receptor mediation is supported by the fact that cholinergic REM sleep enhancement is dose dependent and blocked by pontine injections of the muscarinic cholinergic antagonist atropine (39,40). Figure 1 schematically illustrates the pontine region for, and the polygraphic features of, cholinergically evoked REM sleep. (See color insert.) The excitability of some neurons in medial pontine reticular formation (mPRF) of the cat is increased during REM sleep (41) and in vitro studies show that cholinergic agonists increase neuronal excitability in homologous pontine reticular neurons of the rat (42).

Second, for a molecule to be considered as causing REM sleep, the putatively causal agent should be present during the experimentally induced state (Fig. 1.2). Ten years ago, microdialysis data showed that ACh release in the mPRF increased during the REM sleep-like state caused by microinjecting cholinergic agonists into the contralateral mPRF (43).

Third, during the spontaneously occurring state the putatively causal agent should be present. ACh is synthesized in neurons of the laterodorsal tegmental (LDT) and pedunculopontine tegmental (PPT) nuclei (44). Retrograde tracing studies show that the mPRF receives cholinergic projections from LDT/PPT (45,46). Functional studies found that ACh release in medial pontine reticular regions regulating REM sleep originates from LDT/PPT neurons (47). Figure 1.3A shows polygraphic similarity between REM sleep and REM sleep enhancement caused by mPRF administration of the AChE inhibitor neostigmine (REM-Neo). The histogram in Figure 1.3B shows that compared to waking or NREM sleep,

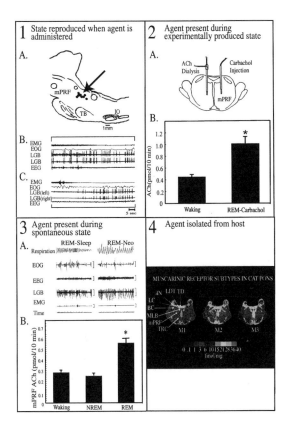

Figure 1 Rapid eye movement sleep generation by pontine cholinergic neurotransmission satisfies Koch's postulates. (1A) Sagittal drawing of cat brain stem (rostral to left) at 1.5 mm from midline. Arrow points to injection sites in the medial pontine reticular formation (mPRF) where cholinergic agonists and acetylcholinesterase inhibitors significantly enhance REM sleep. (From Ref. 39.) (1B) Polygraphic tracings obtained from an animal transitioning from slow wave sleep into REM sleep. (1C) A polygraphic trace showing onset of REM sleep caused by mPRF administration of cholinergic agonists or an acetylcholinesterase inhibitor. (1B,C reprinted from Ref. 172 with permission from Excerpta Medica Inc.) (2A) Schematic diagram of microdialysis (ACh dialysis) in one side of the pontine reticular formation simultaneous with carbachol injection into the contralateral pons. (From Ref. 43.) (2B) ACh release is significantly increased during the REM sleep-like state produced by mPRF injection of carbachol. (Data from Ref. 43.) (3) ACh is significantly enhanced during spontaneous REM sleep. (3A) Polygraphic similarities between REM sleep and REM sleep enhanced by preventing the degradation of the endogenous ACh by mPRF administration of neostigmine. (From Ref. 49.) (3B) mPRF ACh release is significantly enhanced during REM sleep compared to waking and NREM sleep. (Modified from Ref. 49.) (3A,B copyright 1997 by the Society for Neuroscience.) (4) Similar to the neurotransmitter ACh, muscarinic cholinergic receptors have been identified in the medial pontine reticular formation. (From Ref. 52.) (See color insert.)

ACh release in the pontine reticular formation is greatest during spontaneous REM sleep (48,49). Because sleep-dependent alterations in ACh release arise from synaptic release, one would predict enhancement of LDT/PPT activity during REM sleep if ACh were a causal contributor to REM sleep. Electrophysiological data show LDT/PPT cell discharge increases above waking and NREM sleep levels 60 sec before—and throughout—REM sleep (50). Glucose utilization studies show that cellular energy metabolism in LDT/PPT is greater during REM sleep than during waking or NREM sleep (51).

Satisfying Koch's fourth postulate requires that the putatively causal agent be isolated from the host. To differentiate Koch's third and fourth postulates, we add the additional stipulation that in the absence of a viable binding site, a molecule such as ACh is irrelevant. Thus, satisfying postulate four also requires the identification of cholinergic receptors in brain regions regulating sleep. Muscarinic cholinergic receptors have been identified in the same regions of the mPRF (Fig. 1.4) where micro-injection of cholinergic agonists and AChE inhibitors causes REM sleep (52–54).

IV. Upper Airway Muscle Activity Is Modulated by Cholinergic Pontine Mechanisms

In 1989, data from intact, unanesthetized cat showed that the cholinergic model of REM sleep was a powerful tool for studies of sleep and breathing (55,56). Since that time many laboratories have demonstrated the utility of the cholinergic model (reviewed in Refs. 37 and 57). The model has been extended to rodents using intact and surgically reduced adult (57) and neonatal (58) preparations. Studies focusing on breathing during REM sleep are justified by more than 30 years of human data showing that the duration of sleep apnea is greatest during REM sleep (59–61). These data stand in contrast to the rare report that "respiratory disturbance is not greatly affected by sleep stage, in most patients" (62). Obstructive sleep apnea is present in 2% of children (63) and these airway obstructions occur predominantly during the REM phase of sleep (64,65). The number of apneic events per unit of time also is greatest during REM sleep (reviewed in Ref. 66). Increases in REM sleep-related apneas have been demonstrated for many animal models including rat (67,68), English bulldog (69), cat (56), and goat (70). These observations are extensively reviewed in Chapters 8 through 11 of this volume.

Application of the cholinergic model of REM sleep to studies of breathing during sleep began with investigations of upper airway musculature. The posterior cricoarytenoid (PCA) muscles are located bilaterally on the external, posterior larynx (Fig. 2a). These accessory muscles of breathing are not thought to contribute to obstructive sleep apnea, but have provided insights into the effects of sleep on upper airway neuromuscular control (71,72). The PCA muscles function to regulate speech and to open the laryngeal folds during every inspiration. The human PCA muscle comprises vertical/oblique and horizontal compartments that are innervated by two branches of the recurrent laryngeal nerve (73). Recordings of human PCA muscle activity across the sleep–wake cycle (72) reveal muscular hypotonia during the progression from wakefulness to NREM sleep (Fig. 2b).

The state-dependent discharge of laryngeal PCA muscle activity is highly conserved and can be recorded in the cat. PCA muscles in the cat also reveal a diminished discharge during REM sleep compared to wakefulness (71). Intracellular recording of spinal motoneurons revealed that they are actively hyperpolarized during REM sleep and during the cholinergically evoked REM sleep-like state (74). This finding stimulated us to make the first recordings of upper airway muscle activity during the REM sleep-like state caused by pontine injections of carbachol (55). The results of these studies showed that mPRF microinjection of the cholinergic agonist carbachol enhanced REM sleep and caused hypotonia in the PCA muscles of the cat (Fig. 3).

The cellular mechanisms by which pontine cholinergic agonists cause PCA muscle hypotonia remain to be elucidated. The widely distributed pontine reticular formation afferent and efferent projections suggest multiple pathways and mechanisms through which PCA hypotonia might be evoked cholinergically from the mPRF. Neuroanatomical pathway tracing with the transsynaptic labeling protein pseudorabies virus showed that virus injections into the PCA muscle were traceable to mPRF regions that regulated REM sleep (75). Regions of the mPRF known to generate REM sleep have monosynaptic connections with many brain stem respiratory nuclei (40). Additional pathways from the pontine reticular formation activate nucleus gigantocellularis in the medullary reticular formation and inhibit motor tone (76). The muscular hypotonia of REM sleep may contribute to the diminished ability to generate an appropriate ventilatory response to hypercapnia during human REM sleep (61) and during cholinergically enhanced REM sleep (77).

(a)

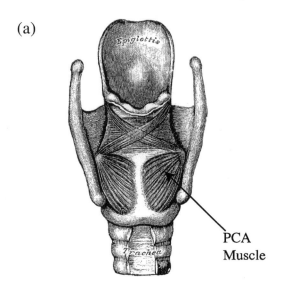

PCA
Muscle

(b)   Human PCA EMG

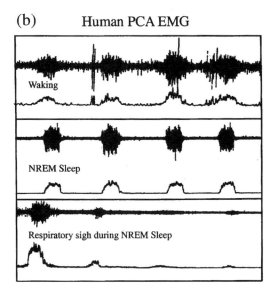

Figure 2 Sleep-dependent changes in upper airway muscle activity. (a) Posterior view of the muscles of the human larynx. Arrow points to the posterior cricoarytenoid (PCA) muscle. The PCA muscle is an accessory respiratory muscle. (Modified from *Gray's Anatomy* by H. Gray, copyright 1966 by permission of Churchill Livingstone.) (b) Electromyographic (EMG) activity recorded from the human PCA muscle during the transition from waking to NREM sleep. Note the state-dependent decrease in inspiratory discharge of the PCA muscle. (From Ref. 72.)

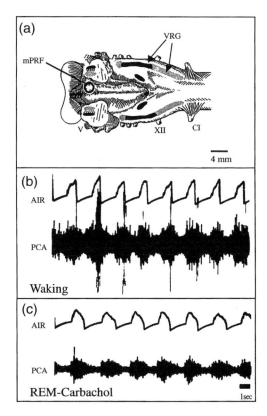

Figure 3 Enhancing pontine cholinergic neurotransmission causes state-dependent upper airway hypotonia. (a) Dorsal view of cat brain stem. In this drawing, the cerebellum has been removed and the perspective is looking into the fourth ventricle. Rostral is to the left. The drawing shows the relationship between the medial pontine reticular formation (mPRF) and the ventral respiratory group (VRG). The fifth (V) and twelfth (XII) cranial nerves and the first cervical nerve (C1) are labeled. (From Ref. 174.) (b) Oscilloscope trace showing air flow (AIR) and discharge of PCA muscle recorded from an awake cat. Note the inspiratory nature of the PCA discharge. (c) A recording from the same animal after carbachol had been microinjected into the mPRF region illustrated in A. Note the PCA hypotonia caused by pontine administration of carbachol. PCA motoneurons are located in the nucleus ambiguus within the VRG. These PCA motoneurons are approximately 9 mm from the mPRF injection site. This distance and the rapid onset of the upper airway muscle hypotonia led us to predict (55) that the cholinergic model of REM sleep could be used to determine whether this sleep-dependent hypotonia of the upper airway muscles was caused by active inhibition or disfacilitation. Evidence has been presented for postsynaptic inhibition of hypoglossal neurons during carbachol-induced REM sleep (115).

V. Cholinergic Pontine Mechanisms After Respiratory Neuron Excitability

The parabrachial region of the dorsolateral pons contains a cluster of premotor neurons that discharge in phase with the respiratory cycle (78). This pontine respiratory group (PRG) is not essential for respiratory rhythm generation, but is able to alter the timing of inspiration and expiration. This respiratory timing or "pneumotaxic" function within the dorsolateral pons first was localized by surgical transection of the brain stem (79). One may note that 40 years later, a similar transection approach was used to localize REM sleep-generating mechanisms to the pons (8). The pneumotaxic center contains the largest cluster of respiratory neurons in closest proximity to the pontine reticular regions that cause cholinergic REM sleep enhancement.

The PRG (as shown in Fig. 4a) comprises medial and lateral parabrachial nuclei (NPBM and NPBL) and the Kölliker-Fuse (KF) nucleus. These three nuclei contain neurons that discharge in phase with inspiration, expiration, or during the interval between breaths. Figures 4b and 4c illustrate that microinjection of the AChE inhibitor neostigmine into the mPRF (39) depressed the discharge of some pontine respiratory neurons (80). Depression of parabrachial cell discharge was present even when microinjections were made into mPRF regions contralateral to parabrachial recording sites. This observation is consistent with enhanced pontine cholinergic neurotransmission altering parabrachial cell discharge via synaptic mechanisms.

Available data show multiple mechanisms by which enhancing cholinergic neurotransmission in the mPRF can alter upper airway muscles. One mechanism for interaction includes monosynaptic and polysynaptic connections between mPRF regions regulating REM sleep and brain regions regulating respiration (40,75). In specific lateral regions of the pons, there also is structural overlap between peribrachial cholinergic neurons in the LDT/PPT nuclei and parabrachial neurons (NPBM, NPBL, KF) comprising the PRG. The distinction between peri- and parabrachial neurons long has been appreciated (1). The peribrachial LDT/PPT neurons synthesize ACh (44), project to the mPRF (45,46), and regulate ACh release in the mPRF (47) by synaptic processes involving negative feedback from muscarinic cholinergic autoreceptors (81). This intermingling of peri- and parabrachial neurons likely provides a second mechanism for pontine cholinergic modulation of breathing. A third mechanism by which mPRF cholinergic neurotransmission can alter upper airway muscles is through the interaction between brain stem respiratory nuclei. For example, this section has described mPRF influences on the PRG, but it also is clear

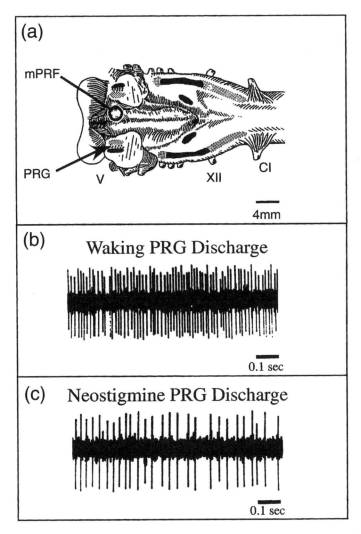

Figure 4 Enhancing pontine cholinergic neurotransmission decreases the discharge of some pontine respiratory neurons. (a) Dorsal view of cat brain stem with cerebellum removed. Perspective is from above looking into the fourth ventricle of the cat brain stem. Rostral is to the left. This drawing illustrates the relationship between the medial pontine reticular formation (mPRF) and the pontine respiratory group (PRG). (b) The extracellular discharge of a cell recorded from the pontine respiratory group of an awake, unanesthetized cat. (c) A recording from the same cell following pontine administration of the acetylcholinesterase inhibitor neostigmine. Note that blocking the degradation of ACh decreases the discharge of the cell in the pontine respiratory group. (b and c from Ref. 80.)

that the PRG can alter medullary hypoglossal nuclei regulating the tongue (82).

VI. Role of the Tongue and Hypoglossal Nucleus in Airway Obstruction

Sleep-dependent hypotonia of the tongue (genioglossus) muscle has been suggested to contribute to the airway obstruction of human sleep apnea (83–85). These studies presented evidence in favor of the tongue blocking the posterior pharyngeal wall when a sleeper assumes the supine position. The genioglossus muscle functions to protrude the tongue and is innervated by the medial branch of the hypoglossal (XII) nerve, whereas the lateral branch of the XIIth nerve innervates the hyoglossus and styloglossus muscles, which retract the tongue (Fig. 5) (reviewed in Ref. 86). Many studies of genioglossal electromyographic (EMG) activity consistently document decrements in tongue muscle tone and hypoglossal nerve activity during sleep (87,88), anesthesia (89), and sedation (90). Studies of sleep apnea patients show that during wakefulness these patients exhibit a compensatory increase in genioglossus muscle EMG that is lost during sleep (91,92). Electrical stimulation of the XIIth nerve in sleep apnea patients increases airflow and decreases apnea frequency (93). Electrical stimulation of tongue protruder or coactivation of protruder and retractor muscles also improves airway flow mechanics in the rat (94). These findings are consistent with earlier reports that contraction of the genioglossus muscle during inspiration contributes to airway dilation (95). The foregoing data encourage exploration of electric stimulation of upper airway muscles as an alternative treatment for patients with obstructive sleep apnea (96).

The data outlined above have stimulated efforts to elucidate the cellular mechanisms regulating genioglossal muscle and excitability of hypoglossal neurons. There is good evidence that hypoglossal neuronal excitability is altered by both serotonin (5-HT) and ACh. The discharge of 5-HT-containing neurons in the midline raphe nuclei is positively correlated with wakefulness, decreases during NREM sleep, and ceases during REM sleep (reviewed in Ref. 3). Caudal raphe neurons project 5-HT-containing terminals to hypoglossal nucleus (97) and 5-HT enhances the excitability of hypoglossal neurons (98). Thus, the REM sleep offset of raphe neuron discharge is consistent with the increased number and duration of apneas during REM sleep. This evidence is more fully reviewed in Chapter 5 of this volume. The possibility that 5-HT can causally contribute to sleep apnea also is suggested by the finding that administration of fluoxetine, a 5-HT reuptake blocker, improves some cases of obstructive sleep apnea (99).

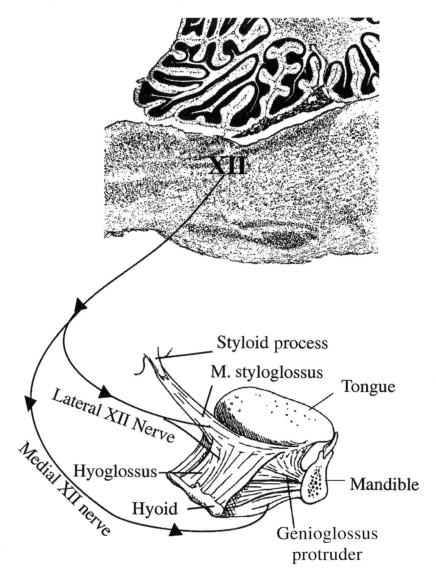

Figure 5 Medullary hypoglossal nucleus (XII) innervation of the tongue muscle. Top photomicrograph is a sagittal view of the medullary brain stem of the cat. Sagittal section is just off midline and illustrates the hypoglossal nucleus as a thin band of cells near the dorsal surface. Rostral is to the right. (From Ref. 175.) The lower half of this figure schematically shows innervation of the tongue muscle by the lateral and medial branches of the hypoglossal nerve. (Modified from Ref. 176 with permission from Elsevier Science.)

Many studies indicate that serotonergic influences on the hypoglossal nucleus are significantly altered by pontine cholinergic neurotransmission. During REM sleep the decreased discharge of 5-HT neurons is accompanied by an increased discharge in putatively cholinergic LDT/PPT neurons (50) and increased ACh release from LDT/PPT terminals in the mPRF (48,49). Microinjection of cholinergic agonists into the mPRF significantly decreases serotonin levels in the hypoglossal nucleus (100; see also Chap. 5 of this volume). It is logical to assume that medullary respiratory neurons might comprise one mechanism influencing the hypoglossal nucleus. Recordings of premotor neurons in the ventral respiratory group (VRG of Fig. 3) projecting to XII suggest that nonrespiratory pathways play a major role in the suppression of XII motoneurons (101). The data reviewed in this chapter support the view that pontine cholinergic and cholinoceptive neurons regulating REM sleep comprise one neuronal substrate that also influences breathing (32).

There also is evidence for intrinsic cholinergic modulation of hypoglossal excitability. In rat dorsal medulla there are three major sources of cholinergic neurons. The dorsal motor nucleus of the vagus, the medial subnucleus and intermediate subnucleus of the nucleus tractus solitarii, and the hypoglossal nuclei all contain cholinergic neurons (102). Cholinergic neurons are phenotypically defined by the ACh synthetic enzyme choline acetyltransferase (ChAT). The distribution of ChAT-positive (ChAT+) neurons in the hypoglossal nucleus is illustrated in Figure 6 (102).

Functional data indicate a role for cholinergic neurotransmission in the regulation of the hypoglossal nucleus. Neurons in the hypoglossal nucleus discharge in phase with the respiratory rhythm (87,103,104) and this discharge pattern persists in brain stem slice preparations (105). In humans, the timing of genioglossal muscle activation is critical to normal breathing. The tongue is activated before peak inspiration and this phase relationship is believed to contribute to upper airway patency (106). In addition to being rhythmically active, tongue muscle excitability is influenced by mechanoreceptor input from the upper airway. Negative upper airway pressure activates human airway dilator muscles (107), including the genioglossus muscle during sleep (108).

Chemoreceptor afferents to the hypoglossal nucleus may be less important than input from tongue mechanoreceptors. In awake humans, hypoxia and hypercapnia do not have the pronounced impact on genioglossal EMG activity that can be evoked even with slowly applied negative pressure (109). The foregoing conclusion stands in contrast to the hypoglossal response to anoxia recorded from mouse brain stem slice. Simultaneous extracellular recordings from hypoglossal neurons and from

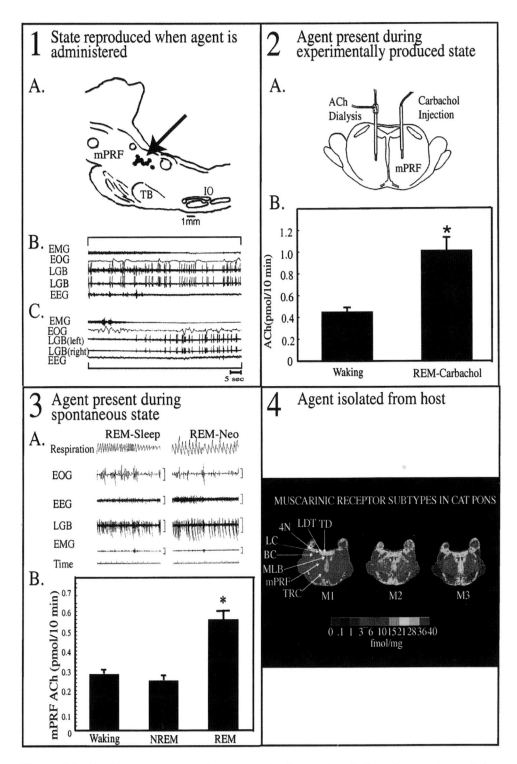

1 State reproduced when agent is administered

A.

mPRF
TB
IO
1mm

B. EMG
EOG
LGB
LGB
EEG

C. EMG
EOG
LGB(left)
LGB(right)
EEG

5 sec

2 Agent present during experimentally produced state

A.

ACh Dialysis
Carbachol Injection
mPRF

B.

ACh(pmol/10 min)

1.2
1.0
0.8
0.6
0.4
0.2
0

Waking   REM-Carbachol
*

3 Agent present during spontaneous state

A.

REM-Sleep   REM-Neo
Respiration
EOG
EEG
LGB
EMG
Time

B.

mPRF ACh (pmol/10 min)

0.7
0.6
0.5
0.4
0.3
0.2
0.1
0

Waking   NREM   REM
*

4 Agent isolated from host

MUSCARINIC RECEPTOR SUBTYPES IN CAT PONS

4N LDT TD
LC
BC
MLB
mPRF
TRC   M1   M2   M3

0 .1 1 3 6 1015212283640
fmol/mg

Figure 3.1 Rapid eye movement sleep generation by pontine cholinergic neurotransmission satisfies Koch's postulates. (See p. 61 for complete legend.)

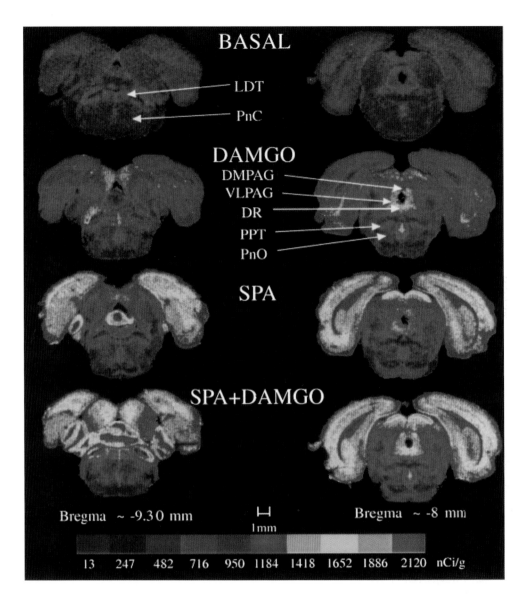

Figure 3.10 Additive activation of G proteins by opioid and adenosine agonists known to alter sleep and breathing. The four rows of coronal rat brain sections correspond to four in vitro treatment conditions. The color code indicates G protein binding (nCi/g) in five brain stem nuclei regulating sleep and breathing. The top row shows G protein activation under basal conditions. The second row shows G protein activation by the mu opioid agonist DAMGO. The third row from the top shows G protein activation by an adenosine A1 agonist N^6-p-sulphophenyladenosine (SPA). The bottom row illustrates greater G protein activation (note color scale) during combined treatments with adenosine and opioid agonists (SPA plus DAMGO). (From Ref. 139.)

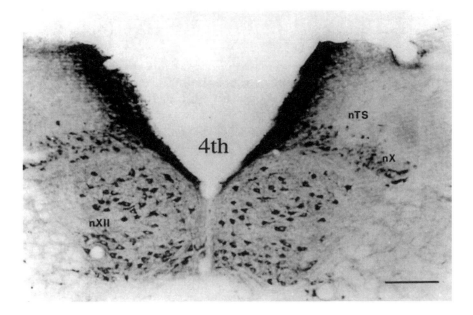

Figure 6 Photomicrograph of a coronal section through the dorsal portion of rat medulla showing the distribution of choline acetyltransferase-positive cells in the hypoglossal (nXII) nucleus. The dorsal vagal (nX) and nucleus of the solitary tract (nTS) also contain choline acetyltransferase positive neurons. The calibration bar in lower right corner equals 300 µm; 4th indicates fourth ventricle. (Modified from Ref. 102 with permission from Elsevier Science.)

respiratory neurons in VRG (Fig. 3) show differential responses to experimentally imposed anoxia (110). The pre-Bötzinger nucleus in the VRG is a leading candidate for the source of respiratory rhythm generation (111). Differential activation of hypoglossal and VRG neurons by anoxia was interpreted (110) as consistent with differential regulation of respiratory rhythm- and motor pattern-generating mechanisms (112). Species-specific differences also may exist because respiratory control of hypoglossal motoneurons appears to be separate from control of phrenic motoneurons in the rat (113) but not the cat (114).

Pontine administration of the cholinergic agonist carbachol activates a glycinergic premotor inhibitory system that causes postsynaptic inhibition of hypoglossal motoneurons (115,116). The source of this strychnine-sensitive premotor inhibition remains to be specified. In addition to containing ChAT+ neurons (Fig. 6) the hypoglossal nucleus contains M2 muscarinic cholinergic receptors (117). M2 receptors mediate presynaptic depression in rat hypoglossal neurons (118). As shown in Figure 7, muscarinic cholinergic mechanisms enhance the discharge of hypoglossal motoneurons (119). Opioids decrease upper airway muscle activity (87) and microdialysis studies indicate that hypoglossal ACh release is significantly decreased by opioids (120). Considered together, the data raise an interesting question. By what differential mechanism is upper airway muscle tone decreased by pontine administration of cholinergic agonists (Figs. 1–3) while opioids decrease hypoglossal (120) and pontine (121) ACh release? Emerging data suggest that one answer to this question will come from differentiating pre- and postsynaptic cholinergic effects on sleep and breathing (122).

VII. Protein Profiling: Proteins Altering Pontine ACh Release and REM Sleep

Protein malfunction now is known to contribute to a large number of human diseases. A goal of protein profiling is to determine which proteins are present in which cells. The expression of these proteins varies with disease states, respiratory stimuli (123), and with different states of behavioral arousal (124,125). One way to characterize the role of cellular proteins is to perturb their function in living animals. These results encourage characterization of pre- and postsynaptic proteins known to participate in cholinergic neurotransmission. This section selectively highlights the results of protein profiling in the context of sleep neurobiology.

There is agreement that REM sleep is associated with the release of ACh from presynaptic LDT/PPT terminals in the mPRF, causing activation of postsynaptic muscarinic cholinergic receptors on mPRF neurons. Prior to being released, ACh is packaged into presynaptic vesicles. Figure 8a schematizes a central cholinergic synapse, and emphasizes proteins in LDT/PPT terminals that accomplish the task of vesicular packaging. Figure 8b shows two proteins contributing to the presynaptic vesicular packaging of ACh (126–128). One component is a vesicular proton pump responsible for bringing hydrogen ions into the vesicle. The second component is an ACh transporter protein that extrudes protons in exchange for molecules of ACh. The ACh transporter contains a binding site that can be blocked by vesamicol [2-(4-phenylpiperidinyl) cyclohexanol] and, hence, is referred to as the vesamicol receptor (129). Vesamicol binding to the ACh transporter inhibits the presynaptic packaging of ACh, thereby decreasing ACh release (128). Vesamicol disrupts central cholinergic neurotransmission (130,131) and intracerebroventricular injections of vesamicol caused a dose-dependent

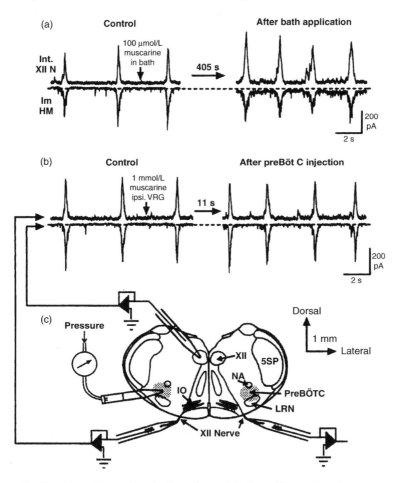

Figure 7 In vitro evidence for cholinergic modulation of hypoglossal motoneurons. (c) Illustrates a brain stem slice from mouse maintained in a bath condition. The dependent measures include recordings of XII nerve activity and intracellular recording of hypoglossal motoneuron under voltage clamp conditions. This figure illustrates two experimental conditions. (a) Muscarine was applied to the bath containing the tissue slice. The effects were to increase the activity of integrated XII nerve discharge (Int. XII N) and reduced holding current (Im HM) of the hypoglossal motoneuron. This change in the inward current is noted by the downward shift from the dashed horizontal line (after bath application). (b) In a second experiment, when muscarine was pressure-injected into the pre-Bötzinger complex (pre-Böt C), there was an increase in inspiratory burst frequency without an increase in amplitude of hypoglossal nerve discharge. In contrast to the bath application, there was no change in the inward current of the voltage clamp hypoglossal motoneuron. (From Ref. 119 with permission from Blackwell Science Ltd.)

(a)

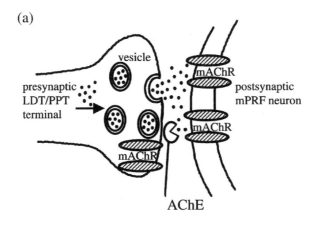

(b)

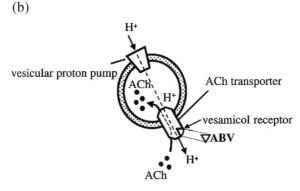

Figure 8 Schematic drawing of a cholinergic synapse and presynaptic cholinergic vesicle. (a) Cholinergic neurons in the pontine LDT/PPT release ACh (dots) into the medial pontine reticular formation (47). Normally, ACh in the synaptic cleft is rapidly degraded by acetylcholinesterase (AChE). Microinjections of acetylcholinesterase inhibitors such as neostigmine into the mPRF block the breakdown of ACh and thereby increase the concentration of ACh available to activate muscarinic cholinergic receptors (mAChR). The synaptic vesicle in the presynaptic LDT/PPT terminal is enlarged below in b. (b) The enlargement schematically illustrates the two main components of the synaptic vesicle. The first is a vesicular proton pump responsible for bringing hydrogen ions into the vesicle. The second component is the ACh transporter, which exchanges protons during the vesicular packaging of ACh. The vesamicol receptor is an allosteric binding site located on the vesicular ACh transporter. This figure also schematizes an analog of vesamicol called aminobenzovesamicol (ABV) binding to the vesamicol receptor. (Modified from Refs. 126, 127, and 129. (Reprinted with permission from Elsevier Science and Academic Press.)

decrease in REM sleep of the rat (132). These findings led us to test the hypothesis that inhibition of presynaptic vesicle proteins within the mPRF would decrease REM sleep.

The compound ($\pm$)-4-aminobenzovesamicol (ABV) is a derivative of vesamicol that selectively binds to the vesamicol receptor, blocking ACh storage and subsequent release (133). Microinjection of ABV alone and ABV as a pretreatment to the AChE inhibitor neostigmine was used to evaluate the effects of ABV on natural REM sleep and on the neostigmine-induced REM sleep-like state. The results (Fig. 9) showed that mPRF

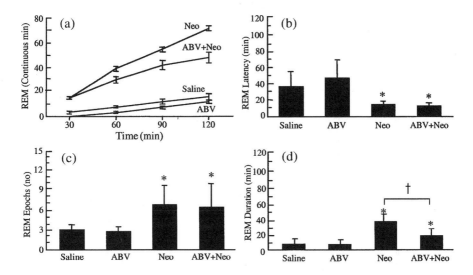

Figure 9 REM sleep is inhibited by microinjection of a vesamicol receptor blocker into the medial pontine reticular formation. (a) The time course of REM sleep enhancement caused by mPRF microinjections of the acetylcholinesterase inhibitor neostigmine (Neo). When neostigmine administration is preceded by microinjection of the vesamicol receptor blocker aminobenzovesamicol (ABV + Neo), the time course of REM sleep accumulation is significantly decreased. (b) mPRF injections of neostigmine significantly decreased the latency to onset of the first REM episode. ABV microinjected into the mPRF did not alter the neostigmine-induced decrease of REM sleep latency. (c) Administration of neostigmine into the mPRF also increased the number of REM sleep epochs recorded during a 2-hr interval. Blocking the vesamicol receptor with ABV (ABV + Neo) did not alter the number of REM sleep epochs. (d) Following mPRF administration of neostigmine, the average duration of each REM epoch was significantly increased. Blocking the vesamicol receptor (ABV + Neo) significantly decreased the neostigmine-induced enhancement of the duration of REM sleep epochs. (From Ref. 134 with permission from Lippincott Williams & Wilkins.)

administration of ABV disrupted REM sleep (134). The vesamicol receptor blocker ABV significantly depressed the time course of both natural REM sleep and the REM sleep-like state caused by mPRF injection of neostigmine (Fig. 9a). Neostigmine significantly reduced the latency to onset of REM sleep (39) and this reduction in latency was not blocked by ABV (Fig. 9b). This latter finding is consistent with the fact that ABV would not be expected to alter vesicular pools of ACh sequestered before ACh transporter blockade. ABV did not alter the number of REM sleep epochs (Fig. 9c) and significantly decreased the duration of REM sleep epochs caused by mPRF microinjection of neostigmine (Fig. 9d). These data suggest differential regulation of the frequency and duration of REM sleep-generating mechanisms.

The ACh transporter is a presynaptic protein with a cytosolic orientation. The Figure 9 data demonstrate REM sleep inhibition caused by blocking a cytosolic protein localized to LDT/PPT terminals releasing ACh (47) within the mPRF (Fig. 8). As noted earlier, the presence of the ACh synthetic enzyme ChAT is the defining phenotype for a cholinergic neuron. Others have noted that the cDNA coding for vesicular ACh transporter (VAChT) protein is contained uninterrupted within the first intron of the ChAT gene locus (135). This proximity between the genes coding for VAChT and ChAT proteins was hypothesized to have regulatory significance for endogenous cholinergic neurotransmission (135). To focus on endogenous ACh, we chose to enhance REM sleep by microinjecting neostigmine, which prevents the degradation of synaptically released ACh. The finding that mPRF blockade of the presynaptic VAChT protein altered REM sleep implies a regulatory role for the VAChT protein in cholinergic LDT/PPT terminals localized to the mPRF.

Data from many laboratories support the conclusion that REM sleep is generated, in part, by mPRF muscarinic cholinergic heteroreceptors (reviewed in Ref. 54). Functional studies show that ACh release in the mPRF is regulated by muscarinic cholinergic receptors of the M2 subtype (81). Thus, mPRF presynaptic and postsynaptic cell surface proteins in the form of M2 muscarinic receptors play a regulatory role in REM sleep generation.

Guanine nucleotide binding proteins (G proteins) in the LDT/PPT and mPRF are activated by the cholinergic agonist carbachol (136). This G protein activation is concentration dependent and blocked by atropine, consistent with mediation by muscarinic cholinergic receptors (136). Additional data are consistent with REM sleep regulation by cholinergic activation of a signal transduction cascade in mPRF neurons. For example, REM sleep and breathing are altered via the M2/M4 muscarinic cholinergic receptor-linked signal transduction pathway in the mPRF. This signal transduction cascade includes a pertussis toxin-sensitive G protein (137), adenylyl cyclase, cAMP, and protein kinase A (138).

Proteomic approaches show great promise for specifying the link between proteins and complex events such as sleep and breathing. These approaches, however, must confront a number of challenges. One complexity is the ability of different neuromodulators to activate common pools of G proteins. For example, sleep is altered both by opioids and adenosine. Recently it was discovered that an agonist of adenosine A1 receptors and an agonist of mu opioid receptors can activate similar pools of G proteins in brain regions known to regulate sleep and breathing (139). These data (Fig. 10) demonstrate that transmembrane signaling from receptor to G protein functions as a complex network rather than as a simple linear pathway (140). (See color insert.) Different receptors can converge on the same G protein pool (141) or diverge to activate multiple G proteins (140).

VIII. Conclusions

Multiple brain regions, neurotransmitters, and signal transduction processes regulate sleep and breathing. The complexity of multiple regulatory mechanisms is daunting and encourages enthusiasm for so-called "simpler" animal models (142–144). It is clear from progress in circadian rhythms research that fruit fly and other invertebrate models can help identify proteins that have been evolutionarily conserved and have a regulatory role in mammals. In addition, it is important to seek mammalian data suggesting common control mechanisms through which a plethora of molecules alter mammalian sleep and breathing. Data are outlined below for a number of molecules which modulate sleep and/or breathing via cholinergic mechanisms.

Peptides such as pituitary adenylate cyclase-activating peptide (PACAP) enhance REM sleep in the rat (145). Notably, the ability of PACAP to enhance REM sleep is blocked by the muscarinic cholinergic antagonist atropine, and REM sleep enhancement by carbachol is prevented by PACAP-27, the antagonist of PACAP (146). Vasoactive intestinal polypeptide (VIP) also alters sleep (147) and VIP-induced REM sleep enhancement is blocked by atropine (148,149), which is consistent with mediation by muscarinic cholinergic receptors. The hypothalamic peptide hypocretin/orexin now is known to participate in the regulation of sleep and wakefulness (150). The hypocretin-1/orexin-A receptor is coupled to G proteins, and hypocretin-1/orexin-A peptide activates G proteins in brain stem nuclei known to regulate sleep (151–153).

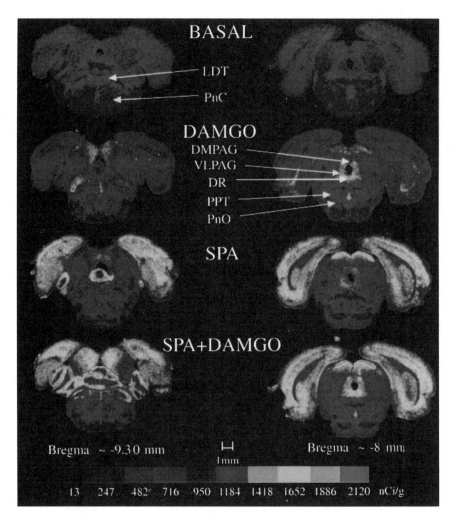

Figure 10 Additive activation of G proteins by opioid and adenosine agonists known to alter sleep and breathing. The four rows of coronal rat brain sections correspond to four in vitro treatment conditions. The color code indicates G protein binding (nCi/g) in five brain stem nuclei regulating sleep and breathing. The top row shows G protein activation under basal conditions. The second row shows G protein activation by the mu opioid agonist DAMGO. The third row from the top shows G protein activation by an adenosine A1 agonist N^6-p-sulphophenyladenosine (SPA). The bottom row illustrates greater G protein activation (note color scale) during combined treatments with adenosine and opioid agonists (SPA plus DAMGO). (From Ref. 139.) (See color insert.)

Neurotrophic proteins such as nerve growth factor (NGF) also modulate sleep (154,155). NGF binds to the cell surface protein trkA receptor kinase located on the basal forebrain (156) and brain stem (157) cholinergic neurons known to regulate sleep (158,159). NGF significantly enhances ACh release from cultured basal forebrain neurons (160). NGF increases ChAT activity and trkA antagonists decrease both ChAT activity and the number of cholinergic synapses (161). Together, these data are consistent with the possibility that REM sleep enhancement caused by NGF microinjection into mPRF (Fig. 1) is cholinergically mediated.

The protein product of the *ob* gene is leptin, a hormone that originates from adipocytes and plays a role in regulating body weight by diminishing food intake. The potential for leptin as a messenger of peripheral fat stores to influence brain ACh comes from the fact that leptin is transported across the blood–brain barrier (162). Leptin has many central nervous system actions, including regulation of neuronal and glial proteins (163). Preclinical and clinical data suggest that leptin may contribute to sleep-disordered breathing. Leptin-deficient *ob/ob* mice are obese and exhibit ventilatory abnormalities that include an altered rate of breathing (164). Treating *ob/ob* mice with leptin replacement attenuates the ventilatory abnormalities (165). Previous sections of this chapter noted the role of pontine neurons in regulating respiratory rate. Breathing frequency is regulated by pontine respiratory neurons and leptin-activated FOS immunoreactive neurons have been localized to the pontine parabrachial nuclei (166). Initial studies of obese male patients with obstructive sleep apnea report increased levels of leptin (167). In vitro data demonstrate that leptin modulates cholinergic neurotransmission and the biosynthesis of VIP expressed in cholinergic neurons (168). These data encourage future studies designed to determine the extent to which the leptin effects on sleep and breathing involve ACh.

Finally, recent evidence suggests that the sleep-enhancing actions of gamma-aminobutyric acid (GABA) may be cholinergically modulated. Rapid eye movement sleep is increased by mPRF administration of the $GABA_A$ antagonist bicuculline (169). The initial part of this chapter noted that ACh release in the mPRF is increased during REM sleep (48,49), and lesions of the LDT/PPT cholinergic neurons that release ACh in the mPRF eliminate REM sleep (170). These data suggest the hypothesis that one mechanism by which pontine GABA regulates REM sleep is by modulation of mPRF ACh release. Emerging data now show that microdialysis delivery to the mPRF of bicuculline causes a significant increase in ACh levels within the mPRF (171). Taken together, these data support the conclusion that many of the molecules that enhance REM sleep do so by modulating pontine cholinergic neurotransmission.

Acknowledgments

Supported by NIH Grants HL40881, MH45361, HL57120, HL65272, and the Department of Anesthesiology, University of Michigan. The authors thank M. A. Norat and C. Lapham for expert assistance.

References

1. Steriade, M. and Biesold, D. Brain Cholinergic Systems. New York: Oxford University Press, 1990.
2. Steriade, M. and McCarley, R. W. Brainstem Control of Wakefulness and Sleep. New York: Plenum, 1990.
3. Lydic, R. and Baghdoyan, H. A. Handbook of Behavioral State Control: Cellular and Molecular Mechanisms. Boca Raton, FL: CRC Press, 1999.
4. Kryger, M. H., Roth, T., and Dement, W. C. Principles and Practice of Sleep Medicine. Philadelphia: W. B. Saunders, 2000.
5. Aserinsky, E. and Kleitman, N. Regularly occurring periods of eye motility, and concomitant phenomena, during sleep. Science 1953; 118:273–274.
6. Dement, W. C. The occurrence of low voltage, fast, electroencephalogram patterns during behavioural sleep in the cat. Electroenceph Clin Neurophysiol 1958; 10:291–296.
7. Campbell, S. S. and Tobler, I. Animal sleep: a review of sleep duration across phylogeny. Neurosci Biobehav Rev 1984; 8:269–300.
8. Jouvet, M. Reserches sur les strucutres nerveuses et les mechanisms responsables des differentes phases du sommeil physiologique. Arch Ital Biol 1962; 100:125–136.
9. Jouvet, M. The role of monoamines and acetylcholine containing neurons in the regulation of the sleep waking cycle. Rev Physiol 1972; 64:1–225.
10. Orem, J., Montplaisir, J., and Dement, W. C. Changes in the activity of respiratory neurons during sleep. Brain Res 1974; 82:309–315.
11. Lin, L., Faraco, J., Li, R., Kadotani, H., Rogers, W., Lin, X., Qiu, X., de Jong, P., Nishino, S., and Mignot, E. The sleep disorder canine narcolepsy is caused by a mutation in the hypocretin (orexin) receptor 2 gene. Cell 1999; 98:365–376.
12. Chemelli, R. M., Willie, J. T., Sinton, C. M., Elmquist, J. K., Scammell, T., Lee, C., Richardson, J. T., Williams, S. C., Xiong, Y., Kisanuki, Y., Fitch, T. E., Nakazato, N., Hammer, R. E., Saper, C. B., and Yanagisawa, M. Narcolepsy in orexin knockout mice: molecular genetics of sleep regulation. Cell 1999; 98:437–451.
13. Thannickal, T., Moore, R. Y., Nienhuis, R., Ramanathan, L., Gulyani, S., Aldrich, M., Cornford, M., and Siegel, J. M. Reduced number of hypocretin neurons in human narcolepsy. Neuron 2000; 27: 469–474.
14. Siegel, J. M. Narcolepsy: a key role for hypocretins (orexins). Cell 1999; 98:409–412.

15. Menotti-Raymond, M., David, V. A., Lyons, L. A., Schaffer, A. A., Tomlin, J. F., Hutton, M. K., and O'Brien, S. J. A genetic linkage map of microsatellites in the domestic cat (*Felis catus*). Genomics 1999; 57:9–23.

16. O'Brien, S. J. and Nash, W. G. Genetic mapping in mammals: chromosome map of the domestic cat. Science 1982; 216:257–265.

17. O'Brien, S. J., Menotti-Raymond, M., Murphy, W. J., Nash, W. G., Wienberg, J., Stanyon, R., Copeland, N. G., Jenkins, N. A., Womack, J. E., and Marshall Graves, J. A. The promise of comparative genomics in mammals. Science 1999; 286:458–481.

18. Murphy, W. J., Sun, S., Chen, Z.-Q., Yuhki, N., Hirschmann, D., Menotti-Raymond, M., and O'Brien, S. J. A radiation hybrid map of the cat genome: implications for comparative mapping. Genome Res 2000; 10:691–702.

19. Longo, V. G. and Silvestrini, B. Action of eserine and amphetamine on the electrical activity of the rabbit brain. J Pharmacol Exp Ther 1957; 120:160–170.

20. Hernandez-Peon, R., Chavez-Ibarra, G., Morgane, P. J., and Timo-Iaria, C. Limbic cholinergic pathways involved in sleep and emotional behavior. Exp Neurol 1963; 8:93–111.

21. Cordeau, J., Moreau, A., Beaulnes, A., and Laurin, C. EEG and behavioral changes following microinjections of acetylcholine and adrenaline in the brain stem of cats. Arch Ital Biol 1963; 101:30–47.

22. Baxter, B. L. Induction of both emotional behavior and a novel form of REM sleep by chemical stimulation applied to cat mesencephalon. Exp Neurol 1969; 23:220–229.

23. George, R., Haslett, W. L., and Jenden, D. L. A cholinergic mechanism in the brain stem reticular formation: induction of paradoxical sleep. Int J Neuropharmacol 1964; 3:541–552.

24. Loizzo, A. and Longo, V. G. A pharmacological approach to paradoxical sleep. Physiol Behav 1968; 3:91–97.

25. Karczmar, A. G., Longo, V. G., and De Carolis, A. S. A pharmacological model of paradoxical sleep: the role of cholinergic and monoamine systems. Physiol Behav 1970; 5:175–182.

26. Domino, E. F., Yamamoto, K., and Dren, A. T. Role of cholinergic mechanisms in states of wakefulness and sleep. Prog Brain Res 1968; 28:113–133.

27. Sagales, T., Erill, S., and Domino, E. F. Differential effects of scopolamine and chlorpromazine on REM and NREM sleep in normal male subjects. Clin Pharmacol Therap 1969; 10:522–529.

28. Sitaram, N., Wyatt, R. J., Dawson, S., and Gillin, J. C. REM sleep induction by physostigmine infusion during sleep. Science 1976; 191:1281–1283.

29. Aquilonius, S.-M. and Gillberg, P.-G. Cholinergic Neurotransmission: Functional and Clinical Aspects. Progress in Brain Research. Vol. 84. Amsterdam: Elsevier, 1990.

30. Cuello, A. C. Cholinergic function and dysfunction. Prog Brain Res 1993; 98:1–462.

31. Baghdoyan, H. A. Cholinergic mechanisms regulating REM sleep. In: Schwartz W. J., ed. Sleep Science: Integrating Basic Research and Clinical Practice. Monographs in Clinical Neuroscience. Vol. 15. Basel: Karger, 1997:88–116.

32. Lydic, R. Respiratory modulation by nonrespiratory neurons. In: Schwartz W. J., ed. Sleep Science: Integrating Basic Research and Clinical Practice. Monographs in Clinical Neuroscience. Vol. 15. Basel: Karger, 1997:117–142.

33. Horner, R. L. and Kubin, L. Pontine carbachol elicits multiple rapid eye movement sleep-like neural events in urethane-anesthetized rats. Neuroscience 1999; 93:215–226.

34. Reinoso-Suárez, F., de Andrés, I., Rodrigo-Angulo, M. L., and Garzón, M. Brain structures and mechanisms involved in the generation of REM sleep. Sleep Med Rev 2000; 5:63–77.

35. Brock, T. D. Robert Koch: A Life in Medicine and Bacteriology. Madison, WI: University of Wisconsin Press, 1999.

36. Lydic, R. and Baghdoyan, H. A. Koch's postulates confirm cholinergic modulation of REM sleep. Behav Brain Sci 2000; 23:966.

37. Lydic, R. and Baghdoyan, H. A. Cholinergic contributions to the control of consciousness. In: Yaksh, T. L., Lynch, C., Zapol, W. M., Maze, M., Biebuyck, J. F., and Saidman, L. J. eds. Anesthesia: Biologic Foundations. Philadelphia: Lippincott-Raven, 1997:433–450.

38. Baghdoyan, H. A., Rodrigo-Angulo, M. L., McCarley, R. W., and Hobson, J. A. Site-specific enhancement and suppression of desynchronized sleep signs following cholinergic stimulation of three brain stem regions. Brain Res 1984; 306:39–52.

39. Baghdoyan, H. A., Monaco, A. P., Rodrigo-Angulo, M. L., Assens, F., McCarley, R. W., and Hobson, J. A. Microinjection of neostigmine into the pontine reticular formation of cats enhances desynchronized sleep signs. J Pharmacol Exp Ther 1984; 231:173–180.

40. Lee, L. H., Friedman, D. B., and Lydic, R. Respiratory nuclei share synaptic connectivity with pontine reticular regions regulating REM sleep. Am J Physiol 1995; 268:L251–L262.

41. Ito, K. and McCarley, R. W. Alterations in membrane potential and excitability of cat medial pontine reticular formation neurons during changes in naturally occurring sleep-wake states. Brain Res 1984; 292:169–175.

42. Greene, R. W., Hass, H. L., Gerber, U., and McCarley, R. W. Cholinergic activation of medial pontine reticular formation neurons in vitro. In: Frotscher, M. and Misgeld, U. eds. Central Cholinergic Synaptic Transmission. Boston: Birkhauser, 1989:123–137.

43. Lydic, R., Baghdoyan, H. A., and Lorinc, Z. Microdialysis of cat pons reveals enhanced acetylcholine release during state-dependent respiratory depression. Am J Physiol 1991; 261:R766–R770.

44. Jones, B. and Beaudet A. Distribution of acetylcholine and catecholamine neurons in the cat brainstem: a choline acetyltransferase and tyrosine hydroxylase immunohistochemical study. J Comp Neurol 1987; 261:15–32.

45. Mitani, A., Ito, K., Hallanger, A. E., Wainer, B. H., Kataoka, K., and McCarley, R. W. Cholinergic projections from the laterodorsal and pedunculopontine tegmental nuclei to the pontine gigantocellular tegmental field in the cat. Brain Res 1988; 451:397–402.

46. Shiromani, P. J., Armstrong, D. M., and Gillin, J. C. Cholinergic neurons from the dorsolateral pons project to the medial pons: a WGA-HRP and choline acetyltransferase immunohistochemical study. Neurosci Lett 1988; 95:19–23.

47. Lydic, R. and Baghdoyan, H. A. Pedunculopontine stimulation alters respiration and increases ACh release in the pontine reticular formation. Am J Physiol 1993; 264:R544–R554.

48. Leonard, T. O. and Lydic, R. Nitric oxide synthase inhibition decreases pontine acetylcholine release. Neuroreport 1995; 6:1525–1529.

49. Leonard, T. O. and Lydic, R. Pontine nitric oxide modulates acetylcholine release, rapid eye movement sleep generation, and respiratory rate. J Neurosci 1997; 17:774–785.

50. El Mansari, M., Sakai, K., and Jouvet, M. Unitary characteristics of presumptive cholinergic tegmental neurons during the sleep-waking cycle in freely moving cats. Exp Brain Res 1989; 76:519–529.

51. Lydic, R., Baghdoyan, H. A., Hibbard, L., Bonyak, E. V., DeJoseph, M. R., and Hawkins, R. A. Regional brain glucose metabolism is altered during rapid eye movement sleep in the cat: a preliminary study. J Comp Neurol 1991; 304:517–529.

52. Baghdoyan, H. A., Mallios, J. V., Duckrow, R. B., and Mash, D. C. Localization of muscarinic receptor subtypes in brain stem areas regulating sleep. Neuroreport 1994; 5:1631–1634.

53. Baghdoyan, H. A. Location and quantification of muscarinic receptor subtypes in rat pons: implications for REM sleep generation. Am J Physiol 1997; 273:R896–R904.

54. Baghdoyan, H. A. and Lydic, R. M2 muscarinic receptor subtype in the feline medial pontine reticular formation modulates the amount of rapid eye movement sleep. Sleep 1999; 22:835–847.

55. Lydic, R., Baghdoyan, H. A., and Zwillich, C. W. State-dependent hypotonia in posterior cricoarytenoid muscles of the larynx caused by cholinergic reticular mechanisms. FASEB J 1989; 3:1625–1631.

56. Lydic, R. and Baghdoyan, H. A. Cholinoceptive pontine reticular mechanisms cause state-dependent respiratory changes in cat. Neurosci Lett 1989; 102:211–216.

57. Kubin, L. Carbachol models of REM sleep: recent developments and new directions. Arch Ital Biol 2001; 139:147–168.

58. Fung, M.-L. and St. John, W. M. Pontine cholinergic respiratory depression in neonatal and young rats. Life Sci 1998; 24:2249–2256.

59. Phillipson, E. A. Control of breathing during sleep. Am Rev Respir Dis 1978; 118:909–939.

60. Deegan, P. C. and McNichols, W. T. Pathophysiology of obstructive sleep apnoea. Eur Respir J 1995; 8:1161–1178.

61. Douglas, N. J. Respiratory physiology: control of ventilation. In: Kryger, M. H., Roth, T., and Dement, W. C. eds. Principles and Practice of Sleep Medicine. Philadelphia: W.B. Saunders, 2000:221–228.

62. Loadsman, J. A. and Wilcox, I. Is obstructive sleep apnoea a rapid eye movement predominant phenomenon? Br J Anaesth 2000; 85:354–358.

63. Redline, S., Tishler, P. V., Schluchter, M., Aylor, J., Clark, K., and Graham, G. Risk factors for sleep-disordered breathing in children. Associations with obesity, race, and respiratory problems. Am J Respir Crit Care Med 1999; 159:1527–1532.

64. Morielli, A., Ladan, S., Ducharme, F. M., and Brouillette, R. T. Can sleep and wakefulness be distinguished in children by cardiorespiratory and videotape recordings? Chest 1996; 109:680–687.

65. Goh D. Y. T. and Galster P. M. C. L. Sleep architecture and respiratory disturbances in children with obstructive sleep apnea. Am J Respir Crit Care Med 2000; 162:682–686.

66. Carley, D. W. and Radulovacki, M. REM sleep and apnea. In: Mallick, B. N. and Inoué, S. eds. REM Sleep. London: Narosa, 1999:286–300.

67. Mendelson, W. B., Martin, J. V., Perlis, M., Giesen, H., Wagner, R., and Rapoport, S. I. Periodic cessation of respiratory effort during sleep in adult rats. Physiol Behav 1988; 43:229–234.

68. Carley, D. W., Trbovic, S., and Radulovacki, M. Effect of REM sleep deprivation on sleep apneas in rats. Exp Neurol 1996; 137:291–293.

69. Hendricks, J. C., Kline, L. R., Kovalski, R. J., O'Brien, J. A., Morrison, A. R., and Pack, A. I. The English bulldog: a natural model of sleep-disordered breathing. J Appl Physiol 1987; 63:1344–1350.

70. Feroah, T. R., Forster, H. V., Pan, L., Wenninger, J., Martino, P., and Rice, T. Effect of slow wave and REM sleep on thyropharyngeus and stylopharyngeus activity during induced central apneas. Respir Physiol 2001; 124:129–140.

71. Orem, J. and Lydic, R. Upper airway function during sleep and wakefulness: Experimental studies on normal and anesthetized cats. Sleep 1978; 1:49–68.

72. Kuna, S. T., Smickley, J. S., and Insalaco, G. Posterior cricoarytenoid muscle activity during wakefulness and sleep in normal adults. J Appl Physiol 1990; 68:1746–1754.

73. Sanders, I., Wu, B. L., Mu, L., and Biller, H. F. The innervation of the human posterior cricoarytenoid muscle: evidence for at least two neuromuscular compartments. Laryngoscope 1994; 104:880–884.

74. Morales, F. R., Englehardt, J. K., Soja, P. A., and Pereda, A. E. Motoneuron properties during motor inhibition produced by microinjection of carbachol into the pontine reticular formation of the decerebrate cat. J Neurophysiol 1987; 57:1118–1129.

75. Fay, R., Gilbert, K. A., and Lydic, R. Pontomedullary neurons transsynaptically labeled by laryngeal pseudorabies virus. Neuroreport 1993; 5:141–144.

76. Lai, Y. Y. and Siegel, J. M. Medullary regions mediating atonia. J Neurosci 1988; 8:4790–4796.

77. Lydic, R., Baghdoyan, H. A., Wertz, R., and White, D. P. Cholinergic reticular mechanisms influence state-dependent ventilatory response to hypercapnia. Am J Physiol 1991; 261:R738–R746.

78. Cohen, M. I. and Wang, S. C. Respiratory neuronal activity in pons of cat. J Neurophysiology 1959; 22:33–50.

79. Lumsden, T. Observations on the respiratory centres in the cat. J Physiol (Lond) 1922; 57:153–160.

80. Gilbert, K. A. and Lydic, R. Pontine cholinergic reticular mechanisms cause state-dependent changes in the discharge of parabrachial neurons. Am J Physiol 1994; 266:R136–R150.

81. Baghdoyan, H. A., Fleegal, M. A., and Lydic, R. M2 muscarinic autoreceptors regulate acetylcholine release in the pontine reticular formation. J Pharmacol Exp Ther 1998; 286:1446–1452.

82. Kuna, S. T. Remmers, J. E. Premotor input to hypoglossal motoneurons from Kolliker-Fuse neurons in decerebrate cats. Respir Physiol 1999; 117:85–95.

83. Sauerland, E. K. and Harper, R. M. The human tongue during sleep: electromyographic activity of the genioglossus muscle. Exp Neurol 1976; 51:160–170.

84. Harper, R. M. and Sauerland, E. K. The role of the tongue in sleep apnea. In: Guilleminault, C. and Dement, W. C. eds. Sleep Apnea Syndromes. New York: Alan R. Liss, 1978:219–234.

85. Remmers, J. E., DeGroot, W. J., Sauerland, E. K., and Anch, M. Pathogenesis of upper airway occlusion during sleep. J Appl Physiol 1978; 44:931–938.

86. Lydic, R., Weigand, L., and Weigand, D. Sleep-dependent changes in upper airway muscle function. In: Lydic, R. and Biebuyck, J. F. eds. Clinical Physiology of Sleep. Bethesda, MD: American Physiological Society, 1988:97–123.

87. Bartlett, D. Upper airway motor systems. In: Cherniack, N. S. and Widdicombe, J. W. eds. Handbook of Physiology: The Respiratory System: Control of Breathing. Vol. II, Section 3, Part 1. Bethesda, MD: American Physiologic Society, 1986:223–245.

88. Megirian, D., Pollard, M. J., and Sherrey, J. H. Respiratory roles of genioglossus, sternothyroid, and sternohyoid muscles during sleep. Exp Neurol 1985; 90:118–128.

89. Bennett, F. M. and St. John, W. M. Anesthesia selectively reduces hypoglossal nerve activity by actions upon the brain stem. Pflugers Arch 1986; 401:421–423.

90. Leiter, J. C., Knuth, S. L., Krol, R. C., and Bartlett, D. The effect of diazepam on genioglossal muscle activity in normal human subjects. Am Rev Respir Dis 1985; 132:216–219.

91. Mezzanotte, W. S., Tangle, D. J., and White, D. P. Waking genioglossal electromyogram in sleep apnea patients versus normal controls: a neuromuscular compensatory mechanism. J Clin Invest 1992; 89:1571–1579.

92. Mezzanotte, W. S., Tangle, D. J., and White, D. P. Influence of sleep onset on upper airway muscle activity in apnea patients versus normal controls. Am J Respir Crit Care Med 1996; 153:1880–1887.

93. Eisele, D. W., Smith, P. L., Alam, D. S., and Schwartz, A. R. Direct hypoglossal nerve stimulation in obstructive sleep apnoea. Arch Otolaryngol Head Neck Surg 1997; 123:57–61.

94. Fuller, D. D., Williams, J. S., Janssen, P. L., and Fregosi, R. F. Effect of co-activation of tongue protrudor and retractor muscles on tongue movements and pharyngeal airflow mechanics in the rat. J Physiol 1999; 519:601–613.

95. Lowe, A. A. The neural regulation of tongue movements. Prog Neurobiol 1980; 15:295–344.

96. Knaack, L. and Podszus, T. Electric stimulation of the upper airway muscle. Curr Opin Pulm Med 1998; 4:370–375.

97. Manaker, S. and Tischler, L. Origin of serotonergic afferents to the hypoglossal nucleus in the rat. J Comp Neurol 1993; 334:466–476.

98. Kubin, L., Tojima, H., Davies, R. O., and Pack, A. I. Serotonergic excitatory drive to hypoglossal motoneurons in the decerebrate cat. Neurosci Lett 1992; 139:243–248.

99. Hudgel, D. W., Gordon, E. A., and Meltzer, H. Y. Abnormal serotonergic stimulation of cortisol production in obstructive sleep apnea. Am J Respir Crit Care Med 1995; 152:186–192.

100. Kubin, L., Reignier, C., Tojima, H., Taguchi, O., Pack, A. I., and Davies, R. O. Changes in serotonin level in the hypoglossal nucleus region during carbachol-induced atonia. Brain Res 1994; 645:291–302.

101. Woch, G., Ogawa, H., Davies, R. O., and Kubin, L. Behavior of hypoglossal inspiratory premotor neurons during the carbachol-induced REM sleep-like suppression of upper airway motoneurons. Exp Brain Res 2000; 130:508–520.

102. Cassell, M. D. and Talman, W. T. Glycine receptor (Gephyrin) immunoreactivity is present on cholinergic neurons in the dorsal vagal complex. Neuroscience 2000; 95:489–497.

103. Hwang, J. C., St. John, W. M., and Bartlett, D. Characterization of respiratory modulated activities of hypoglossal motoneurons. J Appl Physiol 1983; 55:793–798.

104. Whithington-Wray, D. J., Mifflin, S. W., and Spyer, K. W. Intracellular analysis of respiratory modulated hypoglossal motoneurons in the cat. Neuroscience 1988; 25:1041–1051.

105. Funk, G. D., Smith, J. C., and Feldman, J. L. Development of thyrotropin-releasing hormone and norepinephrine potentiation of inspiratory-related hypoglossal motoneuron discharge in neonatal and juvenile mice in vitro. J Neurophysiol 1994; 72:2538–2541.

106. Strohl, K. P., Hensley, M. J., Hallett, M., Saunders, N. A., and Ingram, R. H. Activation of upper airway muscles before onset of inspiration in normal humans. J Appl Physiol 1980; 49:638–642.

107. Horner, R. L., Innes, J. A., Murphy, K., and Guz, R. Evidence for reflex upper airway dilator muscle activation by sudden negative airway pressure in man. J Physiol 1991; 436:31–44.

108. Horner, R. L., Innes, J. A., Morrell, M. J., Shea, S. A., and Guz, R. The effect of sleep on reflex genioglossus muscle activation by stimuli of negative airway pressure in humans. J Physiol 1994; 476:141–151.

109. Shea, S. A., Akahoshi, T., Edwards, J. K., and White, D. P. Influence of chemoreceptor stimuli on genioglossal response to negative pressure in humans. Am J Respir Crit Care Med 2000; 162:559–565.

110. Telgkamp, P. and Ramirez, J. M. Differential responses of respiratory nuclei to anoxia in rhythmic brain stem slices of mice. J Neurophysiol 1999; 82:2163–2170.

111. Smith, J. C., Ellenberger, H. H., Ballayni, K., Richter, D. W., and Feldman, J. L. Pre-Botzinger complex. A brainstem region that may generate respiratory rhythm in mammals. Science 1991; 254:726–729.

112. Feldman, J. L., Smith, J. C., Ellenberger, H. H., Connelly, C. A., Liu, G. S., Greer, J. J., Lindsay, A. D., and Otto, M. R. Neurogenesis of respiratory rhythm and pattern: emerging concepts. Am J Physiol 1990; 259:R879–R886.

113. Peever, J. H., Mateika, J. H., and Duffin, J. Respiratory control of hypoglossal motoneurons in the rat. Pflugers Arch 2001; 442:78–86.

114. Ono, T., Ishiwata, Y., Inaba, N., Kuroda, T., and Nakamura, Y. Hypoglossal premotor neurons with rhythmical inspiratory-related activity in the cat: localization and projection to the phrenic nucleus. Exp Brain Res 1994; 98:1–12.

115. Yamuy, J., Fung, S. J., Xi, M., Morales, F. R., and Chase, M. H. Hypoglossal motoneurons are postsynaptically inhibited during carbachol-induced rapid eye movement sleep. Neuroscience 1999; 94:11–15.

116. Fung, S. J., Yamuy, J., Xi, M., Englehardt, J. K., Morales, F. R., and Chase, M. H. Changes in electrophysiological properties of cat hypoglossal motoneurons during carbachol-induced motor inhibition. Brain Res 2000; 885:262–272.

117. Mallios, V. J., Lydic, R., and Baghdoyan, H. A. Muscarinic receptor subtypes are differentially distributed across brain stem respiratory nuclei. Am J Physiol 1995; 268:L941–L949.

118. Bellingham, M. C. and Berger, A. J. Presynaptic depression of excitatory synaptic inputs to rat hypoglossal motoneuron discharge by muscarinic M2 receptors. J Neurophysiol 1996; 76:3758–3770.

119. Bellingham, M. C. and Funk, G. D. Cholinergic modulation of respiratory brain-stem neurons and its function in sleep-wake state determination. Clin Exp Pharmacol Physiol 2000; 27:132–137.

120. Lydic, R., Baghdoyan, H. A., and McGinley, J. Hypoglossal nucleus acetylcholine release is decreased by systemically administered morphine. Soc Neurosci Abstr 2000; 26:1757.

121. Mortazavi, S., Thompson, J., Baghdoyan, H. A., and Lydic, R. Fentanyl and morphine, but not remifentanil, inhibit acetylcholine release in pontine regions modulating arousal. Anesthesiology 1999; 90:1070–1077.

122. Capece, M. L., Baghdoyan, H. A., and Lydic, R. New directions for the study of cholinergic REM sleep generation: specifying presynaptic and postsynaptic mechanisms. In: Mallick, B. N. and Inoué, S. eds. REM Sleep. London: Narosa Press, 1999:123–141.

123. Gozal, D., Gozal, E., and Simakajornboon, N. Signaling pathways of the acute hypoxic ventilatory response in the nucleus tractus solitarius. Respir Physiol 2000; 121:209–221.

124. Cirelli, C., Pompeiano, M., and Tononi, G. Neuronal gene expression in the waking state: a role for the locus coeruleus. Science 1996; 274:1211–1215.

125. Cirelli, C. and Tononi, G. Differential expression of plasticity-related genes in waking and sleep and their regulation by the noradrenergic system. J Neurosci 2000; 20:9187–9194.

126. Parsons, S. M., Bahr, B. A., Rogers, G. A., Clarkson, E. D., Noremberg, K., and Hicks, B. W. Acetylcholine transporter-vesamicol receptor pharmacology and structure. Prog Brain Res 1993; 98:175–181.

127. Parsons, S. M., Prior, C., and Marshall, I. G. Acetylcholine transport, storage, and release. Int Rev Neurobiol 1993; 35:279–390.

128. Prior, C., Marshall, I. G., and Parsons, S. M. The pharmacology of vesamicol: an inhibitor of the vesicular acetylcholine transporter. Gen Pharmacol 1992; 23:1017–1022.

129. Marshall, I. G. and Parsons, S. M. The vesicular acetylcholine transport system. Trends Neurosci 1987; 10:174–177.

130. Buccafusco, J. L., Wei, J., and Kraft, K. L. The effect of the acetylcholine transport blocker vesamicol on central cholinergic pressor neurons. Synapse 1991; 8:301–306.

131. Marien, M. R., Richard, J. W., Allaire, C., and Altar, C. A. Suppression of in vivo neostriatal acetylcholine release by vesamicol: evidence for a functional role of vesamicol receptors in brain. J Neurochem 1991; 57:1878–1883.

132. Salin-Pascual, R. J. and Jimenez-Anguiano A. Vesamicol, an acetylcholine uptake blocker in presynaptic vesicles, suppresses rapid eye movement (REM) sleep in the rat. Psychopharmacology 1995; 121:485–487.

133. Rogers, G. A., Kornreich, W. D., Hand, K., and Parsons, S. M. Kinetic and equilibrium characterization of vesamicol receptor-ligand complexes with picomolar dissociation constants. Mol Pharmacol 1993; 44:633–641.

134. Capece, M., Efange, S., and Lydic, R. Vesicular acetylcholine transport inhibitor suppresses REM sleep. Neuroreport 1997; 8:481–484.

135. Erickson, J. D., Varoqui, H., Shafer, M., Modi, W., Diebler, M. F., Weihe, E., Rand, J., Eiden, L. E., Bonner, T. I., and Usdin, T. B. Functional identification of a vesicular acetylcholine transporter and its expression from a "cholinergic" gene locus. J Biol Chem 1994; 269:21929–21932.

136. Capece, M. L., Baghdoyan, H. A., and Lydic, R. Carbachol stimulates [^{35}S]guanylyl 5'-(γ-thio)triphosphate binding in REM sleep-related brain stem nuclei of rat. J Neurosci 1998; 18:3779–3785.

137. Shuman, S. L., Capece, M. L., Baghdoyan, H. A., and Lydic, R. Pertussis toxin-sensitive G proteins mediate cholinergic regulation of sleep and breathing. Am J Physiol 1995; 269:R308–R317.

138. Capece, M. L. and Lydic, R. Cyclic AMP and protein kinase A modulate cholinergic rapid eye movement (REM) sleep generation. Am J Physiol 1997; 273:R1430–R1440.

139. Tanase, D., Martin, W. A., Baghdoyan, H. A., and Lydic, R. G protein activation in rat ponto-mesencephalic nuclei is enhanced by combined treatment with a mu opioid and an adenosine A1 receptor agonist. Sleep 2001; 24:52–62.

140. Spiegel, A. M. G proteins in cellular control. Curr Opin Neurobiol 1992; 4:203–211.

141. Olianas, M. C. and Onali, P. Synergistic interaction of muscarinic and opioid receptors with Gs-linked neurotransmitter receptors to stimulate adenylyl cyclase activity in rat olfactory bulb. J Neurochem 1993; 61:2183–2190.

142. Kilduff, T. S. What rest in flies can tell us about sleep in mammals. Neuron 2000; 26:295–298.

143. Hendricks, J., Sehgal, A., and Pack, A. The need for a simple animal model to understand sleep. Prog Neurobiol 2000; 61:339–351.

144. Greenspan, R. J., Tononi, G., Cirelli, C., and Shaw, P. J. Sleep and fruit fly. Trends Neurosci 2001; 24:142–145.

145. Fang, J., Payne, L., and Krueger, J. M. Pituitary adenylate cyclase-activating peptide enhances REM sleep in rats. Brain Res 1995; 686:23–28.

146. Ahnaou, A., Laporte, A. M., Ballet, S., Escourrou, P., Hamon, M., Adrien, J., and Bourgin, P. Muscarinic and PACAP receptor interactions at pontine levels in the rat: significance for REM sleep regulation. Eur J Neurosci 2000; 12:4496–4504.

147. Drucker-Colin, R., Bernal-Pedraza, J., Fernandez-Cancino, F., and Oksenberg, A. Is vasoactive intestinal polypeptide (VIP) a sleep factor? Peptides 1984; 5:837–840.

148. Bourgin, P., Lebrand, C., Escourrou, P., Gaultier, C., Franc, B., Hamon, M., and Adrien, J. Vasoactive intestinal polypeptide microinjections into the oral pontine tegmentum enhance rapid eye movement sleep in the rat. Neuroscience 1997; 77:351–360.

149. Bourgin, P., Ahnaou, A., Laporte, A. M., Hamon, M., and Adrien, J. Rapid eye movement sleep induction by vasoactive intestinal peptide infused into the oral pontine tegmentum of the rat may involve muscarinic receptors. Neuroscience 1999; 89:291–302.

150. Kilduff T. S. and Peyron C. The hypocretin/orexin ligand-receptor system: implications for sleep and sleep disorders. Trends Neurosci 2000; 23:359–365.

151. Bernard, R., Norat, M., Tanase, D., Lydic, R., and Baghdoyan, H. A. Hypocretin-1/orexin-A (hcrt-1/OX-A) activates G proteins in locus coeruleus and pontine reticular nucleus, oral part (PNO). FASEB J 2001; 15:A231.

152. Bernard, R., Lydic, R., and Baghdoyan, H. A. Hypocretin-1/orexin-A (hcrt-1/ OX-A) induced G protein activation in rat locus coeruleus (LC) varies as a function of the 24 hr light-dark cycle. Sleep 2001; 24:A136.

153. Bernard, R., Lydic, R., and Baghdoyan, H. A. Hypocretin-1 activates G proteins in arousal-related brain stem nuclei of rat. Neuroreport 2002; 13:447–450.

154. Yamuy, J., Morales, F. R., and Chase, M. H. Induction of rapid eye movement sleep by the microinjection of nerve growth factor into the pontine reticular formation of the cat. Neuroscience 1995; 66:9–13.

155. Takahashi, S. and Krueger, J. M. Nerve growth factor enhances sleep in rabbits. Neurosci Lett 1999; 264:149–152.

156. Steininger, T. L., Wainer, B. H., Klein, R., Barbacid, M., and Palfrey, H. C. High-affinity nerve growth factor receptor (Trk) immunoreactivity is localized in cholinergic neurons of the basal forebrain and striatum in the adult rat brain. Brain Res 1993; 612:330–335.

157. Holtzman, D. M., Killbridge, J., Li, Y., Cunningham, E. T., Lenn, N. J., Clary, D. O., Reichardt, L. F., and Mobley, W. C. TrkA expression in the CNS: evidence for the existence of several novel NGF responsive CNS neurons. J Neurosci 1995; 15:1567–1576.

158. Vazquez, J. and Baghdoyan, H. A. Basal forebrain acetylcholine release during REM sleep is significantly greater than during waking. Am J Physiol 2001; 49:R598–R601.

159. Thakkar, M., Portas, C., and McCarley, R. W. Chronic low-amplitude electrical stimulation of the laterodorsal tegmental nucleus of freely moving cats increases REM sleep. Brain Res 1996; 723:223–227.

160. Auld, D. S., Mennicken, F., and Quirion, R. Nerve growth factor rapidly induces acetylcholine release from cultured basal forebrain neurons: differentiation between neuromodulatory and neurotrophic influences. J Neurosci 2001; 21:3375–3382.

161. Debeir, T., Saragovi, H. U., and Cuello, A. C. TrkA antagonists decrease NGF-induced ChAT activity in vitro and modulate cholinergic synaptic number in vivo. J Physiol (Paris) 1998; 92:205–208.

162. Banks, W. A., Kastin, A. J., Huang, W., Jaspan, J. B., and Maness, L. M. Leptin enters the brain by a saturable system independent of insulin. Peptides 1996; 17:305–311.

163. Ahima, R. S., Bforbaek, C., Osei, S., and Flier, J. S. Regulation of neuronal and glial proteins by leptin: implications for brain development. Endocrinology 1999; 140:2755–2762.

164. Tankersley, C. G., Kleeberger, S., Russ, B., Schwartz, A., and Smith, P. Modified control of breathing in genetically obese (ob/ob) mice. J Appl Physiol 1996; 81:716–723.

165. Tankersley, C. G., O'Donnell, C., Daood, M. J., Watchko, J. F., Mitzner, W., Schwartz, A., and Smith, P. Leptin attenuates respiratory complications associated with the obese phenotype. J Appl Physiol 1998; 85:2261–2269.

166. Elias, C. F., Kelly, J. F., Lee, C. E., Ahima, R. S., Drucker, D. J., Saper, C. B., and Elmquist, J. K. Chemical characterization of leptin-activated neurons in rat brain. J Comp Neurol 2000; 423:261–281.

167. Phillips, B. G., Kato, M., Narkiewicz, K., Choe, I., and Somers, V. K. Increases in leptin levels, sympathetic drive, and weight gain in obstructive sleep apnea. Am J Physiol 2000; 279:H234–H237.

168. DiMarco, A., Demartis, A., Gloaguen, I., Lazzaro, D., Delmastro, P., Ciliberto, G., and Laufer, R. Leptin receptor-mediated regulation of cholinergic neurotransmitter phenotype in cells of central nervous system origin. Eur J Biochem 2000; 267:2939–2944.

169. Xi, M.-C., Morales, F. R., and Chase, M. C. Evidence that wakefulness and REM sleep are controlled by a GABAergic pontine mechanism. J Neurophysiol 1999; 82:2015–2019.

170. Webster, H. H. and Jones, B. E. Neurotoxic lesions of the dorsolateral pontomesencephalic tegmentum-cholinergic cell area in cat. II. Effects upon sleep-waking states. Brain Res 1988; 458:285–302.

171. Baghdoyan, H. A. and Vazquez, J. GABA$_A$ receptors modulate ACh release in the medial pontine reticular formation. Soc Neurosci Abstr 2000; 26:1757.

172. Baghdoyan, H. A., Rodrigo-Angulo, M. L., McCarley, R. W., and Hobson, J. A. A neuroanatomical gradient in the pontine tegmentum for the cholino-ceptive induction of desynchronized sleep signs. Brain Res 1987; 414:245–261.

173. Goss, C. M. Gray's Anatomy. Philadelphia: Lea & Febiger, 1966.

174. Feldman, J. L. Neurobiology of breathing in mammals. In: Bloom F. E., ed. Handbook of Physiology. The Nervous System: Intrinsic Regulatory Systems of the Brain. Vol. IV. Bethesda: American Physiological Society, 1986:463–525.

175. Berman, A. L. The Brain Stem of the Cat. Madison: University of Wisconsin Press, 1968.

176. Fregosi, R. F. and Fuller, D. D. Respiratory-related control of extrinsic tongue muscle activity. Respir Physiol 1997; 110:295–306.

4

Functional Anatomical Analysis of Respiratory Circuitry

NANCY L. CHAMBERLIN and CLIFFORD B. SAPER

Harvard Medical School and
Beth Israel Deaconess Medical Center
Boston, Massachusetts, U.S.A.

I. Introduction

Physiological investigators have developed a wide range of powerful tools that allow the functional analysis of biological systems. In the nervous system, these methods allow the analysis of the activity patterns of individual nerve cells, and can be used to measure the effects of manipulating those nerve cells on system output. However, a complete understanding of the regulation of a function requires knowledge of the full range of cell groups that are involved in its control, and the ways in which those populations of neurons interact. The analysis of neural connectivity, then, becomes a critical component of understanding how a neural system works.

Fortunately, methods have improved in the last few years for analyzing the functional neuroanatomy of neural control of functions such as breathing. Methods currently are available that allow large-scale analysis of neuronal circuitry and its functional significance, at a cellular level of detail. This chapter reviews how the application of these methods to a classic problem in neurophysiology, the mechanisms for reflex apnea, has allowed us to elucidate a putative neural circuit for regulating this critical response.

Normal respiratory control is essential for life and well being. Therefore, it is not surprising that reflexes aimed at protection of the airway are among the most powerful in the nervous system. For example, reflexive apnea occurs in response to a host of airway stimuli that might threaten the airway, ranging from chemical to mechanical irritation, to invasion by foreign organisms. Noxious stimulation of the nasal mucosa is a particularly potent stimulus for producing apnea. The combined apneic, hypotensive, and bradycardic response to nasal stimulation, termed the diving response, is mediated by primary afferents carried by the ethmoidal branch of the trigeminal nerve (1–5). Thus, trigeminal apnea may have evolved as a portion of a coordinated autonomic response to facial immersion to prevent aspiration of water and drowning. Sensory input causing transient cessation of breathing is also conveyed by the branches of the glossopharyngeal and vagal nerves that supply the oropharynx, larynx, and lung (6,7). The most well known of these responses is the Hering-Breuer reflex, in which apnea is caused by activation of slowly adapting pulmonary stretch receptors.

Central projections of the trigeminal, facial, glossopharyngeal, and vagus nerves convey somatic sensory information from the upper airway to both the spinal trigeminal nucleus caudalis (Sp5c) and the nucleus tracti solitarii (NTS). The NTS is the main recipient of the visceral sensory afferents from the respiratory tree. Ramon y Cajal (7a) traced fibers from the respiratory tree through the vagus and glossopharyngeal nerves into the solitary tract and finally the to NTS. Subsequent to Cajal, numerous investigators have focused their attention on the intramedullary course of vagal, glossopharyngeal, and trigeminal afferent fibers (8,9). Slowly adapting vagal afferents responding to pulmonary stretch terminate primarily in the intermediate and ventral lateral NTS subnuclei, where they make monosynaptic excitatory connections with inspiratory beta neurons (10–14). Laryngeal and pharyngeal vagal afferents carried by the superior laryngeal and pharyngeal branches innervate the interstitial NTS (15–17). Finally, pharyngeal afferents in the glossopharyngeal nerve also terminate in the NTS (18,19). Autoradiographic tracing indicates that the NTS receives ophthalmic trigeminal inputs (20), although the ethmoidal branch does not project to the NTS (21,22).

The Sp5c receives a convergence of noci-, chemo-, and thermoceptive sensory information from different upper airway structures that include the tongue, oropharyngeal, and nasal mucosa (21,23–26). These airway inputs arrive via the trigeminal, facial, glossopharyngeal, and vagal nerves (19,21,27–31). The trigeminal diving reflex is mediated by the ethmoidal nerve, a branch of the ophthalmic division of the trigeminal nerve which innervates the nasal mucosa and projects to the ventral parts of lamina I and II in the medullary dorsal horn, most densely in the transition zone at the border of Sp5c and interpolaris. Electrical stimulation of the ethmoidal nerve can cause apnea and also sneezing (32,33). Injections of excitatory amino acid antagonists into this region of the Sp5c blocks apnea produced by ethmoidal nerve stimulation (34). The central pathways for transmission of sensory input from secondary sensory neurons in the Sp5c and NTS nuclei to the respiratory control neurons that ultimately suppress breathing remain undefined. Presumably, the sensory information must reach the ventrolateral medulla, which contains the rhythm-generating and respiratory muscle premotor neurons (35). This may be via direct projections of secondary sensory neurons (36). However, a number of lines of evidence suggest that a relay or integrative site in the pons may also participate in airway defensive reflexes. The parabrachial complex (PB), located in the rostral, dorsolateral pons, receives the bulk of the ascending output of the NTS (37–39) as well as substantial input from the spinal trigeminal nucleus (40,41). Evidence that these inputs are functionally related to the respiratory system comes from studies showing that slowly adapting NTS neurons that respond to pulmonary stretch stimuli (pump cells) project to the PB (42). Sensory NTS neurons that receive input from rapidly adapting pulmonary receptors also project to the dorsolateral rostral pons including the medial PB and Kölliker-Fuse (KF) subnuclei (43). Single-unit recordings in these PB regions have demonstrated a collection of neurons, now known as the pontine respiratory group, the activity of which is patterned by the respiratory rhythm (44–52).

II. Microstimulation Experiments

PB neurons not only receive respiratory-related sensory input and exhibit firing activity patterned by the respiratory rhythm, but also activation of PB neurons by electrical or chemical stimulation can produce a variety of changes in the breathing pattern that are similar to those seen when airway afferents are stimulated, including respiratory phase transitions and apnea. Electrical stimulation in the medial PB or KF subnuclei causes inspiratory termination and apnea, whereas stimulation at more dorsal sites in the lateral PB facilitates inspiration (53–57). At some sites chemical activation with excitatory amino acids has the same effect as electrical stimulation. Chemical stimulation in the lateral PB produces increases in respiratory rate and tidal volume in cats (58,59) and rats (60,61) (Fig. 1A,B). In addition, stimulation of the medial PB and KF causes characteristic changes in the

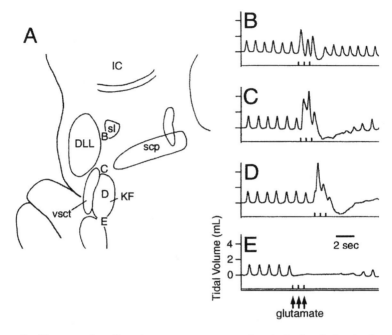

Figure 1 Topography of respiratory responses to chemical stimulation in the pons. A camera lucida drawing of a coronal section through the rostral end of the parabrachial complex where glutamate (10 nL; 1 mM) was injected at four sites denoted by the letters B–E. (B) Stimulation at the most dorsal site in the lateral PB produced hyperpnea. (C,D) Stimulation in or near the dorsal KF produced the inspiratory-facilitatory response we termed apneusis. (E) Activation of cells at the ventral border of KF caused apnea. DLL, dorsal nucleus of the lateral lemniscus; IC, inferior colliculus; KF, Kölliker-Fuse nucleus; scp, superior cerebellar peduncle; sl, superior lateral parabrachial subnucleus; vsct, ventral spinocerebellar tract. (From Ref. 61.)

breathing pattern. Injections of relatively large amounts of glutamate (200–3000 pmol) into the medial PB or KF decreases the respiratory rate (60,62). However, injections of smaller doses of glutamate (5–100 pmol) into the KF has mainly inspiratory facilitatory effects, which we have observed in two qualitatively different forms (61) (Fig. 1A–D). An increase in respiratory rate, tidal volume, or both, which we termed hyperpnea, occurred following glutamate injections into the caudal KF nucleus; these were indistinguishable from the types of responses seen in the lateral PB (Fig. 1B). In contrast, rostral KF responses consisted of a series of augmented breaths that occurred in close succession without complete expiration (Fig. 1C,D).

Because we have not recorded phrenic nerve activity during this response, we do not know if the phrenic response includes silent periods (expiration). However, the peaks in the respiratory flow signal suggest that the phrenic discharge is not constant, but rather waxes and wanes during the response. We termed these types of responses apneusis mainly to emphasize the qualitative difference from the other inspiratory–facilitatory responses.

To examine medullary inputs to hyperpneic sites in the PB, we conducted microstimulation experiments in rats that had previously received injections of retrograde tracers into the ventrolateral medulla or the nucleus of the solitary tract, which are sites that contain the ventral and dorsal respiratory groups, respectively. Comparisons of the stimulation sites with the locations of retrogradely labeled neurons revealed that hyperpneic and apneustic sites both contained neurons projecting to the ventral respiratory group, but only the apneustic sites also contained a dense population of neurons that project to the NTS (61). We hypothesized that the observed respiratory responses may be mediated by direct effects of pontine neurons on the cells that generate the respiratory rhythm (63) or the premotor neurons that drive the respiratory pump muscles. Furthermore, the production of apneusis may be dependent not only on effects on the ventral respiratory group, but also concomitant actions at the level of the nucleus of the solitary tract, perhaps affecting processing of airway sensory information. For example, simultaneous increases in inspiratory drive and inhibition of pulmonary stretch receptor feedback (the Hering-Breuer reflex) may cause apneusis. These pathways may be engaged in, for example, sneezing or coughing, which require deep preparatory inspiration.

Whereas others have reported decreases in respiratory rate in response to stimulation of the medial PB or KF, we found apneic responses to glutamate injected only into the most ventral part of the KF (Fig. 1E; see also Fig. 5 in Ref. 61) and nearly all the effective sites were located between the principal sensory and motor trigeminal nuclei (Fig. 2–3). This area, termed the intertrigeminal region (ITR), contains medium to large multipolar neurons scattered among the motor rootlets of the trigeminal nerve (64). Doses of glutamate as low as 1 pmol in this region prolonged expiration. Owing to the sensitivity of the apneic response, it is possible that previous reports of apnea following injections of glutamate into the KF or medial PB were due to spread of large volumes into the adjacent ITR. If so, pontine apneic responses must override hyperpneic responses when both cell groups are activated simultaneously. Why this might be so should become clearer once the cellular mechanism of each type of response is elucidated.

These microstimulation results suggest that there is an inspiratory off-switch in the ITR. However, a physiological role for this switch depends upon its ability to be engaged by neural inputs as well as by exogenous

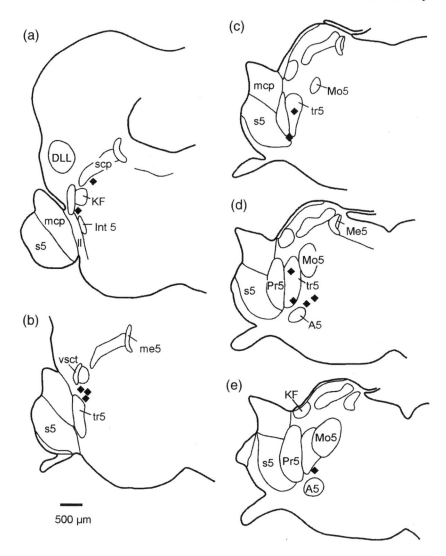

Figure 2 Distribution of pontine apneic sites. (A–E) Representative coronal sections through the rat brain at 160 µM intervals. Each diamond represents the location where microinjection of glutamate (0.5 mM) caused a decrease in respiratory rate in one rat. A5, noradrenergic cell group; DLL, dorsal nucleus of the lateral lemniscus; Int 5, intertrigeminal nucleus; KF, Kölliker-Fuse nucleus; ll, lateral lemniscus; mcp, middle cerebellar peduncle; Me5, mesencephalic trigeminal nucleus; me5, mesencephalic trigeminal tract; Mo5, motor trigeminal nucleus; Pr5, principal sensory trigeminal nucleus; s5, sensory root of the trigeminal nerve; scp, superior cerebellar peduncle; tr5, motor roots of the trigeminal nerve; vsct, ventral spinocerebellar tract. (From Ref. 76.)

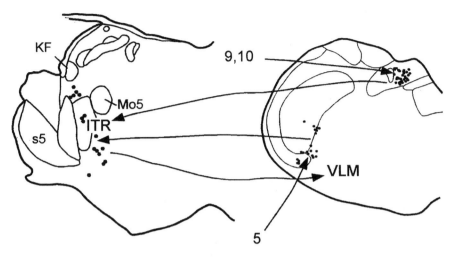

Figure 3 Summary diagram illustrating the proposed apneic pathways. Sensory information from the upper airway carried by the trigeminal nerve (5) terminates in the spinal trigeminal nucleus caudalis, which in turn projects to the intertrigeminal region (ITR). Vagal (10) and glossopharyngeal (9) afferents terminate in the nucleus of the solitary tract, which also projects to the ITR. The ITR causes apnea via a projection to the ventral respiratory group in the ventrolateral medulla (VLM). Dots on the left drawing, a coronal section through the rostral pons, represent neurons retrogradely labeled following an injection into the VLM. Dots on the right side, a coronal section through the medulla, show locations of neurons retrogradely labeled from cholera toxin b subunit injections into an apneic site in the ITR. KF, Kölliker-Fuse nucleus; Mo5, motor trigeminal nucleus; s5, sensory root of the trigeminal nerve. (From Ref. 76.)

glutamate. Markwald (1887) first demonstrated that synaptic activation of pontine neurons can produce apnea by showing that transection of the brain caudal to the inferior colliculus caused a marked prolongation of the inspiratory phase of the respiratory cycle, whereas more rostral transections between the pons and midbrain had no effect on breathing (65). In a landmark study, Lumsden (1923) also reported that transections at midpontine levels caused inspiratory cramps, which he termed apneusis, in vagotomized cats (66). Subsequent studies in both cats and rats have confirmed Lumsden's original observation, showing that apneusis can occur not only after transections, but also following pontine kainic acid lesions or injections of muscimol or N-methyl-D-aspartate (NMDA) receptor antagonists into the rostral pons of vagotomized animals (57,67–70). Thus, there appears to be an inspiratory off-switch in the pons that is capable of terminating prolonged inspiration in the absence of (and perhaps over-riding) vagal inputs. We hypothesized that the normal physiological role of this apneic response may be airway protection (61). Strong evidence for this idea was provided by Dutschmann et al., who showed that blockade of synaptic transmission with large injections of cobalt or NMDA receptor antagonists aimed at the KF attenuates the apneic response to ethmoidal nerve stimulation. Furthermore, injections of gamma-aminobutyric acid (GABA$_A$) receptor antagonists potentiate trigeminal apnea (71). They proposed that the KF mediates trigeminal apnea, because effective injections were centered in this nucleus. However, they did not place control injections into more ventral regions, and hence it is not clear whether their injections may have also affected the ITR.

The aforementioned microstimulation, blocking, and single-unit recording experiments suggest that cells in the rostral pons in the vicinity of the caudal KF and the ITR mediate trigeminal reflex apnea; however, the specific neurons and pathways involved remain to be identified. One strategy aimed at bringing a cellular level of resolution to this problem is the Fos technique. The Fos protein is expressed in neurons following prolonged stimulation (72), and this has been exploited by neuroscientists to uncover collections of neurons that are candidates for involvement in specific behaviors. The principal limitation of this technique is that, like single-unit recording, it can only correlate activation with the behavior and cannot determine causality. Another limitation is that as a metabolic marker of neuronal activation, Fos will not reveal cells that are inhibited. Nonetheless, it can be a valuable means to identify specific neurons that may participate in a given behavior. It is particularly useful to combine tract tracing with Fos labeling to elucidate the connections of neurons activated by a specific stimulus. These experiments consist of placing retrograde tracers into hypothesized target regions and subsequently looking for the occurrence of retrogradely labeled, Fos-positive cells. Neurons that express Fos following stimulation of the ethmoidal nerve or noxious nasal stimulation in rats are found in the pons, specifically in the KF and lateral parabrachial complex, and in addition in the NTS, Sp5c, and upper cervical spinal cord (73,74). These results are consistent with the idea that these pontine neurons are active during apneic reflex responses, which is one criterion for mediating them. Furthermore, neurons in the Sp5c that project to the PB are activated in response to subcutaneous formalin injection into the perioral region in the rat, suggesting that the PB receives nociceptive information from trigeminal afferents (75), although it is not known if these are the same afferents that mediate reflex apnea.

III. Combined Microstimulation and Tract-Tracing Methods

We have approached the problem of connections of neurons responsible for pontine-mediated apnea by combining chemical microstimulation with tract tracing (76). We hypothesized that apneic sites may mediate airway protective reflexes, and therefore may receive sensory information via the trigeminal complex, the NTS, or both. Furthermore, because we found that the ITR contains scattered neurons that may be retrogradely labeled from the ventral lateral medullary reticular formation, which contains the ventral respiratory group, we hypothesized that apneic sites may have connections with neurons that control the respiratory rhythm, which reside in the ventrolateral medulla.

To examine the inputs and outputs of the apneic region, we injected apneic sites in the ITR with a solution containing threshold doses of glutamate combined with the retrograde tracer, cholera toxin b subunit. In addition, we included the anterograde tracer, biotinylated dextranamine, to examine the pattern of the efferent connections of the neurons that caused apnea (76). Very small (nanoliter) injection sizes were used to maximize the anatomical specificity of these tracing experiments. Examination of the locations of anterogradely labeled nerve terminals in these experiments showed that the apneic zone in the ITR of the pons projects heavily to the entire rostrocaudal extent of the ventrolateral medulla (which contains the ventral respiratory group). We therefore hypothesize that apnea is a result in changes in activity of some of these neurons. Although it is not clear which subsets of neurons mediate the response, the densest terminal fields were located rostrally, in the vicinity of the pre-Bötzinger complex, suggesting a direct effect on neurons that generate the respiratory rhythm (63). Testing this hypothesis will require determination of synaptic contact of ITR neurons with pre-Bötzinger complex neurons, which can now be identified by their expression of neurokinin 1 and mu opioid receptors (77). In contrast to the ventral medulla, there were few projections to the NTS, consistent with our earlier findings that neurons in apneustic, but not apneic sites project to the NTS (61). In fact, only those injections that included the KF nucleus contained terminals in the NTS, suggesting that connections with this nucleus are not critical for producing apnea. Retrogradely labeled cells following injections of cholera toxin b subunit into the intertrigeminal apneic zone were seen in the same region of the Sp5 where injections of excitatory amino acid antagonists block trigeminal apneic reflexes (Fig. 3) (34,76). We found retrogradely labeled cells in medial and interstitial subnuclei of the NTS as well. These two regions are known to receive vagal, glossopharyngeal, and trigeminal sensory input from the upper airway. We therefore hypothesized that the ITR may be the target of secondary sensory neurons in the Sp5 that receive trigeminal apneic signals, and also of neurons in the interstitial NTS that receive inputs from the superior laryngeal nerve, which mediates apnea during swallowing and in response to chemical or mechanical laryngeal stimulation (78–80).

IV. Conclusion

In conclusion, we propose that the ITR could represent a key relay for several airway-protective apneic reflexes via the neural pathways revealed by combining microstimulation and tract-tracing methodologies (Fig. 3).

References

1. McCulloch, P. F., Faber, K. M., and Panneton, W. M. Electrical stimulation of the anterior ethmoidal nerve produces the diving response. Brain Res 1999; 830:24–31.
2. James, J. E., De Burgh, and Daly, M. Reflex respiratory and cardiovascular effects of stimulation of receptors in the nose of the dog. J Physiol (Lond) 1972; 220:673–696.
3. Yavari, P., McCulloch, P. F., and Panneton, W. M. Trigeminally-mediated alteration of cardiorespiratory rhythms during nasal application of carbon dioxide in the rat. J Auton Nerv Syst 1996; 61:195–200.
4. Ho, C. L. and Kou, Y. R. Protective and defensive airway reflexes evoked by nasal exposure to wood smoke in anesthetized rats. J Appl Physiol 2000; 88:863–870.
5. Kratschmer, F. On reflexes from the nasal mucous membrane on respiration and circulation. Respir Physiol 2001; 127:93–104.
6. Sant'Ambrogio, G., Tsubone, H., and Sant'Ambrogio, F. B. Sensory information from the upper airway: role in the control of breathing. Respir Physiol 1995; 102:1–16.
7. Lucier, G. E., Daynes, J., and Sessle, B. J. Laryngeal reflex regulation: peripheral and central neural analyses. Exp Neurol 1978; 62:200–213.
7a. Ramón y Cajal, S. Histology of the Nervous System. N. Swanson and L.W. Swanson, tr. Oxford Univ Press, 1995.
8. Kalia, M. and Mesulam, M. M. Brain stem projections of sensory and motor components of the vagus complex in the cat: II. Laryngeal, tracheobronchial, pulmonary, cardiac, and gastrointestinal branches. J Comp Neurol 1980; 193:467–508.

9. Kalia, M. and Mesulam, M. M. Brain stem projections of sensory and motor components of the vagus complex in the cat: I. The cervical vagus and nodose ganglion. J Comp Neurol 1980; 193:435–465.

10. Kalia, M. and Richter, D. Morphology of physiologically identified slowly adapting lung stretch receptor afferents stained with intra-axonal horseradish peroxidase in the nucleus of the tractus solitarius of the cat. II. An ultrastructural analysis. J Comp Neurol 1985; 241:521–535.

11. Kalia, M. and Richter, D. Morphology of physiologically identified slowly adapting lung stretch receptor afferents stained with intra-axonal horseradish peroxidase in the nucleus of the tractus solitarius of the cat. I. A light microscopic analysis. J Comp Neurol 1985; 241:503–520.

12. Kalia, M. and Richter, D. Rapidly adapting pulmonary receptor afferents: II. Fine structure and synaptic organization of central terminal processes in the nucleus of the tractus solitarius. J Comp Neurol 1988; 274:574–594.

13. Kalia, M. and Richter, D. Rapidly adapting pulmonary receptor afferents: I. Arborization in the nucleus of the tractus solitarius. J Comp Neurol 1988; 274:560–573.

14. Anders, K., Ohndorf, W., Dermietzel, R., and Richter D. W. Synapses between slowly adapting lung stretch receptor afferents and inspiratory beta-neurons in the nucleus of the solitary tract of cats: a light and electron microscopic analysis. J Comp Neurol 1993; 335:163–172.

15. Lucier, G. E., Egizii, R., and Dostrovsky, J. O. Projections of the internal branch of the superior laryngeal nerve of the cat. Brain Res Bull 1986; 16:713–721.

16. Mrini, A. and Jean, A. Synaptic organization of the interstitial subdivision of the nucleus tractus solitarii and of its laryngeal afferents in the rat. J Comp Neurol 1995; 355:221–236.

17. Furusawa, K., Yasuda, K., Okuda, D., Tanaka, M., and Yamaoka, M. Central distribution and peripheral functional properties of afferent and efferent components of the superior laryngeal nerve: morphological and electrophysiological studies in the rat. J Comp Neurol 1996; 375:147–156.

18. Grelot, L., Barillot, J. C., and Bianchi, A. L. Central distributions of the efferent and afferent components of the pharyngeal branches of the vagus and glossopharyngeal nerves: an HRP study in the cat. Exp Brain Res 1989; 78:327–335.

19. Normura, S. and Mizuno, N. Central distribution of afferent and efferent components of the glossopharyngeal nerve: an HRP study in the cat. Brain Res 1982; 236:1–13.

20. Beckstead, R. M. and Norgren, R. An autoradiographic examination of the central distribution of the trigeminal, facial, glossopharyngeal, and vagal nerves in the monkey. J Comp Neurol 1979; 184:455–472.

21. Panneton, W. M. Primary afferent projections from the upper respiratory tract in the muskrat. J Comp Neurol 1991; 308:51–65.

22. Lucier, G. E. and Egizii, R. Central projections of the ethmoidal nerve of the cat as determined by the horseradish peroxidase tracer technique. J Comp Neurol 1986; 247:123–132.

23. Kerr, F. W. L. The divisional organization of afferent fibres of the trigeminal nerve. Brain 1963; 85:721–732.
24. Bereiter, D. A., Bereiter, D. F., Hirata, H., and Hu, J. W. c-fos expression in trigeminal spinal nucleus after electrical stimulation of the hypoglossal nerve in the rat. Somatosens Mot Res 2000; 17:229–237.
25. Shigenaga, Y., Chen, I. C., Suemune, S., et al. Oral and facial representation within the medullary and upper cervical dorsal horns in the cat. J Comp Neurol 1986; 243:388–408.
26. Anton, F. and Peppel, P. Central projections of trigeminal primary afferents innervating the nasal mucosa: a horseradish peroxidase study in the rat. Neuroscience 1991; 41:617–628.
27. Contreras, R. J., Beckstead, R. M., and Norgren, R. The central projections of the trigeminal, facial, glossopharyngeal and vagus nerves: an autoradiographic study in the rat. J Auton Nerv Syst 1982; 6:303–322.
28. Kerr, F. W. L. Facial, vagal, and glossopharyngeal nerves in the cat. Afferent connections. Arch Neurol 1962; 6:264–281.
29. Nomura, S. and Mizuno, N. Central distribution of afferent fibers in the intermediate nerve: a transganglionic HRP study in the cat. Neurosci Lett 1983; 41:227–231.
30. Nomura, S. and Mizuno, N. Central distribution of efferent and afferent components of the cervical branches of the vagus nerve. A HRP study in the cat. Anat Embryol 1983; 166:1–18.
31. Brining, S. K. and Smith, D. V. Distribution and synaptology of glossopharyngeal afferent nerve terminals in the nucleus of the solitary tract of the hamster. J Comp Neurol 1996; 365:556–574.
32. Batsel, H. L. and Lines, A. J. Discharge of respiratory neurons in sneezes resulting from ethmoidal nerve stimulation. Exp Neurol 1978; 58:410–424.
33. Angell James, J. E. and Daly, M. Nasal reflexes. Proc R Soc Med 1969; 62:1287–1293.
34. Panneton, W. M. and Yavari, P. A medullary dorsal horn relay for the cardiorespiratory responses evoked by stimulation of the nasal mucosa in the muskrat *Ondatra zibethicus*: Evidence for excitatory amino acid transmission. Brain Res 1995; 691:37–45.
35. Feldman, J. L. Neurophysiology of breathing in mammals. In: Handbook of Physiology. Vol. 4. Bethesda, MD: American Physiological Society, 1986:463–524.
36. Zheng, Y., Riche, D., Rekling, J. C., Foutz, A. S., and Denavit-Saubie, M. Brainstem neurons projecting to the rostral ventral respiratory group (VRG) in the medulla oblongata of the rat revealed by co-application of NMDA and biocytin. Brain Res 1998; 782:113–125.
37. Norgren, R. Projections from the nucleus of the solitary tract in the rat. Neuroscience 1978; 3:207–218.
38. Ricardo, J. A. and Koh, E. T. Anatomical evidence of direct projections from the nucleus of the solitary tract to the hypothalamus, amygdala, and other forebrain structures in the rat. Brain Res 1978; 1553:1–26.

39. Loewy, A. D. and Burton H. Nuclei of the solitary tract: efferent projections to the lower brain stem and spinal cord of the cat. J Comp Neurol 1978; 181:421–449.
40. Cechetto, D. F., Standaert, D. G., and Saper, C. B. Spinal and trigeminal dorsal horn projections to the parabrachial nucleus in the rat. J Comp Neurol 1985; 240:153–160.
41. Feil, K. and Herbert, H. Topographic organization of spinal and trigeminal somatosensory pathways to the rat parabrachial and Kolliker-Fuse nuclei. J Comp Neurol 1995; 353:506–528.
42. Ezure, K., Tanaka, I., and Miyazaki, M. Pontine projections of pulmonary slowly adapting receptor relay neurons in the cat. Neuroreport 1998; 9:411–414.
43. Ezure, K., Otake, K., Lipski, J., and Wong She, R. B. Efferent projections of pulmonary rapidly adapting receptor relay neurons in the cat. Brain Res 1991; 564:268–278.
44. Bertrand, F. and Hugelin, A. Respiratory synchronizing function of nucleus parabrachialis medialis: pneumotaxic mechanisms. J Neurophysiol 1971; 34:189–207.
45. Bertrand, F., Hugelin, A., and Vibert, J. F. Quantitative study of anatomical distribution of respiration related neurons in the pons. Exp Brain Res 1973; 16:383–399.
46. Bertrand, F., Hugelin, A., and Vibert, J. F. A stereologic model of pneumotaxic oscillator based on spatial and temporal distributions of neuronal bursts. J Neurophysiol 1974; 37:91–107.
47. Feldman, J. L. A network model for control of inspiratory cutoff by the pneumotaxic center with supportive experimental data in cats. Biol Cybern 1976; 21:131–138.
48. St. John, W. M. Influence of pulmonary inflations on discharge of pontile respiratory neurons. J Appl Physiol 1987; 63:2231–2239.
49. Dick, T. E., Bellingham, M. C., and Richter, D. W. Pontine respiratory neurons in anesthetized cats. Brain Res 1994; 636:259–269.
50. Lydic, R. and Orem, J. Respiratory neurons of the pneumotaxic center during sleep and wakefulness. Neurosci Lett 1979; 15:187–192.
51. Sieck, G. C. and Harper, R. M. Pneumotaxic area neuronal discharge during sleep-waking states in the cat. Exp Neurol 1980; 67:79–102.
52. Sieck, G. C. and Harper, R. M. Absence of high-frequency oscillations in the discharge of pneumotaxic neurons in intact, unanesthetized cats. Brain Res 1981; 221:397–401.
53. Cohen, M. I. Switching of the respiratory phases and evoked phrenic responses produced by rostral pontine electrical stimulation. J Physiol 1971; 217:133–158.
54. Bassal, M. and Bianchi, A. L. Inspiratory onset or termination induced by electrical stimulation of the brain. Respir Physiol 1982; 50:23–40.
55. Younes, M., Baker, J., and Remmers, J. E. Temporal changes in effectiveness of an inspiratory inhibitory electrical pontine stimulus. J Appl Physiol 1987; 62:1502–1512.

56. von Euler, C. and Trippenbach T. Excitability changes of the inspiratory "off-switch" mechanism tested by electrical stimulation in nucleus parabrachialis in the cat. Acta Physiol Scand 1976; 97:175–188.

57. Wang, W., Fung, M. L., and St. John, W. M. Pontile regulation of ventilatory activity in the adult rat. J Appl Physiol 1993; 74:2801–2811.

58. Miura, M. and Takayama, K. Circulatory and respiratory responses to glutamate stimulation of the lateral parabrachial nucleus of the cat. J Auton Nerv Syst 1991; 32:121–133.

59. Takayama, K. and Miura, M. Respiratory responses to microinjection of excitatory amino acid agonists in ventrolateral regions of the lateral parabrachial nucleus in the cat. Brain Res 1993; 604:217–223.

60. Lara, J. P., Parkes, M. J., Silva-Carvhalo, L., Izzo, P., Dawid-Milner, M. S., and Spyer, K. M. Cardiovascular and respiratory effects of stimulation of cell bodies of the parabrachial nuclei in the anaesthetized rat. J Physiol 1994; 477:321–329.

61. Chamberlin, N. L. and Saper, C. B. Topographic organization of respiratory responses to glutamate microstimulation of the parabrachial nucleus in the rat. J Neurosci 1994; 14:6500–6510.

62. Dutschmann, M. and Herbert, H. The Kolliker-Fuse nucleus mediates the trigeminally induced apnoea in the rat. Neuroreport 1996; 7:1432–1436.

63. Smith, J. C., Ellenberger, H. H., Ballanyi, K., Richter, D. W., and Feldman, J. L. Pre-Botzinger complex: a brainstem region that may generate respiratory rhythm in mammals. Science 1991; 254:726–729.

64. Brodal, A. Neurological Anatomy. New York, Oxford: Oxford University Press, 1981:520.

65. Marckwald, M. Die athembewegungen und deren innervation beim kaninchen. Z Biol 1887; 23:149–283.

66. Lumsden, T. Observations on the respiratory centres. J Physiol 1923; 57:354–367.

67. Denavit-Saubie, M., Riche, D., Champagnat, J., and Velluti, J. C. Functional and morphological consequences of kainic acid microinjections into a pontine respiratory area of the cat. Neuroscience 1980; 5:1609–1620.

68. Ling, L., Karius, D. R., and Speck, D. F. Role of N-methyl-D-aspartate receptors in the pontine pneumotaxic mechanism in the cat. J Appl Physiol 1994; 76:1138–1143.

69. Jodkowski, J. S., Coles, S. K., and Dick, T. E. A 'pneumotaxic centre' in rats. Neurosci Lett 1994; 172:67–72.

70. Jodkowski, J. S., Coles, S. K., and Dick, T. E. Prolongation in expiration evoked from ventrolateral pons of adult rats [see comments]. J Appl Physiol 1997; 82:377–381.

71. Dutschmann, M. and Herbert, H. NMDA and GABAA receptors in the rat Kolliker-Fuse area control cardiorespiratory responses evoked by trigeminal ethmoidal nerve stimulation [in process citation]. J Physiol (Lond) 1998; 510:793–804.

72. Sagar, S. M., Sharp, F. R., and Curran, T. Expression of c-fos protein in brain: Metabolic mapping at the cellular level. Science 1988; 240:1328–1331.
73. Takeda, M., Matsumoto, S., and Tanimoto, T. C-Fos-like immunoreactivity in the upper cervical spinal dorsal horn neurons following noxious chemical stimulation of the nasal mucosa in pentobarbital-anesthetized rats. Arch Histol Cytol 1998; 61:83–87.
74. Dutschmann, M. and Herbert, H. Fos expression in the rat parabrachial and Kolliker-Fuse nuclei after electrical stimulation of the trigeminal ethmoidal nerve and water stimulation of the nasal mucosa. Exp Brain Res 1997; 117:97–110.
75. Wang, L. G., Li, H. M., and Li, J. S. Formalin induced FOS-like immunoreactive neurons in the trigeminal spinal caudal subnucleus project to contralateral parabrachial nucleus in the rat. Brain Res 1994; 649:62–70.
76. Chamberlin, N. L. and Saper, C. B. A brainstem network mediating apneic reflexes in the rat. J Neurosci 1998; 18:6048–6056.
77. Gray, P. A., Rekling, J. C., Bocchiaro, C. M., and Feldman, J. L. Modulation of respiratory frequency by peptidergic input to rhythmogenic neurons in the preBotzinger complex. Science 1999; 286:1566–1568.
78. Sant'Ambrogio, G., Anderson, J. W., Sant'Ambrogio, F. B., and Mathew, O. P. Response of laryngeal receptors to water solutions of different osmolality and ionic composition. Respir Med 1991; 85:57–60.
79. Ryan, S., McNicholas, W. T., O'Regan, R. G., and Nolan, P. Reflex respiratory response to changes in upper airway pressure in the anaesthetized rat. J Physiol 2001; 537:251–265.
80. Ootani, S., Umezaki, T., Shin, T., and Murata, Y. Convergence of afferents from the SLN and GPN in cat medullary swallowing neurons. Brain Res Bull 1995; 37:397–404.

5

Gene and Protein Expression and Regulation in the Central Nervous System

LESZEK KUBIN

University of Pennsylvania
Philadelphia, Pennsylvania, U.S.A.

MARIA F. CZYŻYK-KRZESKA

University of Cincinnati
Cincinnati, Ohio, U.S.A.

DAVID GOZAL

Kosair Children's Hospital Research
    Institute
University of Louisville School of Medicine
Louisville, Kentucky, U.S.A.

I. Introduction

Respiratory disorders during sleep are common and present problems, the full understanding and resolution of which is to physiologists both a formidable challenge and an exciting opportunity. Sleep-disordered breathing occurs at the interface between two physiologic processes essential for survival; one regulating gas exchange and the other ensuring adequate amounts of rest and activity. Thus, the problems posed by obstructive sleep apnea (OSA) require interdisciplinary expertise.

Periodic nocturnal apneic episodes acutely disrupt and limit sleep, produce recurring blood oxygen desaturations, and lead to large swings in the airway and arterial blood pressures. One night of sleep disrupted by apneic events is sufficient to cause a measurable decrement in daytime functioning (sleepiness) (1–3) and elevated arterial blood pressure on the subsequent day (4–6). These immediate consequences of the disorder further accumulate from night to night. Obstructive sleep apnea is a distinct risk factor for arterial hypertension (7,8), with episodic hypoxia, and probably also the large variations in arterial pressure and frequent arousal, making distinct contributions to the daytime blood pressure elevation (see Chap. 6) and obstructive sleep apnea is also associated with detrimental changes in cognitive functions and mood disorders (1,9–11). These long-term changes are most likely accompanied by complex alterations in gene expression that involve many regulatory systems, including those residing in the central nervous system (CNS).

The mechanisms involved in OSA engage both central and peripheral regulatory systems. To better understand this complexity, it is useful to design experiments mimicking individual components of the disorder and study their consequences at distinct outputs. Accordingly, acute and chronic-intermittent upper airway occlusions, acute and chronic-episodic hypoxia, and sleep deprivation/fragmentation are produced in suitable experimental animal models to model distinct aspects of the disorder. The impact of these manipulations and the mechanisms they activate can then be investigated at different levels ranging from individual cells to the whole organism, with a focus on different functional systems such as the respiratory, cardiovascular, cognitive, or affective (Fig. 1).

At least three distinct vicious cycles, each operating on a different time scale, determine the pattern, severity, and progression of the sleep-disordered breathing (SDB). On the time scale of minutes, i.e., within a single obstructive cycle, anatomically narrow airway causes larger than normal negative inspiratory pressures. This increases the centripetal forces that collapse the airway; the narrower the airway, the higher the negative inspiratory pressure, and the more likely an airway obstruction. Those segments of the airway that lack rigid support and sufficient opposing force generated by upper airway dilating muscles are most vulnerable. The response to individual obstructive episodes is unlikely to involve lasting changes in gene and protein expression, but the same disturbance occuring repeatedly does involve such lasting changes. Therefore, the aim of the two most common treatments for OSA, the continuous positive airway pressure (CPAP) treatment and surgical intervention (uvulopalatopharyngoplasty), is to prevent the obstructions by enlarging the narrowest and most collapsible segments of the upper airway.

On an intermediate time scale of days, recurring nocturnal sleep disruptions lead to sleepiness. An increased pressure for sleep accelerates the occurrence of obstructive episodes after the sleep onset (12). The obstructions also last longer in sleep-deprived than in adequately rested subjects because the threshold for the arousal needed to resolve the apnea is higher. Thus, the more sleep-deprived is the patient, the more severe are respiratory disorders and the lower are the nadirs of blood oxygen level, with a parallel increase in sleep loss, cognitive deficits, and mood disorders.

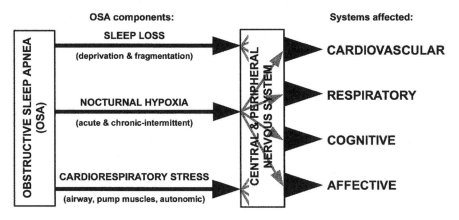

Figure 1 Each of the three principal pathophysiologic components of OSA (hypoxia, sleep loss, and cardiorespiratory stress) are likely to produce distinct changes in gene and protein expression in the nervous system, provided that they occur in a chronic or chronic-intermittent, manner. Each of these components may have adverse impact on each of the four major homeostatic subsystems: cardiovascular, respiratory, cognitive, and affective. To dissect and understand the possible interactions associated with OSA, experiments are performed in which the effects of one selected pathophysiologic component are observed in a selected output and at levels ranging from molecular to systemic.

The third vicious cycle is related to the extreme demand imposed on upper airway muscles at the time of arousals that terminate airway obstructions. As upper airway muscles repeatedly generate large forces and are subjected to large loads, upper airway muscles sustain injuries (13,14), and additional changes occur in the connective tissue and afferent innervation of the affected muscles (15–17). The larger are the forces generated in upper airway muscles, the more severe are the resulting injuries and the less effective are muscle contractions. Both the central and reflex control of the muscles become impaired.

In this chapter, following a brief review of the methods used to study gene and protein expression in the CNS used in studies of OSA, we provide examples of animal and cellular model-based research concerned with distinct regulatory mechanisms affected by SDB. First, we show how studies of neurotransmitter receptor mRNA and protein expression in upper airway motoneurons help elucidate the mechanisms underlying sleep-related upper airway hypotonia. We then review the molecular regulatory mechanisms activated at the cellular level by acute hypoxia. Finally, we present examples of the impact of a chronic, episodic hypoxia on protein expression in respiratory brain regions and regions relevant for cognitive deficits consequent to hypoxic stress.

II. Application of Genetic and Molecular Studies to OSA

Chronic hypoxia or hypercapnia and total or selective sleep deprivation have been used to assess changes in gene expression in the CNS (see Refs. 18–20 for earlier references). Each of these conditions results in altered transcriptional activity in many brain regions. However, the methodologies used did not adequately capture one extremely important feature of the cardiorespiratory and sleep disturbances typical of OSA—their repetitive and intermittent nature. Therefore, the results of those earlier studies may not be fully applicable to the pathophysiology of OSA.

Recurring nocturnal obstructive episodes, leading to sleep fragmentation, frequent arousals, intermittent hypoxia, and unusual stimulation of the cardiorespiratory system, are unique to OSA. The disturbances are chronic, but intermittent, and occur in a manner that distinctly ties two homeostatic systems, one controlling sleep and the other controlling cardiorespiratory functions. The importance of the intermittent nature of the disorder is underscored by recent findings that chronic-intermittent hypoxia leads to a sustained elevation of arterial blood pressure, whereas neither acute nor long-lasting chronic hypoxia has such an effect (this volume, Chap. 6). Analogously, chronic sleep fragmentation, as well as an intermittent stimulation of the respiratory system, most likely elicit changes in sleep regulation, cognitive performance, and central and reflex cardiorespiratory regulation different from those caused by long periods of sleep limitation or steady loads imposed on breathing. Although experimental paradigms modeling these two distinct aspects of OSA have been used in animal studies (21–23), so far, they have been applied to the investigation of changes in gene expression in the CNS to a very limited extent (24,25). Thus, molecular and cellular approaches are only just entering this field, thereby offering abundant new research opportunities.

Another area in which genetic studies are needed and should enhance our understanding of OSA is concerned with factors that predispose for the disorder. Here, the craniofacial anatomy, body fat distribution and metabolism, vulnerability to cognitive impairments caused by sleep loss, and the magnitude and pattern of cardiorespiratory response to airway obstruction show large intersubject variability in both humans and different strains of experimental animals (26,27). These differences have their origin, at least in part, in the polymorphism of relevant genes. Population studies demonstrate that hereditary factors contribute to OSA (28–30). However, to understand the relationships of these complex traits to the occurrence and severity of OSA and its consequences will require large population studies. This will be the next logical step following the recent findings that OSA is a defined risk factor in the development of arterial hypertension (7,31). Relevant examples of large-scale animal research are offered in the fields concerned with primary hypertension (32,33) and psychiatric disorders (34).

III. Methods of Assessing Gene Expression in the CNS

The complex structure and cellular heterogeneity of the brain pose particular challenges to the studies of gene expression and regulation in the CNS when compared to many other organs or in vitro systems. Standard methods, such as Northern blots, RNAse protection assay, and microarray technology, require relatively large amounts of total RNA (10–50 µg) or 0.2–1.0 µg of poly(A) RNA (about 3% of the total). To obtain this amount, one needs to start from a 5 to 25 mg sample of the relevant biological material. The CNS tissue samples of this size will usually include several functionally distinct brain regions and many cell types (neurons, astrocytes, microvasculature). This is acceptable for global screening of changes in gene expression and may help identify new genes, albeit with a relatively low detection sensitivity. The detection will be limited to those genes in which the basal mRNA levels are high and which undergo large changes with the studied conditions. The interpretation is also limited by the inability to determine which cell populations are the source of the observed changes. In some cases, the latter can be overcome by cellular localization of the transcripts of interest through complementary techniques such as *in situ* hybridization or immunohistochemistry (see below).

The sensitivity of mRNA detection can be greatly increased by amplification of the cDNA produced by reverse transcription (RT) of the RNA extracted from the tissue sample of interest. Common to all work with RNA that includes the RT step is the caveat that the RT efficiency is difficult to determine and variable, and therefore, often remains unknown. This makes a complete quantification of the results difficult. Fortunately, in many applications, the information about the absolute starting mRNA amount is not necessary. Following RT, 10–50 µg of total RNA will yield 0.05–0.25 µg of total cDNA. The polymerase chain reaction (PCR) is then commonly used to amplify specific sequences of interest (amplicons). An alternative method of RNA amplification using T7 polymerase (35–37) is less popular because of its complexity, except in the preparation of complementary RNA for display on microarrays. For the latter, the ability of T7 polymerase to faithfully amplify long transcripts (thousands of base pairs [bp]) 50- to 200-fold is very useful. In contrast, the amplifying power of PCR is almost limitless, but the targets need to be relatively short (several hundreds of bp) and only a few can be amplified and detected in one reaction. With appropriate quality control, one copy of the sequence of interest (about 0.17×10^{-6} pg for a typical 300 bp amplicon) can be amplified 10^{10}–10^{12} times, i.e., to obtain of the order of 85 pg/μL of cDNA needed to visualize the product and assess its amount using sensitive radioactive or fluorescent detection systems. Such an ultimate amplification and high detection sensitivity, although not routinely achieved or needed, are possible and demonstrate the tremendous power of the technique (as well as its potential to generate false-positive results).

Through PCR, one can detect rare mRNA species in tissue samples (micropunches) having volumes as small as 50 nL and containing only several hundreds neurons (38,39). Tissue samples this small can be obtained from distinct brain nuclei in rodents. Notably, following RNA extraction and RT, the available amount of cDNA is sufficiently large to investigate the expression of hundreds of genes by running multiple PCRs with specific primers. Thus, using the micropunch approach, one can combine a high degree of spatial (but not cellular) selectivity with the ability to screen for many genes. Further reduction of the sample size is limited by the RNA extraction step that requires a direct observation of the processed sample.

The ability to detect, following PCR, multiple targets in even very small amounts of total cDNA provides the basis for a convenient method of relative quantification of gene expression by "normalizing" the amount of the specific cDNA of interest relative to the expression of housekeeping genes, i.e., those coding for proteins controlling cellular structure or metabolism, and whose levels of expression are assumed to be stable under most experimental conditions (e.g., actins, albumin, cyclophillin, glyceraldehyde-3-phosphate dehydrogenase [GAPDH], neuron-specific enolase, tubulins, and 18S ribosomal RNA). This approach is useful for studies of regional differences (40,41), but less so for quantification of changes induced by varied experimental conditions because the expression of many housekeeping genes may be also altered (42,43). With the introduction of the real-time, quantitative PCR techniques (Sec. V. A), one can quantify each amplified target without the need to refer to the expression of other genes. Thus, the methods in which the results are expressed relative to the expression of housekeeping genes should soon become obsolete. With the quantitative, real-time PCR, the changes in gene expression induced by experimental conditions (such as exposure to intermittent hypoxia or sleep fragmentation), or specific to the host (e.g., different animal strains or animals at different stages of development) can be studied quantitatively and with a single-cell resolution.

Samples of mRNA can be extracted from single cells and then subjected to RT and PCR (see Refs. 44–47 for reviews). Through direct microscopic observation of slices in vitro, one can obtain mRNA samples from identified cells (48,49). Alternatively, cells may be labeled *in vivo* by retrogradely transported fluorescent dyes, acutely dissociated, and then collected, one at a time, for further processing (46,50). Cells may be also extracted from fixed brain sections by means of laser-assisted cell dissection (51–53), provided that the fixation method is optimized to minimize mRNA degradation (54). Immunohistochemical labeling combined with laser-assisted dissection is an established and powerful diagnostic tool of anatomic pathology (55). The single-cell approach minimizes or eliminates the problems caused by cellular heterogeneity of the brain tissue, while still allowing for the detection of multiple genes expressed in individual, identified cells acutely extracted from their environment. By monitoring "on line" the PCR amplification process (real-time PCR), one can ensure high quality and efficiency of the reaction, expedite the quantification process, and measure the amount of even very rare targets present in single cells in absolute numbers of cDNA copies. Examples of the application of single-cell RT-PCR are presented in more detail in Section V.B.

In situ hybridization techniques, in contrast to the methods involving RNA extraction, allow one to assess regional distribution of gene expression in thin brain sections and to screen large regions of the brain. Thus, a major strength of this approach is its high regional, and often also substantial cellular, resolution. The latter, however, is reliably achieved only in those regions where hybridization density is high, so that the pattern of labeling can be related to the morphological boundaries of underlying cells. To enhance the sensitivity, in situ hybridization can be combined with PCR (56,57). The in situ hybridization technique is compatible with double labeling. Thus, one can simultaneously visualize the distribution of two genes (58,59) or, by combining in situ hybridization with immunohistochemistry, one gene and one protein (60). Double labeling can help localize the in situ hybridization signal to distinct cells types, or may be used to observe changes in the expression of a gene and its corresponding, or functionally related, protein. Cells may also be physiologically characterized in an in vivo experiment, labeled juxtacellularly (61), and then one of their mRNA visualized by in situ hybridization. Following juxtacellular labeling and immunohistochemistry, one can extract the labeled cell using laser-assisted cell dissection, thus bringing together in vivo physiology with the study of gene and protein expression at the cellular level.

The ability to quantify the in situ hybridization data is limited. Most commonly, the density of labeling is visually graded into three to five levels, while the level of background staining is taken into consideration. The method has a low dynamic range, and is more suitable for revealing regional differences than for quantification of changes in gene expression caused by different experimental conditions (except when the changes are large). A more sophisticated quantification involves "grain counting" within regions delineated by outlines of individual cells or anatomic nuclei. The latter approach is more amenable to statistical analysis, but is tedious, so it is usually applied to few regions targeted for such an analysis by earlier, more global screening.

The interpretation of in situ hybridization data may be difficult in those regions where the level of expression is low. Negative results have to be treated with caution, and should not be used as the evidence of absence of a given mRNA. In regions of low labeling density, it is particularly difficult to ascertain that it is localized to neurons, rather than adjacent nonneuronal cells that are usually not visible without specific staining. Although there are examples of a proportional relationship between the level of mRNA expression and functional effects (49,62,63), generally the relationship between the level of mRNA expression and the production and stability of the corresponding protein may be nonlinear and regulated by a host of posttranscriptional processes (e.g., Sec. VI.C). Consequently, low levels of mRNA expression do not necessarily indicate low activity of the corresponding protein and vice versa. Thus, to fully evaluate a given pathway, gene expression studies need to be combined with a mapping of the distribution and functional assessment of the corresponding protein.

Another common method of screening large brain regions for changes in transcriptional activity is based on the detection of immediate-early genes (IEGs) such as *c-fos* or *Jun B* (64,65). The proteins coded by these genes (c-Fos and Jun B, respectively) are induced within minutes following the appropriate stimulus and can be detected by immunohistochemistry. Thus, the expression of IEGs can be visualized using specific and sensitive antibodies, instead of the more laborious in situ hybridization. Observations of regional changes in the distribution of IEGs have been used to identify brain regions and cell types affected by various perturbations of the normal sleep–wake behavior (Sec. IV), and localize in the CNS sites affected by chronic-intermittent hypoxia applied in a manner mimicking OSA (24,25) (see also Chap. 6).

IV. Gene Expression Changes with the Sleep–Wake Cycle

Changes in gene expression in the CNS have not been studied following sleep fragmentation similar to that in OSA. Rather, the main questions addressed to date the following:

- Regional differences in transcriptional activity between sleep and wakefulness, as assessed by observations of IEGs (66–68); reviewed in Refs. 20,69;
- Changes in the IEG transcriptional activity in selected brain regions following a total or selective (e.g., REM sleep only) sleep deprivation (64,70–72) or pharmacologically stimulated wakefulness (65,73–75);
- Changes with the sleep–wake cycle and following sleep deprivation in the expression of specific genes (e.g., tyrosine hydroxylase [*TH*], neurogranin) in selected brain regions (40,66,74–79);
- Sleep–wake-related changes in IEGs (mainly c-Fos protein) in immunohistochemically identified cellular populations (65,80–82);
- Identification of known and new genes, the expression of which in brain tissue (cortex) is correlated with distinct phases of the sleep–wake cycle or altered following sleep deprivation (83–85).

Many lines of evidence indicate that intense mRNA and protein synthesis take place during both slow-wave and REM sleep (86–89). In a striking contrast with these observations, the expression of IEGs (c-Fos) is much higher during wakefulness than during sleep in most brain regions (reviewed in Ref. 20). A moderate sleep deprivation (3–6 hr in rats) results in a further enhancement of c-Fos expression, whereas longer sleep deprivation periods produce no additional increase or even a reduction (64,73). Another IEG protein, Jun B, also shows a wakefulness-related and sleep deprivation-stimulated increase in many brain regions (64). Notably, the basal levels of Jun B protein appear to be higher than those of c-Fos. Because in order to stimulate transcription of other downstream genes, c-Fos has to heterodimerize with other IEG proteins, its relatively low basal levels may limit the wakefulness-related transcription. So far, however, double-labeling studies of the coexpression of pairs of IEG proteins across the sleep-wake cycle and following sleep deprivation were not performed.

Thus, it appears that the c-Fos level in the brain is proportional to the amount of sensorimotor activity during wakefulness. This is consistent with the common view that, parallel to its functioning as a transcription factor, c-Fos is a marker of high electrical activity in neurons regardless of the nature of the stimulus responsible for the increased firing. Accordingly, the enhanced expression of c-Fos (and other IEGs) in the CNS during wakefulness suggests that one function of c-Fos is to regulate transcription in those pathways that are essential for cellular homeostasis. There is, however, also evidence that c-Fos protein is involved in cell-specific protein synthesis (e.g., tyrosine hydroxylase in catecholaminergic cells), and many neurons and glia cells do not express detectable c-Fos levels under most physiologic conditions (e.g., motoneurons). Thus, c-Fos expression may be closely related to an increased metabolic demand in some cells, whereas in others it may serve other specific functions, the intracellular pathways of which rely on c-Fos synthesis. For example, endogenous norepinephrine is a very powerful stimulus of c-Fos expression (90) and other IEGs, such as phosphorylated cyclic AMP-responsive element-binding protein (CREB), Arc, and brain-derived neurotrophic factor (BDNF) (79). Notably, some of these factors may play a role in memory formation. It is, however, noteworthy that the activity of central noradrenergic neurons is very low or absent during sleep, is high during wakefulness, and probably increases further during sleep deprivation. Thus, the relationship between c-Fos expression during wakefulness, memory formation processes during the sleep–wake cycle, and noradrenergic activity is complex and may require a sequential activation of relevant cellular and molecular processes. Such sequences are likely to be disrupted in OSA. In addition, in contrast to the studies involving sleep deprivation in which great attention is paid to minimize stress, sleep disruption in OSA is a stressful condition. Thus, stress-activated genes probably play an important role in the pathophysiological processes affecting the sleep–wake regulation, as well as cognitive and affective functions in OSA.

The recent global screening for genes differentially expressed in the cortex across the sleep–wake cycle revealed an increased expression during wakefulness of at least 7 IEGs, 2 nuclear and 2 mitochondrial genes related to increased cellular metabolism, 10 genes for neurotransmitter receptors or neurotransmitter transporters, and at least 16 other genes (84,85). The mRNA levels for two genes, neuroganin and dendrin, decreased during a prolonged (24 hr) sleep deprivation (83). Notably, another 10 genes were upregulated during sleep, but only one of them has been identified (85). Thus, it again appears that, at least in the cortex, sleep is characterized by a low transcriptional activity. However, if relatively rare transcripts are preferentially expressed during sleep, whereas the enhanced expression of highly abundant transcripts dominates during wakefulness, the current microarray and differential display technologies may not be sensitive enough to detect sleep-related transcriptional activity.

All the methods of gene expression studies considered so far are suitable for the detection of known genes, but are very inefficient as tools for the discovery of new genes involved in sleep–wake and cardiorespiratory regulation. In addition, recent data show that transcripts of noncoding gene regions may cause diseases (91), although the mechanisms leading to activation of such transcripts remain largely unknown. Thus, new methodologies are needed that will enable a broad ("open-system") screening and identification of new genes (92). They will require powerful bioinformatic analysis provided through core facilities possessing the resources and data processing capabilities larger than those typically available in individual laboratories.

In contrast to global screening, neuroanatomical approaches in which selected genes were investigated with the due consideration to the cellular heterogeneity of the CNS show sleep-related c-Fos increases in at least two distinct groups of inhibitory neurons. The gamma-amino butyric acid (GABA)- and galanin-containing neurons of the anterior hypothalamic ventrolateral preoptic nucleus are activated during slow-wave sleep (93), and GABAergic neurons of the dorsal mesopontine tegmentum show increased c-Fos expression during intense REM sleep following selective REM sleep deprivation (80,81). These findings highlight the need for studies of transcriptional changes targeting selected genes and selected neuronal populations whose major role in sleep–wake regulation is well established through physiological studies. Among such "candidate genes," those related to the function of the recently discovered orexin-containing hypothalamic neurons may be of particular interest. Orexins are two peptides produced by a distinct group of hypothalamic cells implicated in mediating wakefulness-related excitatory effects (reviewed in Refs. 94,95). The cells are located in the perifornical hypothalamic region having a well-established role in the regulation of energy balance, as well as the cardiovascular and respiratory functions. The region receives important afferent connections from the insular cortex (96,97), brain regions that express c-Fos following chronic-intermittent hypoxia (98), and pontine and hypothalamic neuronal groups involved in sleep–wake control (99,100). The efferent projections of orexin-containing neurons are widespread, and include the classical wakefulness and arousal-related regions (noradrenergic, serotonergic, histaminergic, and cholinergic), as well as output neurons of both the somatic and autonomic nervous systems (101–103). Thus, sleep disruptions, stress, and cardiorespiratory perturbations characteristic of OSA are likely to have a strong impact on the hypothalamic orexin-containing neurons and their major downstream targets.

V. Neurotransmitter Receptor mRNA and Proteins Expressed in Upper Airway Motoneurons

Many of the wakefulness and arousal related-neurons of the brainstem and posterior hypothalamus (serotonergic, noradrenergic, cholinergic, orexinergic, histaminergic) have direct projections to motor nuclei, including those that innervate upper airway muscles, and motoneurons have receptors that mediate excitatory effects of these transmitters (see Ref. 104 for a review). The withdrawal of excitatory effects mediated by aminergic transmitters such as serotonin (5-HT) and norepinephrine (NE) is a major cause of the sleep-related hypotonia of upper airway muscles (105–108). On the basis of pharmacological studies, aminergic excitatory effects in motoneurons could be mediated by type 2A, 2C, and possibly other serotonergic subtypes, as well as α_{1A}, α_{1B}, α_{1D}, and some of the three known β-adrenergic subtypes. In addition, inhibitory effects may be produced in motoneurons by 1B-serotonergic and α_{2A}- or α_{2C}-adrenergic receptors (see Refs. 109 for a review of respiratory motoneuron pharmacology, and Refs. 110 and 111 for reviews of aminergic receptors). However, the information as to which of these receptors are expressed in upper airway motoneurons and, therefore, mediate postsynaptic effects of 5-HT and NE became available only recently, and largely through the use of gene expression studies in identified upper airway motoneurons (see Sec. V.B).

A. Quantitative Real-Time RT-PCR at the Single-Cell Level

The amplification by PCR of specific cDNAs obtained through the reverse transcription (RT) of mRNAs from single cells poses a particular challenge because of a very small amount of the starting material. For example, if following RT there are 100 copies the cDNA of interest and PCR occurs with a maximal efficiency (i.e., the amount of the product is doubled after each cycle), it will take nearly 30 PCR cycles to generate a sufficient number of copies of the amplicon (about 10^{11}) to allow visualization and measurement of the amount of the amplified product. In practice, PCR efficiency is lower than the theoretical maximum, and only a fraction of the material obtained from each cell is usually amplified in each reaction so that the presence of several mRNAs can be assessed. Moreover, in order to be able to interpret negative PCRs as the evidence of absence of the target, one needs to establish the PCR conditions at which a single copy of the target is sufficiently amplified to make the product detectable. Consequently, PCRs often need to be longer than 40 cycles. The optimization of the conditions for such long PCRs is difficult, especially when done using a standard thermal cycler.

The first attempts to amplify DNA obtained from single cells using PCR were performed in two rounds of what is called a nested or seminested approach (46,48,50,112,113). In this method, intracellular material from a single cell is treated with DNAse (if mRNA is investigated) and initially amplified with one set of specific primers ("external" primers). Subsequently, a portion of the products from the first round is reamplified in a second PCR with a second set or primers ("internal" primers) designed to recognize a segment enclosed within the sequence obtained from the first round. Such a two-stage procedure is more likely to result in a specific amplification of the target than is one long reaction (114). If the first round is performed with multiple sets of primer pairs (multiplex PCR), one can preamplify many cDNAs and then detect their presence in the starting material in multiple second-round PCRs with primers specific for distinct targets (115–117). The presence in single-cell samples of as many as 40 distinct mRNA species can be assessed using this method. However, individual targets may not amplify as efficiently as they would in separate reactions precisely optimized for only one pair of primers. Thus, the multiplex PCR in which dozens of targets are amplified simultaneously followed by specific amplification of individual cDNAs is an effective and sensitive screening tool. However, the efficiency of the first round of a nested PCR cannot be directly assessed when the starting amount of cDNA originates in a single cell. Consequently, the entire amplification process cannot be quantified.

In the same manner as the introduction of PCR revolutionized molecular biology by offering a dramatic increase in sensitivity of DNA and RNA detection, the quantitative, real-time PCR represents a major advancement toward PCR monitoring, quality control, and quantification. The real-time PCR allows one to visualize "on line" the progress of the cDNA amplification process by measuring the amount of fluorescence emitted by double-stranded DNA-sensitive dyes (e.g., SYBR Green I), by specific hybridization probes that bind to the product and generate fluorescence through fluorescence resonance energy transfer (FRET), or by oligonucleotide probes containing a fluorescent reporter and quencher dyes that become separated during second strand generation. The reactions with specific probes allow one to amplify and detect simultaneously several targets and offer an improved detection specificity, although their efficiency appears to be lower than that of real-time PCRs with DNA-sensitive dyes. However, specific probes are being continuously improved. Currently, four principal designs are used: "molecular beacons" that take advantage of the by 5′ nuclease activity of the *Taq* DNA polymerase (118), TaqMan® probes (Roche Molecular Systems, Inc., Indianapolis, IN) (119–121), "scorpions" (122), and "cyclicons" (123). Through its simplicity, the real-time PCR replaces the nested competitive PCR techniques used in the past for the detection and quantification of rare targets (124).

The real-time PCR offers the following major advantages over the standard PCR technology (see Figs. 2 and 3):

- The ability to monitor the accumulation of PCR products during the reaction. This allows one to use the PCR cycle number (c_T) at which fluorescence reaches a user-selected threshold as a measure of the starting amount of the sequence of interest in the sample. The c_T values of unknown samples can then be compared directly to a standard or, with additional calibration procedures, converted to the absolute number of copies of the amplicon. Direct monitoring makes it also possible to prevent the reaction from running past its saturation point, thus helping reduce the amount of incorrect products (e.g., primer dimers).
- The ability to calibrate the reaction using a standard curve constructed by amplifying known starting amounts of the amplicon. When performed properly, with appropriate care to eliminate any differences in the amplification rate of the standard and the unknown sample, a satisfactorily accurate, absolute quantification can be obtained in a cost- and effort-effective way. Through this feature, real-time PCR can take the full advantage of the inherently quantitative nature of PCR, and can be used as any other quantitative biochemical assay.
- The ability to assess the PCR quality prior to, or without, gel electrophoresis. This is achieved by "melting" the products at the end of the reaction by slow, controlled heating during which the decrease in the amount of double-stranded DNA is displayed as a function of temperature. Following a successful and specific amplification, the negative derivative of the resulting melting curve should show a distinct peak at the temperature characteristic of the amplicon. Faulty PCRs can be identified, thus helping to expedite optimization of the primers and reaction conditions. Melting also can be used to detect mutations.
- About a seven-fold increase in the speed of the reaction compared to a standard PCR. This is achieved by performing the reaction in glass capillaries (with the LightCycler® from Roche Diagnostics) that allow for a much faster heat exchange than standard polyethylene PCR tubes; a typical 35-cycle-long reaction that would take about 3 hr on a standard thermal cycler can be completed in less than 25 min (Fig. 2B).

- The ability to monitor the accumulation of two or three distinct targets (multiplex PCR) with the use of specific fluorescent hybridization probes that emit lights at different wavelengths. The use of specific probes also improves the monitoring of product accumulation by excluding from monitoring incorrect products.

The insights into the progress and quality of PCR offered by the real-time PCR and improvements in primer designing software make it practically possible to optimize long PCRs so that the reactions can be run for more than 40 cycles without a loss of specificity (Fig. 3a and b). Single-cell PCR and RT-PCR can be performed in one run, thus allowing for quantification and a mathematical analysis of the reaction (49,125). Figure 3 illustrates the application of quantitative PCR to the study in which developmental changes in the level of orexin 2 receptor mRNA expression were determined in single XII motoneurons.

B. Aminergic Receptor mRNAs in Upper Airway Motoneurons

The single-cell RT-PCR allows for a very specific and sensitive detection of mRNA for distinct neurotransmitter receptors and/or receptor or channel subunit composition in identified central neurons (113,116,125–129).

To determine which serotonergic and adrenergic receptors may contribute to postsynaptic effects of 5-HT and NE in motoneurons innervating the genioglossus muscle of the tongue, an important upper airway dilator, we recently studied aminergic neurotransmitter mRNA expression in hypoglossal (XII) motoneurons using the single-cell RT-PCR technique (50,129). XII motoneurons were retrogradely labeled by injecting a fluorescent dye, rhodamine, into the tongue muscle of juvenile and young adult rats. Several days later, the animals were sacrificed and XII motoneurons were acutely dissociated from micropunches of tissue extracted from fresh medullary slices containing the XII motor nucleus. Dissociated cells were plated and XII motoneurons were identified by the presence of retrogradely transported rhodamine (Fig. 2A). Individual motoneurons were collected, treated with DNAse, and subjected to RT. Subsequently, the cDNA from each cell was divided into three to four aliquots and each was subjected to two rounds of seminested PCR with primers for the receptors of interest (see Ref. 50 for details). Because many motoneurons were studied, the mRNA expression patterns were characterized by the frequency of occurrence of distinct mRNA species.

In contrast to earlier pharmacological and in situ hybridization results implicating many adrenoceptors in the control of upper airway motoneurons, the single-cell RT-PCR studies show that only one adrenoceptor, the α_{1B} subtype, plays a major role in mediating postsynaptic excitatory effects

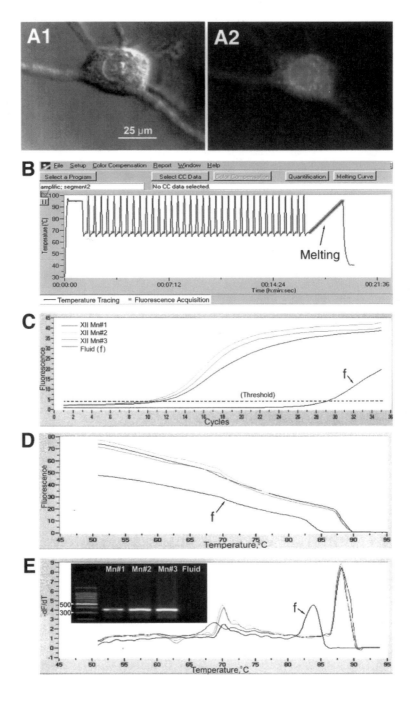

in XII motoneurons (Fig. 4a). The mRNA for other α_1 subtypes was expressed in very few XII motoneurons, and the remaining adrenoceptors were expressed in nearly none. These findings help clarify recent functional pharmacological studies which suggested that α_{1A} subtypes are not involved but, because of limited selectivity of the available drugs, could not conclusively resolve whether the excitation of XII motoneurons by phenylephrine was mediated by α_{1B} or α_{1D} or both receptors (132).

Additional single-cell RT-PCR studies demonstrated that, in contrast to the involvement of only one adrenoceptor, the postsynaptic effects mediated in XII motoneurons by 5-HT may involve several receptor subtypes. In mature rats, the mRNA for 5-HT_{2A} receptors is present in all XII motoneurons (129). These receptors mediated excitatory effects, and 5-HT_{2A} receptor-like protein is also strongly expressed in XII (Fig. 4b) and other orofacial motoneurons (131). About 35% of XII motoneurons express mRNA for the fully functional splice variant of another excitatory

---

Figure 2 Application of real-time PCR to the detection of distinct mRNA species in identified, single central neurons. (A) Hypoglossal (XII) motoneuron (Mn) acutely dissociated and plated prior to collection for single-cell RT-PCR procedures. The presence of rhodamine in the cell (A2) indicates that it is a XII motoneuron (the tracer was injected into the genioglossus muscle a few days before cell dissociation). (B–E) examples of the outputs generated during a real-time PCR in which, following reverse transcription and the first round of amplification, cDNA from single XII Mns was reamplified with primers specific for neuron-specific enolase, a neuronal marker. (B) The time course of temperature changes during the reaction. After 35 amplification cycles, the resulting cDNA is subjected to a linear "melting" and then allowed to reassemble during the subsequent cooling. The entire process is completed in less than 20 min. (C) the increasing level of fluorescence (proportional to the amount of cDNA) detected during the PCR portion of the reaction shown in B with three cDNA samples from Mns and one sample of the fluid (f) in which the cells were plated (control). The fluorescence curves for the three neurons cross the threshold near cycle 11, whereas for the control sample the threshold is not reached until cycle 29. (D) the relationship between fluorescence emitted by each sample and temperature during the period of melting shown in B. (E) the negative derivatives ($-dF/dT$) of the fluorescence versus temperature curves shown in D. The peak at 88°C is characteristic of the amplified target. The inset shows gel display of PCR products obtained in this experiment. Consistent with the outcome of the melting curve analysis, only the samples from the three Mns yield specific product of the expected size. (The data from Ref. 50 were obtained using a LightCycler and SYBR green I as the indicator dye.)

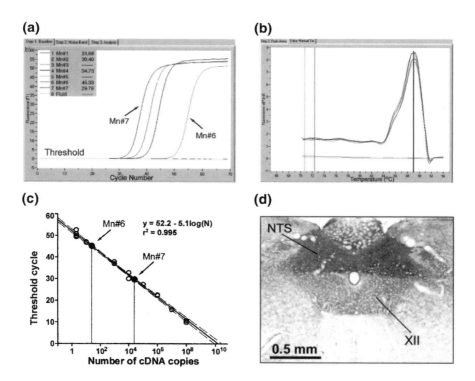

Figure 3 Example of a quantitative PCR in which samples containing 1/5 of cDNA from seven hypoglossal Mns and one control sample (f) were amplified with primers specific for orexin 2 receptor. (a) The level of fluorescence emitted by the samples during the amplification (proportional to the amount of cDNA). Amplification occurs for Mns 1, 2, 4, 6, and 7, whereas Mns 3 and 5 and the control sample yield no cDNA. (b) the negative derivative of the melting curves for the products of the PCR shown in (a) confirms that the cDNA amplified from Mns 1, 2, 4, 6, and 7 has the melting peak characteristic of the expected amplicon. (c) The cycle numbers at which the fluorescence from Mns 6 and 7 crossed the threshold in (a) (filled circles) are superimposed on an external calibration curve generated by amplifying known copy numbers of the target cDNA (the regression line with 95% confidence interval constructed from points shown by open circles). The vertical lines point on the abscissa to the orexin 2 receptor cDNA copy numbers present before the PCR in Mns 6 and 7. (d) Immunohistochemical labeling shows that the XII nucleus contains the orexin 2 receptor-like protein, although the staining is considerably stronger in the NTS. Thus, the orexin 2 receptor mRNA detected in individual XII motoneurons is translated into the corresponding protein. (Data from Ref. 125.)

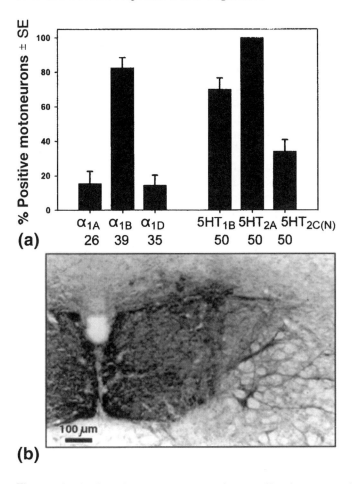

Figure 4 Aminergic receptor expression profiles in upper airway dilator Mns innervating the genioglossus muscle obtained from the RT-PCR experiments in which distinct mRNA species were detected in single hypoglossal (XII) motoneurons dissociated from juvenile rats. (a) The frequency of occurrence of XII motoneurons containing cDNAs for distinct receptors. Most motoneurons express the adrenergic α_{1B}, and serotonergic 5-HT$_{1B}$ and 5-HT$_{2A}$ receptor mRNAs (85%, 70%, and 100%, respectively); the mRNAs for the remaining receptors studied are relatively rare (adrenergic α_{1A}, and α_{1B}, and serotonergic 5-HT$_{2C(N)}$ receptor-normal splice variant), or absent (adrenergic α_{2A-C} and β_{1-3}; data not shown). The numbers of studied motoneurons are shown under the columns. (Data from Refs. 129 and 130.) (b) The 5-HT$_{2A}$ receptor-like protein in the XII nucleus, as detected by immunohistochemistry. The strong labeling of the entire nucleus is consistent with the presence of the mRNA for this receptor in 100% of XII motoneurons. (From Ref. 131.)

serotonergic receptor, the 5-HT$_{2C}$ subtype. Notably, nearly 70% of XII motoneurons also have 5-HT$_{1B}$ mRNA. This is an inhibitory receptor that often occurs presynaptically (133,134), and regulates the release of many transmitters (135,136). The presence of the 5-HT$_{1B}$ receptor mRNA in XII motoneurons suggests that this receptor mediates in motoneurons additional postsynaptic inhibitory effects, consistent with earlier in vivo pharmacological results (137). Thus, 5-HT controls upper airway motoneurons through both pre- and postsynaptic actions mediated by multiple receptors.

These data exemplify how mRNA detection at the single-cell level can provide new information about the neurochemical mechanisms of upper airway control across the sleep–wake cycle. Both chronic and intermittent loads imposed on upper airway muscles (e.g., secondary to obesity or repetitive airway obstructions), as well as aging, are likely to result in distinct changes in neural control of upper airway motoneurons. For example, the density of serotonergic innervation of upper airway motoneurons decreases with age (138). Such changes must be accompanied by altered expression of receptors and other proteins relevant for sleep–wake-related control of upper airway patency. Studies of these changes at the mRNA level in identified cells offer a precise and sensitive method for their detection and quantification. This should help relate the pathophysiological conditions characteristic of OSA to distinct cellular events and mechanisms, and help researchers devise pharmacological treatments that would enhance the activity of upper airway dilating muscles during sleep. Such treatments are not yet available, but their viability is the subject of animal research (139–142) and limited-scale clinical trials (143,144).

VI. Molecular Regulatory Mechanisms Activated by Hypoxia in Model Systems In Vitro

Nocturnal episodes of upper airway obstruction characteristic of OSA lead to repetitive reductions in blood oxygen level, i.e., intermittent hypoxia. Reduced oxygen tension (pO$_2$) in blood is detected by the type I O$_2$-sensitive cells in the arterial chemoreceptors of the carotid body, which is the main oxygen-sensing organ. An acute activation of arterial chemoreceptors elicits reflex respiratory and cardiovascular responses—hyperventilation and increased activity of the sympathetic nervous system. Stimulation of arterial chemoreceptors over extended periods (days) results in, or at least contributes to, a sustained augmentation of sympathetic activity (145–147). It appears that an intermittent, rather than continuous, occurrence of hypoxia is necessary for the development of clinically serious consequences of OSA—systemic arterial hypertension (146). The increased activity of sympathetic neurons and adrenal medulla cells accompanies the intermittent hypoxia-induced arterial hypertension (147).

A. Responses of Catecholaminergic Cells to Hypoxia

Catecholamines are essential neurotransmitters expressed and released by neurons regulating cardiorespiratory systems. Because physiologic and pathophysiologic adaptation to hypoxia involves gene regulation, the regulation of gene expression for TH, the rate-limiting enzyme in catecholamine biosynthesis (Fig. 5) has been the subject of extensive investigation.

The following neuronal groups participating in the arterial chemoreceptor pathway and control of sympathetic activity synthesize catecholamines:

- O_2-sensitive type I cells in the carotid body that detect reduced O_2 tension in the blood (148);
- Sensory neurons of petrosal ganglion that convey signals from the carotid body to the nucleus tractus solitarii (NTS) in the caudal brainstem (149);
- Interneurons within the commissural and medial subnuclei of the caudal NTS (150–156);
- Interneurons in the ventrolateral medulla, a major central site responsible for generation of sympathetic activity (150–156);
- Postganglionic sympathetic neurons (148); and
- Adrenal medulla cells that release catecholamines into the bloodstream (148,157,158).

The sustained augmentation of sympathetic activity in rats exposed to repetitive intermittent hypoxia is dependent on the presence of intact chemoreceptors (146). Although it is clear that sympathetic neurons and carotid body cells are critical for development of the intermittent hypoxia-induced arterial hypertension, the molecular mechanisms underlying this phenomenon are only beginning to be unraveled. These mechanisms involve biochemical and genetic changes activated at cellular levels by both a decrease in oxygen supply and reoxygenation, and operate not only in the specialized sensory cells of the carotid body and the output cells of the sympathetic systems, but potentially also in other cells and tissues.

The regulation of the *TH* gene expression by hypoxia in catecholaminergic cells provides a good example of hypoxic regulation of gene expression and may be relevant for the molecular and cellular events occurring in OSA patients. This regulation has been primarily investigated

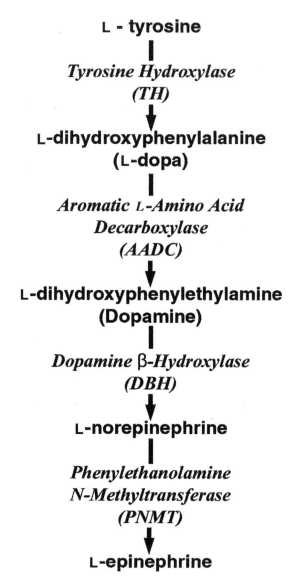

Figure 5 Biosynthetic pathway of catecholamines.

in dopaminergic type I cells of carotid body (148) and in pheochromocytoma PC12 cells, which are used as an experimental model for type I chemoreceptor cells (159).

Stimulation of the carotid body by hypoxia (1–48 hr; 10% O_2) causes a several-fold (three- to six-fold) increase in TH mRNA levels (148), increases enzymatic activity of TH protein (160,161), and augments dopamine synthesis and release from type I cells (162,163). This dopamine release is believed to attenuate the responsiveness of carotid body cells to hypoxia, thus contributing to the long-term adaptation to changes in O_2 level. The entire chain of events is intrinsic to type I cells, because it requires no neural or hormonal inputs (148). It is also specific for hypoxia in that it does not occur with hypercapnia, another physiologic stimulus for carotid body chemoreceptors (148). Regulation of the *TH* gene expression by short-term hypoxia (6 hr, 10% O_2) was not observed in postganglionic sympathetic neurons or adrenal medulla cells (148), but an increase in TH enzyme activity has been reported (157,160). In contrast, a long-term hypoxia (2–3 weeks of 10% O_2) increases TH protein content in adrenal medullary cells, with the induction being dependent on the neural input to the adrenal medulla (157,158). Likewise, similar long-term hypoxia augments *TH* gene expression, protein synthesis, and catecholamine release in the C2/A2 neurons of the NTS (152–156) and increases the TH protein level in the ventrolateral medulla, the caudal part of the dorsomedial medulla (NTS), and the locus coeruleus (153). In contrast, the TH protein content of dopaminergic neurons of substantia nigra is not affected (153).

Studies of the regulation of the *TH* gene expression by hypoxia allow identification of the molecular mechanisms by which decreased level of oxygen regulates the hypoxia-responsive genes. Hypoxic induction of the *TH* gene expression occurs at the level of gene transcription and stability of the TH mRNA (159,164–168). The activation of the *TH* gene transcription involves interaction of specific sites on the *TH* gene promoter with transcription factors activated in response to hypoxic stimulus. Regulation of the *TH* gene expression by hypoxia occurs in a dual transcriptional and posttranscriptional mechanism. These mechanisms will be described below.

B. Regulation of *TH* Gene Expression by Hypoxia in PC12 Cells: Transcriptional Regulation

The molecular regulatory mechanisms of hypoxia-mediated *TH* gene expression can be more efficiently studied in cultured cells in vitro than in currently available in vivo models. A dopaminergic, pheochromocytoma-derived cell line, PC12, has been extensively used for this purpose (159). Hypoxia induces *TH* gene expression in these cells (159), augments their TH protein level, and increases enzymatic activity of the TH protein (169). The sensitivity, magnitude, and time course of PC12 cell response to hypoxia are very similar to those measured in the carotid body O_2-sensitive type I cells (148). The increase in accumulation of TH mRNA starts within the first hour of hypoxia, is maximal at 6 hr, and then somewhat declines but remains at the elevated level for as long as 48 hr, which was the longest exposure studied (Czyżyk-Krzeska, unpublished results). When exposed to hypoxia, PC12 cells depolarize and release dopamine (170).

The rat *TH* gene is a single-copy gene (7.3 kb) located on chromosome 11. The gene comprises 13 exons and 12 introns (171,172). Most of the regulatory cis-acting elements are located within the first −300 bp of the *TH* gene promoter region (Fig. 6). The promoter contains a potential hypoxia-responsive element (HRE)-like site (5′TCGTG3′) located at position −225 to −221 bp from the transcription start site. This is followed by cis-acting elements such as the activating protein 2 (AP2) motif at −220 to −214 bp, the AP1 motif (−206 to −200 bp; 5′TGACTCA3′) with an overlapping E box/dyad at −212 to −185 bp, a POU/octamer (OCT) site at −176 to −169 bp, a heptamer (HEPTA) site at −159 to −165 bp, an Sp1 site at −120 to −113 bp, and two cyclic AMP-responsive element (CRE) sites (5′TGACGTCA3′). The main site, CRE1, is at position −45 to −38 bp, and CRE2 is at position −97 to −90 bp.

The AP1 and CRE motifs appear to be the major elements involved in both the constitutive and regulated expression of *TH* transcription (173–184). The tissue-specific expression of the *TH* gene in a transgenic mouse model additionally requires distal sequences from −9 to −4.8 kb of the *TH* promoter (175,176). In the case of the human *TH* gene, additional sequences in the 3′ flanking region are important for *TH* expression in catecholaminergic cells of the peripheral, but not the central, nervous system (177).

The effects of hypoxia on the *TH* gene promoter were studied in PC12 cells using different deletions of the 5′ region of the *TH* promoter–reporter gene construct in transient transfection assays (164,168,184). The −284 to −150 bp fragment of the *TH* promoter containing the AP1/E box/dyad

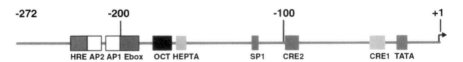

Figure 6 Schematic representation of the rat TH promoter. HRE, hypoxia-responsive element; AP1/AP2, activating proteins binding sites; OCT, octamer; HEPTA, heptamer; SP1, specificity protein element; CRE, cyclic AMP-responsive elements.

motifs and the putative HRE element is critical for activation of *TH* expression (164,168). Hypoxia induces binding of c-Fos and Jun B to this element (164,168). Consistent with the presence of the HRE site, our recent results show that hypoxia-inducible factors (HIFs) regulate *TH* promoter activity (Czyżyk-Krzeska, unpublished results). The transcription factors binding to both AP1 and HRE sites may interact in PC12 cells to confer full hypoxic response onto the *TH* gene. Such interaction occurs between the HRE and AP1 site-binding proteins in the process of hypoxia-activated transcription of vascular endothelial growth factor (VEGF) (185).

The signaling pathways activated by low oxygen leading to increased gene expression for *TH* are only somewhat understood. First, stimulation of glomus cells or PC12 cells with hypoxia results in inhibition of potassium channels (170,186) and depolarization of the cell membrane. This activates voltage-gated calcium channels leading to calcium influx, and activation of calcium-activated signaling. Notably, when PC12 cells are grown in calcium-free medium, attenuation of hypoxic inducibility of the *TH* gene results. In that respect, both depolarization and Ca^{+2} influx, when not associated with hypoxia, strongly induce *TH* gene transcription (178–180). This effect is mediated by the binding of CRE-binding protein (CREB) phosphorylated on serine 133 to the CRE1 motif, and/or possibly other CREBs (174,179,181,182,184). Mutations of the CRE motif attenuate hypoxia-induced activation of the −272 bp *TH* promoter (184). Indeed, hypoxia induces phosphorylation of CREB (184), but this event is not sufficient to induce *TH* gene transcription. Site-directed mutagenesis of the AP1 site or the CRE1 element shows that both elements are necessary for Ca^{+2}-mediated regulation of *TH* transcription (179). An increase in intracellular Ca^{+2} leads to increased binding of c-Fos, c-Jun, Jun B, and Jun D to the AP1 site (175). Thus, the increased activity of the AP1 site during hypoxia results from the hypoxia-induced depolarization and Ca^{+2} influx. The intracellular pathway leading to accumulation of HIF1α protein in PC12 cells during hypoxia is not well understood. It appears to be unrelated to changes in the intracellular calcium concentration, but is likely to result, similarly as in other tissues in accumulation of HIF1α subunit during hypoxia, from the inhibition of proteasomal degradation of HIF1α (186).

Ubiquitination is a biochemical pathway by which many different transcription factors are targeted for proteasomal degradation. Ubiquitination is a complex enzymatic process that requires adenosine triphosphate (ATP) (for a review, see Ref. 187). In the first step, the C-terminal glycine of the 76 amino acid protein, ubiquitin (Ub), is activated by ATP to a high-energy intermediate in a reaction catalyzed by Ub-activating enzyme (E1). In the next step, Ub-conjugating enzyme (E2) transfers Ub from E1 to the substrate. A third enzyme, ubiquitin ligase (E3), forms the isopeptide bond between the activated C-terminal glycine of Ub and $\varepsilon - NH_2$ group of lysine residue to the substrate, and the substrate is presented to 26 proteasome for degradation (Fig. 7).

In the next section we will discuss the specific upstream transcription factors and their coactivators that contribute to stimulation of *TH* gene transcription by hypoxia.

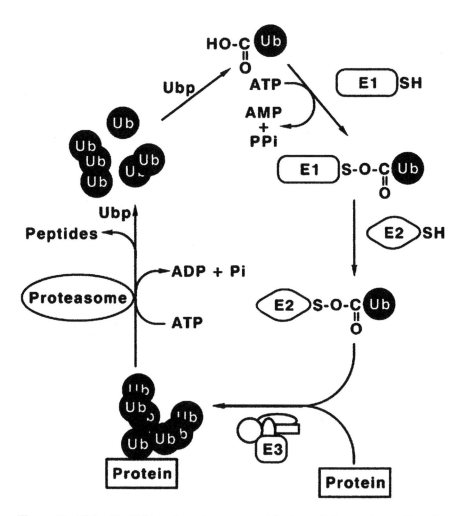

Figure 7   Ubiquitin (Ub) and proteasome protein degradation pathway. Proteins covalently bound to polyubiquitin chains are degraded by proteasome in enzymatic reactions involving enzymes E1, E2, and E3.

AP1 Transcription Factors

In PC12 cells, environmental hypoxia (10% O_2) stimulates accumulation of c-Fos and Jun B proteins and induces the binding of c-Fos–Jun B heterodimers to the AP1 site on the *TH* promoter (164,168). This binding facilitates activation of the *TH* promoter activity (164,168). AP1 activators comprise a family of basic region leucine zipper transcription factors that are homo- or heterodimers of Jun (v-Jun, c-Jun, Jun B, Jun D) and Fos (v-Fos, c-Fos, Fos B, Fra1, Fra2) or activating transcription factors (ATF2, ATF3, leukemia/lymphoma-related factor 1 [LRF1], B-ATF). Jun-Jun and Jun-Fos dimers preferentially bind to the AP1 site, whereas ATF-ATF or Jun-ATF dimers bind to CRE elements (Fos proteins heterodimerize only with members of the Jun family proteins). The activity of the AP1 complex depends on its composition and is subject to posttranslational modifications. Extracellular stimuli can change the composition of the AP1 complex from Jun-Jun homodimers to Jun-Fos heterodimers (188). Because heterodimers have higher DNA binding affinity, they may more strongly stimulate transcription (188). The activity of the AP1 proteins depends on their redox potential. DNA binding activity of Jun and Fos is inhibited by oxidizing reagents and is partially mimicked by reducing agents (189–191). A single cysteine residue within Fos and Jun binding domains of DNA is subject to redox regulation (189). A bifunctional protein, Ref-1, physiologically maintains the reduced state of cystine residues in the absence of reducing agents (191,192). The activity of the AP1 factors is also coregulated by CREB-binding protein (CBP)/p300 (193). For example, phosphorylated c-Jun binds CBP (193).

The members of the AP1 family have short half-lives. At least some of them (c-Fos, c-Jun, ATF2, and Jun B) are regulated at the level of protein degradation, which involves ubiquitination (194,195). c-Jun is targeted for ubiquitination by c-Jun kinase (JNK). c-Jun kinase binds to c-Jun, but under constitutive conditions is inactive and, consequently, c-Jun is not phosphorylated (196). Activation of JNK by extracellular stimuli results in phosphorylation of c-Jun, which protects it from degradation (196,197). The specific Ub-conjugating and ubiquitin ligase enzymes involved in ubiquitination of Fos and Jun are not known (195).

Hypoxia-Inducible Factors

Hypoxia-inducible factors (for a review, see Ref. 198) are heterodimers consisting of the 120 kDa alpha and 90 kDa beta subunits. Both subunits contain a basic helix–loop–helix (bHLH) domain in their N-terminals, followed by the PAS (PER-arylhydrocarbon nuclear translocation [ARNT]-SIM) homology domain. These domains are important for the dimerization of the two subunits and their interaction with DNA (Fig. 8). Hypoxia-inducible transcription factor-1α and HIF1β (also known as ARNT) are prototypic HIFs that were purified based on their ability to bind to DNA (199). They are both members of the bHLH-PAS family, and both contain several amino- and carboxyl-terminal transactivation domains. Hypoxia-inducible transcription factor-1α, a class II bHLH-PAS protein, contains in its C-terminal transactivating domain that interacts with the CPB/p300 coactivators (200–202). Its other regulatory sites include proline–glutamic acid–serine–threonine-rich protein stabilization domains (PEST-like motifs, at amino acids 499–518 and 581–600) and N- and C-terminal nuclear localization signals (198,203). Recently, two new types of HIFα were identified: HIF2α (204–206) and HIF3α (207). Similar to HIF1α, these proteins dimerize with the HIF1β subunit. Hypoxia-induced transcription factor-2α (also known as endothelial PAS domain protein 1 [EPAS1] or HIF1α-like factor [MOP2]) is highly expressed in endothelial cells (205), fetal lung, and in catecholamine-producing cells, including the carotid body (206), suggesting that this transcription factor has specific function in these tissues. The expression of HIF3α is not known. HIF1β belongs to the class I of bHLH-PAS proteins. It binds the aryl hydrocarbon receptor (AHR), which is also a member the class II of bHLH-PAS proteins, and this dimer activates transcription of genes encoding cytochrome P-450 (198).

Activation of HIFs by hypoxia involves changes in the accumulation and activity of the HIF1α subunit. The primary level of regulation, at least in the cell culture model system, is inhibition of proteasomal degradation of the HIF1α subunit during hypoxia (186,208–210). During normoxia, the

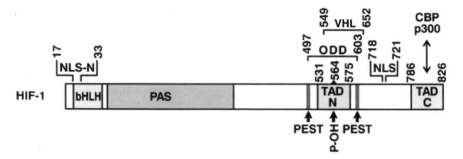

Figure 8 Structure of HIF1α. bHLH, basic helix-loop-helix domain; PAS, (PER-ARNT-SIM) homology domain; NLS, nuclear localization signal; TAD, transactivation domain (N/C-amino/carboxy terminal); PEST, protein stabilization domains; ODD, oxygen degradation domain; P-OH, hydroxylation of proline 564; VHL, VHL protein binding site, CBP p300, protein p300/CBP binding site.

level of the HIF1α subunit is usually very low because of the ongoing ubiquitination and proteasomal degradation (186,208–210). During hypoxia, or treatment with iron chelators (desferrioxamine) or $CoCl_2$, which mimic the effects of hypoxia, ubiquitination and proteasomal degradation of HIFα are inhibited. This results in the cytosolic accumulation of HIF1α and formation of dimers with the HIF1β subunit. The dimer translocates to the nucleus and transactivates HIF-sensitive genes by binding to the HRE sites in their promoter, enhancer, or intervening regions. HIF activity is also regulated at the level of nuclear translocation, posttranslational modifications (e.g., phosphorylation by mitogen-activated protein [MAP] kinases) (211,212) and, at least in some tissues, by induction of HIFα mRNA (198). Transactivation of specific genes by HIFs requires their interaction with additional transcription coactivators, such as p300 and CBP (200–202,213,214) (see next section). In addition, the HRE constitutively binds the ATF1 and CREB-1 transcription factors (215). These data indicate that regulation of gene expression by HIFs is a complex process that involves multiprotein complexes with different activities.

The major ubiquitin ligase demonstrated in ubiquitination of HIFα subunits during normoxia is the multiprotein complex associated with the von Hippel-Lindau (pVHL) tumor suppressor protein (216–222) (see Sec. VI.C, Von Hippel-Lindau Protein). Another E3 implicated in ubiquitination of HIFs is MDM2 (223). HIFα molecules contain a region recognized as an oxygen-dependent degradation (ODD) domain (208), which contains two PEST-like domains between amino acids 401 and 603 (208). This region is necessary for ODD of HIFα during normoxia. It contains a conserved proline residue (Pro[564]) that becomes enzymatically hydroxylated during normoxia, by thus-far unidentified O_2-and iron-dependent prolyl-4 hydroxylase (221,222). The hydroxylated proline is recognized by the pVHL complex and HIFα is ubiquitinated and targeted for degradation (221,222).

Transcriptional Coactivators: CBP and p300

CBP (CREB-binding protein) and the adenovirus E1A-associated 300 kDa protein (p300) are structurally similar and share important cellular functions (224). They have histone acetyltransferase activity and create a physical bridge between various transcription factors and the basal transcriptional machinery. Both proteins have three cysteine–histidine-rich zinc finger domains (C/H). The most N-terminal domain (C/H1) binds CREB, Jun, MYB, ELK1, and HIF, whereas the most carboxy-terminal domain (C/H3) binds E1A, transcription factor IIB (TFIIB), and Fos. Notably, CBP and p300 are present at limiting concentrations, so that their interaction with one group of regulators reduces their ability to interact with other regulators

(224–226). Thus, they may serve as integrators of multiple signal transduction pathways within the nucleus (224–226). The HIF–p300/CBP interaction can be blocked by a hypoxia-inducible p35srj protein interacting with the C/H1 domain. This may additionally modulate HIF activity (213). HIF1α also interacts with steroid receptor coactivator-1 (SRC-1)/p160 transcriptional coactivators harboring histone acetyltransferase activity and transcription intermediary factor 2 (TIF2) (214). The complex also includes the Ref-1, a dual-function protein that has DNA repair endonuclease and cysteine-reducing activities (214). These protein factors seem to act in synergy with CBP. Although little is known about regulation of *TH* gene expression by transcriptional coactivators at present, it is possible that binding of p300/CBP or SRC-1/p160 to the AP1 and HIF proteins to the *TH* promoter might play a role in the hypoxic induction of that gene.

Von Hippel-Lindau Protein

Von Hippel-Lindau protein (PVHL) was originally discovered as a tumor suppressor protein of which function was lost in sporadic and familial renal clear-cell carcinomas, hemangioblastomas, and pheochromocytomas (reviewed in Ref. 227). Additional tumors arising from extra-adrenal chromaffin cells, paragangliomas, including carotid body tumors, are also encountered in VHL disease (228,229). The human *VHL* gene is located on chromosome 3p25–26, and includes three exons (230). The human pVHL contains 213 amino acid residues (28–30 kDa molecular weight) (231). The rodent pVHL is shorter (19 kDa), as it does not have a pentameric acidic repeat in the N-terminus (232). The C-terminus of human pVHL is highly conserved among different species.

Von Hippel-Lindau Protein regulates constitutive and hypoxia-inducible *TH* gene expression in PC12 cells (233). Overexpression of the wild-type pVHL in PC12 cells results in a five-fold repression of TH mRNA and TH protein (233). In contrast, overexpression of the pVHL mutant (1–115) results in three-fold induction of TH mRNA and protein (233). The response is specific for *TH*, because other genes, such as tubulin or GAPDH, are not affected. The regulation of constitutive *TH* gene expression by overexpressed pVHL is transcriptional, and results from a block in *TH* transcript elongation that occurs in the distal part of the *TH* gene (after exon 7) as demonstrated in nuclear runoff assays (233). Regulation of the *TH* promoter activity during normoxia by overexpressed pVHL is relatively small, probably because the endogenous pVHL already saturates the pathway. A truncated pVHL mutant, pVHL (1–115), stimulates *TH* gene expression by increasing the efficiency of *TH* transcript elongation. Hypoxia, a physiological stimulus for *TH* gene expression, alleviates the elongation block, but inhibits hypoxic stimulation of the *TH* promoter activity. The specific data regarding the molecular mechanism by which pVHL inhibits hypoxic induction of the *TH* promoter are currently being studied. It is possible that one of the mechanisms by which pVHL inhibits the hypoxic activation of the *TH* promoter is targeting the HIF1α subunit for ubiquitination and proteasomal degradation.

Von Hippel-Lindau Protein functions in the context of a multiprotein complex (232,234,235). At the present time some components of the pVHL complex have been identified (Fig. 9). Von Hippel-Lindau Protein binds elongins C and B, the two regulatory subunits of the elongation trimeric factor elongin, SIII, containing elongins A, B, and C (236). Von Hippel-Lindau Protein complex includes also CUL2 (a member of cullin protein family) (237) and RING-H2 finger protein RBX-1 (a RING box protein with E3 activity) (238). (237). RBX-1 is a subunit that has the E3 ubiquitin ligase activity and strongly activates ubiquitination of the E1/E2 ubiquitin activating and conjugating enzymes (238). The role of pVHL in multiprotein complexes is to recognize specific substrates for ubiquitination and subsequent degradation. Consistent with this, pVHL-associated protein complex has ubiquitin ligase activity toward the HIF1α subunit (216–222), and loss of VHL gene function leads to high levels of HIF and upregulation of the hypoxia-inducible genes during normoxia, such as VEGF and platelet-derived growth factor (PDGF) (239). Tumors from patients with VHL disease produce high amounts of VEGF and erythropoietin (EPO) (240–242).

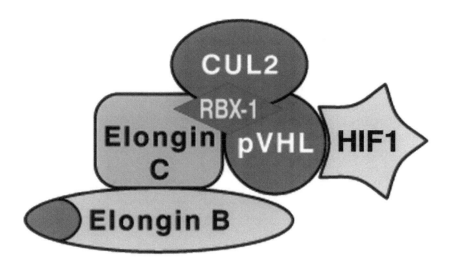

Figure 9   Von Hippel-Lindau protein-associated E3 ligase complex.

C. Regulation of *TH* Gene Expression by Hypoxia in PC12 Cells: Posttranscriptional Regulation

The hypoxia-inducible genes are often regulated by hypoxia in a dual fashion that, in addition to transcription, involves an increase in mRNA stability. Such regulation occurs in the case of mRNAs for TH, VEGF, EPO, and glucose transporter 1 (Glut-1) (243). The increase in gene transcription is a fast event that allows for rapid generation of new mRNA. However, prolonged exposure to hypoxia, at least in the cell culture models, results in a general decrease in transcription. In that case, an increase in mRNA half-life helps to maintain the necessary mRNAs at the high level. In the case of TH mRNA, the half-life of which is on the order of several hours, alterations in mRNA stability may meaningfully contribute to mRNA accumulation in response to hypoxia after approximately 24 hr of exposure. Regulation of mRNA stability involves interactions of specific regulatory factors with *cis*-acting elements within the mRNA, which are often located in the 3' or 5' untranslated regions (UTRs), but also in the coding region of the mRNA. These protein–nucleic acid interactions regulate secondary structure of mRNA and the interactions of specific RNA with degrading nucleases. TH mRNA has a 27-base-long pyrimidine-rich sequence within the 3'UTR of TH mRNA that binds protein factors in a hypoxia-inducible manner (hypoxia-inducible protein binding sequence [HIPBS]). One such site is represented by the motif (U/C)(C/U)CCCU within the pyrimidine-rich sequence; it is conserved in TH mRNAs from different species (166). Hypoxia induces protein binding to this sequence in cytoplasmic extracts from PC12 cells, catecholaminergic cells of superior cervical ganglia, and dopaminergic cells of the carotid body, but not in extracts from the adrenal medulla cells (244). Thus, the formation of the protein complex associated with the HIPBS site in the 3'UTR of TH mRNA occurs in some, but not all, populations of catecholaminergic cells. HIPBS regulates both the constitutive and hypoxia-regulated stability of the TH mRNA. A four-point mutation that abolishes the protein binding site within the full-length TH mRNA results in a two-fold destabilization of the mutated mRNA, and the corresponding two-fold decrease in mRNA steady-state levels (164). In addition, mutation of HIPBS abolishes the O_2-dependent regulation of TH mRNA stability (167). A short fragment of the TH 3'UTR containing the wild type HIPBS is sufficient to confer augmented mRNA stability on a heterologous mRNA, which in turn results in augmented steady-state levels of the chimeric mRNA and its derived protein. Conversely, the mutated HIPBS confers destabilization to the chimeric TH mRNA (167).

Analysis of the hypoxia-inducible protein–RNA complexes formed with the HIPBS element revealed the presence of two approximately 40 kDa poly(C)-binding proteins (PCBP1 and PCBP2) (167). The level of the PCBP1, but not PCBP2, is doubled in cytoplasmic extracts from hypoxic PC12 cells. This correlates with a similar enrichment of PCBP1 in the electroeluates from the ribonucleoprotein complexes formed with the hypoxic protein extracts, and is similar to the quantitative increase in the complex formation (167). This induction in the PCBP1 levels results from an absolute enrichment for the PCBP1, as similar increases were measured using total cellular lysates, and immunocytochemistry did not show any intracellular translocation of PCBP1 (Czyżyk-Krzeska, unpublished results). The difference in the hypoxic inducibility between the two isoforms suggests that although PCBP1 and PCBP2 have a high degree of sequence homology, they show some specific functional differences. The PCBPs participate also in regulating stability of other mRNAs, including EPO (245). The 3'UTR of mRNA for EPO contains poly-cytidine elements that bind both PCBPs. However, in cell lines that express EPO, *i.e.*, Hep3B or HepG2, hypoxia neither induces expression of PCBPs nor formation of the ribonucleoprotein complex associated with EPO mRNA that would involve PCBPs. This indicates that some tissue-specific mechanisms are involved in regulation of mRNA stability by PCBPs (245).

The upregulation of mRNA stability during hypoxia through binding of PCBP to the HIPBS element may be caused by protection of a nuclease cleavage site within the region associated with HIPBS in the TH mRNA, because mutation of the HIPBS region confers decreased mRNA stability to the chimeric mRNA (167). However, HIPBS is necessary, although not sufficient, for the O_2-dependent stabilization of TH mRNA. Although HIPBS binds protein factors in a hypoxia-inducible manner, it does not alone confer hypoxic regulation to the heterologous mRNA. Additional necessary regulatory elements must be located within other regions of the TH mRNA. In that respect, the regulation of VEGF mRNA stability by hypoxia involves elements located within UTRs and the coding region of the VEGF mRNA (246). Thus, both the TH and VEGF example show that the regulation of mRNA stability is complex and involves multiple factors.

VII. Effects of Acute and Chronic-Intermittent Hypoxia on Brain Regions Relevant for Cognitive Functions and Respiratory Control

As mentioned in the introduction, the major cognitive manifestations of SDB in both adults and children include excessive daytime sleepiness

(247,248), and a variety of personality and psychosocial maladjustments along with thought processing, perception, memory, communication, or learning ability disruptions (249,250). However, the sleep restriction and/ or fragmentation associated with the SDB may not be the sole mechanism leading to excessive daytime sleepiness. Indeed, the ability to maintain wakefulness was found to be extremely affected in patients with SDB and linearly correlated with both the degree of nocturnal hypoxemia and the magnitude of sleep deprivation. Thus, hypoxemia, hypercapnia, and sleep disruption, the three major hallmarks of SDB, seem to interact and impose both isolated, additive, and possibly synergistic effects on daytime neurocognitive functioning. However, to examine the individual roles played by each of these factors on neurocognitive morbidity, and the interactions of the roles, animal models need to be developed that specifically include one of the putative disruptors of neuronal integrity without interfering with the other parameters. Several other important considerations have also been included in the simplistic model of neural injury as it relates to SDB, as shown in Fig. 10. The figure depicts neural injury as the result of a balance between injurious processes occurring during SDB, the intrinsic vulnerability of the system, and the capability for repair. It also shows the potential interactions among the three major factors potentially involved in neural deficits exhibited by SDB patients. These factors can be counteracted by mechanisms that are either normally present or are recruited in response to the injury. The magnitude of any one of these elements will determine to what extent the arrow will move toward injury. The duration of the detrimental process(es) may further impose additional injurious effects.

Although the neurocognitive morbidity of SDB is irrefutable, the neural elements underlying each component of such dysfunction are unknown. Of particular interest is the assumption of differential susceptibility of neural functions and corresponding regions mediating such functions to each of the elements underlying SDB. Thus, with the clear understanding that extrapolation from human studies to animal models may be inherently hampered by a variety of limitations, assessment of changes in protein expression induced by intermittent hypoxia, sleep disruption, episodic hypercapnia, or a combination thereof in brain regions with defined neurobehavioral functions could provide important insights into pathophysiological correlates of neural dysfunction brought about by each of the disrupted elements associated with SDB. In this section, we will address initially the consequences of hypoxia on brain tissue, the potential differences between chronic-sustained hypoxia and chronic-intermittent hypoxia relating to their effects on particular neural substrates, and finally,

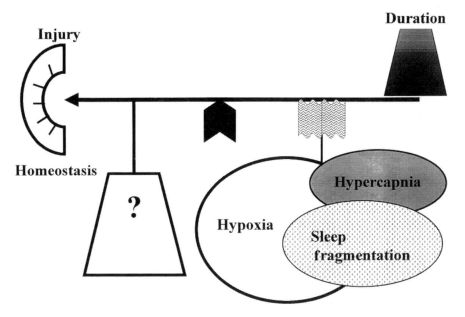

Figure 10 Hypothetical model of neuronal injury in SDB. Intermittent hypoxia, hypercapnia, and sleep fragmentation exert not only their own deleterious effect on neural viability and function, but also impose additional effects resulting from their interactions. These effects are further compounded by their prolonged duration. The inherent vulnerability of the individual and the ability to mount a defense response by yet-unknown homeostatic mechanisms further determine the overall magnitude of functional impairment.

we will describe how novel strategies involving high-throughput techniques in protein analysis can facilitate this a priori formidable task.

A. Chronic-Sustained Hypoxia

The effects of chronic hypoxia on cognitive function have not been examined in great detail. From the experience accumulated over the years during sojourns at high altitude, such as those studies performed on mountain climbers, alterations in psychological mood, personality, behavior, and cognitive functioning associated with hypobaric hypoxia have been recognized (251,252). Psychological and behavioral changes resulting from the effects of hypoxia often include increases in euphoria, irritability, hostility, and impairment of neuropsychological functions such as vision and memory (253). The long-term persistence of such decrements is unclear, but they may persist for long periods of time after return to sea level (254)

Monkeys exposed to a short hypoxic stimulus (6% O_2) exhibited significant decrements in their ability to acquire or retain attention-dependent tasks (255). Similarly, short daily severe hypoxic exposures (3.5% O_2) for 10 min markedly disrupted a learned behavioral task in rats (256). Analogous findings have been reported in humans, where administration of 10% O_2 to naive subjects was associated with electroencephalogram (EEG) changes indicative of deterioration of vigilance, memory, and attention variability, all of which were mitigated by administration of the calcium channel blocker/antiglutamatergic caroverine (257). However, hypobaric hypoxia or acute ischemia has variable effects on these measures (258–261).

Chronic exposure to hypoxia is associated with increased seizure susceptibility in animals (262), and this, in turn, may be related to alterations in neurotransmitter receptor expression and/or function. In support of this, recent studies in rats reveal that chronic (2–10 weeks) exposures to hypobaric hypoxia (−12.5% O_2) are associated with impaired mitochondrial respiration in the cerebral cortex (263), and demonstrate alterations in neurotransmitter receptor binding for a variety of substances such as substance P, met-enkephalin, dopamine, and GABA even as early as after 14 days of hypoxia in distinct brain regions (264–266). Pichiule et al. showed that mild hypobaric hypoxia resulted in decreased [^{3}H]MK-801 binding and affinity to the *N*-methyl-D-aspartate (NMDA) receptor in membranes prepared from cerebral cortex, hippocampus, and corpus striatum of juvenile (3 weeks old) rats (267). Recent data from our laboratory confirm a decreased expression of NMDA receptors in the prefrontal cortex of young adult rats (8–10 weeks old) exposed to 3 weeks of sustained hypoxia (10% O_2) (D. Gozal and N. Simakajornboon, unpublished observations).

B. Differential Regional Susceptibility to Hypoxia

The hippocampal formation has been long recognized as a critical region underlying learning and memory functions. Furthermore, subregions of the hippocampus display preferential functional roles, some of which are more likely to be affected by SDB. The CA1 region of the hippocampus has been identified as being intimately involved in spatial learning and memory functions. Despite substantial overlap, the hippocampus area CA3 performs the tasks of recent declarative memory including recovery of complete traces from partial cues and recognition of familiarity (268,269). The differences between CA3 and CA1 pyramidal neurons further extend to their susceptibility to hypoxia. Indeed, mammalian neurons are sensitive to hypoxia to a variable degree, but the mechanisms underlying this heterogeneous sensitivity are not well understood. Regional variability in hypoxic sensitivity has been reported in the brain during conditions of oxygen deprivation such as hypoxic ischemia (270,271), malonate-induced mitochondrial metabolic disruption (272), and during oxidant stress following ischemia (273). However, despite the wealth of information regarding heterotopic vulnerability to ischemic hypoxia, there is a relative paucity of information on the temporal and spatial characteristics of selective vulnerability of CNS neurons during mild hypoxic challenges typical of SDB. Such mild hypoxic events, if chronic or sustained, would be analogous to high-altitude exposure, whereas, if intermittent, they would resemble the oxygenation profiles seen in patients with SDB. Notably, in this latter situation, CNS neurons have to cope with two challenges, hypoxia and subsequent reoxygenation, the latter being associated with extensive oxidant stress that may induce neuronal injury and further lead to amplification of the hypoxia-induced injury.

As an example of selective vulnerability within a well-defined brain structure, two regions of the hippocampus display different susceptibilities to hypoxia. For example, a severe hypoxia for 3 hr in organotypic hippocampal slice cultures increased the delayed neuronal cell death in the CA1 hippocampal region but failed to do so in the CA3 hippocampal region when assessed using morphological criteria as well as propidium iodide fluorescence at 24 hr post-hypoxia (274). The extent of neuronal damage was linearly correlated with the duration of hypoxia. In this model, both NMDA and non-NMDA glutamate receptor antagonists (MK-801 and CNQX, respectively) were highly neuroprotective, suggesting that both types of glutamate receptors are involved in the generation of hypoxia/ischemia-induced neuronal damage (274,275). These findings implicate glutamate in the oxygen deprivation-related neurotoxicity, although the interplay between the two stimuli remains to be fully elucidated, and the excitotoxicity attributable to one cannot be used as a model for the other (276). Notably, much milder levels of long-term hypoxia also result in spatially selective changes. Neuronal cultures from cortical or CA1 hippocampal regions revealed that CA1-derived neurons were more vulnerable to a relatively mild hypoxic challenge (5% O_2 balance N_2 for 12 or 24 hr) (277). In addition, application of several protective strategies such as protein synthesis or nitric oxide synthase inhibitors, or alternatively platelet-activating factor and NMDA receptor antagonists, were all neuroprotective (277). Similarly, neuronal cell cultures from the CA1 hippocampal region were more susceptible to glutamate-induced neurotoxicity than were neurons from the CA3 and CA2 regions or from the dentate gyrus, and a treatment with either

NMDA or non-NMDA glutamate receptor antagonists attenuated gluta-mate-induced excitotoxicity (278). Thus, in the context of mild or even severe chronic anoxia/ischemia, neurons from the CA1 region of the hippocampus clearly display enhanced susceptibility when compared to the those from CA3 region.

When shorter periods of severe hypoxia are applied to these hippocampal regions, a similar pattern emerges. Indeed, neuronal damage assessed by recording population spikes in the pyramidal layer of CA1 and CA3 areas in hippocampal slices exposed to severe hypoxia for 30–60 min shows enhanced vulnerability as well as slower recovery in the CA1 than in the CA3 region (279). Furthermore, measurements of hypoxic depolariza-tion and swelling, both contributing to hypoxic damage in hippocampal slices subjected to severe hypoxia for 5–15 min, indicate higher vulnerability in the CA1 region, whereas neurons within the CA3 hippocampal region are clearly more resistant (280,281). Similarly, brief periods of severe hypoxia lasting 5–60 sec induced electrographic seizures in the rat hippocampal slice that were primarily restricted to the CA1 (282).

CA1 region vulnerability was also noticeable when regional suscept-ibility to hypoxia/ischemia was examined as the extent of neuronal apoptosis. The latter was significantly suppressed in the dentate granule cell layer, but not in the CA1 area of adult transgenic mice over expressing Bcl-2 when compared to wild-type littermates, indicating that different pathways may regulate apoptotic susceptibility within these regions (283). The protooncogene Bcl-2, which was isolated originally from the t(14;18) chromosomal translocation in follicular lymphoma (284), has been shown to prevent apoptotic cell death in a wide variety of cell types (285). Several studies have shown that overexpression of Bcl-2 prevent neurons from undergoing cell death induced by free radicals (286), hypoxia (287), and glutamate toxicity (288). Conversely, Bcl-2 attenuation using antisense strategies markedly reduced neuronal survival during severe hypoxic challenges (289) in neuronal cell cultures obtained from rat neocortex. However, it must be stressed that multiple pathways exist for inducing apoptosis. Thus, it is highly likely that a multiplicity of regulatory proteins and transcription factors are involved in survival mechanisms during hypoxic stress. For example, the tumor suppressor gene *p53* exhibits expression-dependent regulation by hypoxia (290), and has also been implicated in cell-related survival pathways. Although originally identified as a tumor suppressor gene, the inactivation of which is a common event in the development of human neoplasia (291), the product of the *p53* gene has been shown recently to play an important role in the regulation of apoptosis in a large number of cell types. The level of *p53* expression increases after treatments that cause an increased DNA damage (292). Depending on the cell type, elevated *p53* after DNA damage can result in either growth arrest or apoptosis (293,294). Consistent with these observations, downregulation of *p53* increased the proportion of surviving neurons exposed to severe hypoxia in culture (295). All of these studies suggest that regional hypoxic vulnerability is heterotopically distributed and that multiple mechanisms may underlie the differences in hypoxic susceptibility or tolerance.

C. Intermittent Hypoxia

In a great majority of in vivo experiments with sustained hypoxia described heretofore, sleep recordings were not obtained, which may lead to an impression that sleep was not affected by the hypoxic exposure. Moreover, a chronic sustained hypoxia does not represent an adequate model of SDB. Therefore, it was necessary to establish a suitable model of intermittent hypoxia, in which the sleep disturbance would be minimized. Indeed, sleep disturbances are a very frequent occurrence in sustained hypobaric hypoxia, as seen during mountain climbing, even though they are not present in high-altitude natives (296,297). Therefore, we have taken a methodic approach aiming to expose rodents to intermittent hypoxia, while reducing the degree of sleep disturbance as much as possible, and thereby allowing an unbiased and unconfounded determination of the effect of intermittent hypoxia during sleep on neural function and protein expression (298). In these studies, application of intermittent hypoxic challenges in Sprague Dawley rats during sleep elicited marked changes in the hippocampal CA1 region and cortex without evidence of major sleep disruption.

In our studies, the animals are housed from 0 to 14 days in environmental chambers (Oxycycler model A44XO, Reming Bioinstruments, Redfield, NY) that are operated under a 12 hr light–dark cycle (6:00 AM to 6:00 PM). Gas is circulated through each chamber at $60 \, 1 \cdot min^{-1}$ (one complete change per 10 sec). The O_2 concentration is continuously measured by an O_2 analyzer, and is cyclically altered throughout the 12 hr of the light period (the rats' sleep time) by a computerized system controlling the gas valve outlets, with the moment-to-moment O_2 concentration in each chamber adjusted automatically to a preprogrammed level. Deviations from the target concentration are corrected by addition of N_2 or O_2 through solenoid valves. For the remaining 12 hr, O_2 concentration is kept at 21% and the gas flow follows a pattern similar to that occurring during oscillation. Ambient CO_2 in the chamber is periodically monitored and maintained at <0.01% by adjusting the overall chamber ventilation. The humidity is maintained at 40–50% by circulating the gas through a freezer and silica gel, and the ambient temperature is maintained at 22–24°C.

The optimal intermittent hypoxia profile consists of alternating room air and 10% oxygen every 90 sec during the light phase. A small sleep deprivation was apparent during the initial 24 hr from which the animals recovered over the subsequent days of the protocol. Using this exposure pattern, we mimicked the oxygenation pattern of patients with moderate to severe OSA, in whom oxyhemoglobin desaturations to 70–75% are frequent. The exposure to this intermittent hypoxia protocol for 14 days was associated with learning impairments during acquisition of a spatial memory task in a water maze that were only partially reversed after a period of recovery (298). Immunohistochemical correlates for the markedly altered maze performance showed temporally defined increases in apoptosis within the cortex and CA1 region of the hippocampus, with little effect on the CA3 region. The increase in cell loss within this region was associated with marked changes in tissue distribution of NMDA-harboring cells within the affected regions, and increased c-Fos protein expression in surviving cells. Similar increases in c-Fos protein expression were recently reported by Sica et al. using a different intermittent hypoxia profile (24,25,98). This group of investigators found that regions involved in the behavioral responses to chronic stress, such as the thalamus and epithalamus, exhibited marked increases in early gene expression (24). Similarly, multiple cortical regions displayed similar c-Fos enhancements, and included the medial prefrontal, cingulate, retrosplenial, and insular cortices (25), suggesting that these regions may be particularly vulnerable to intermittent hypoxia. Finally, increased c-Fos expression was also found in caudal brainstem regions such as the nucleus of the solitary tract and ventral medulla, indicating potential relationships between these sites and the characteristically increased sympathetic outflow that develops over time with intermittent hypoxic exposures (98).

Thus, the changes in neural substrates associated with intermittent hypoxia during sleep are compatible with the concept of a gradually progressing excitotoxic process that may occur as a consequence of impaired cellular energy metabolism, free radical production, and/or modifications in glutamate ion/receptor complexes (299–301), and may lead to neuronal cell death (295) in the cortex and CA1 region but not in the CA3 region of the hippocampus. In the context of intermittent hypoxia, careful consideration needs to be given to the fact that alternating short periods of hypoxia with reoxygenation may result in generation of free radicals and oxidant injury. Although the molecular mechanisms underlying the differential susceptibility of these neighboring brain regions to intermittent hypoxia are unknown, they clearly involve a multiplicity of pathways. Elucidation of such pathways and their naturally occurring interactions cannot be examined one protein or gene at a time, but requires higher throughput techniques that permit such an assessment.

VIII. Changes in Protein Expression Following Brain Hypoxia

Variations in protein expression have been reported at different levels of hypoxia in a variety of tissues. In guinea pig heart, nucleic acids and protein syntheses were induced by intermittent normobaric hypoxia (302), but were reduced in the brain after 80 hr of chronic hypoxia (303). In rats exposed to 7% O_2 for up to 2 hr, protein and mRNA levels of heme oxygenase-1 were increased (304). In cultured human pulmonary cells, severe hypoxia (3% O_2) induced growth factors, cytokines, and inflammatory mediators expression, including PDGF, platelet-activating factor, and interleukins 6 and 8 (305). In cultured fetal rat forebrain neurons, proteins such as the pro-apoptotic gene products Bax and ICE were induced by hypoxia–reoxygenation, as well as the early gene products Jun and Fos (306,307). In the rat NTS, c-Fos protein expression was induced by mild hypoxia, and neuronal nitric oxide synthase expression was increased by cycles consisting of 5 min hypoxia–10 min normoxia (308,309). Neuronal nitric oxide synthase mRNA and protein expression were increased in central and peripheral neurons of rats exposed to 4–24 hr of hypobaric hypoxia (310). Similarly, Millhorn et al. showed that both acute and sustained hypoxia elicit the recruitment of multiple signaling cascades in the PC12 cell line (311–313). Activation of specific signaling pathways can further recruit downstream transcription factors and lead to gene upregulation. For example, mild hypoxia (5% O_2) for up to 24 hr increased VEGF mRNA and protein expression in astroglial cultures (314) and in rat C6 glioma cells (315). VEGF induction was due to both transcriptional activation and increased stability of VEGF mRNA, indicating that protein expression was regulated at both the transcriptional and the translational level (315).

Alterations in protein synthesis contribute to the impact of hypoxia on central neurons (306,316,317). The rates of protein synthesis, measured in vivo in several tissues from rats exposed for 6 hr to 10% O_2, were depressed by 15–35% when compared to normoxic rat tissue, with the greatest decreases being found in the brain and skin (316). In contrast, cultured neurons from fetal rat forebrain exhibited peak protein synthesis 1 hr after the onset of 6 hr hypoxia and 48 hr post-reoxygenation, when an increased rate of apoptosis was apparent (306). Both the increases in protein synthesis and in apoptosis were prevented by the addition of the protein synthesis inhibitor cyclohexamide (306), suggesting that both hypoxia and reoxygenation induce apoptosis via changes in synthesis of specific proteins.

In addition to reoxygenation injury, brief exposure to hypoxia induces adaptive mechanisms that may also depend on newly synthesized proteins. Supporting this hypothesis, pre-exposure of hippocampal slices to brief periods of hypoxia has been reported to increase their resistance to longer periods of hypoxia and this preconditioning was blocked by inhibition of protein synthesis (cyclohexamide) or mRNA synthesis (actinomycin D), but not by AMPA or NMDA glutamate receptor blockade (317). These observations suggest that the adaptation to hypoxia may be triggered by the induction of newly expressed proteins mediating adaptation and tolerance.

A. Overview of Proteomic Analysis

Recent advances in genomic analytical techniques have permitted the efficient characterization of cellular genotypes. Molecular biology offers high-throughput techniques with which to characterize the full complement of genes and their expression in cells, tissues, and organisms. Several yeast, bacterial, and mammalian genomes have been completely or almost completely sequenced, including a complete sequencing of the human genome announced on February 9, 2001. However, knowledge of the genomic sequence does not reveal a great deal about function. The efficiency of DNA analysis has resulted in a wealth of data concerning the genomic message, but little information about the proteins that are the product of that message. Therefore, new approaches that examine mechanisms of genomic *function* must be applied in the postgenomic era. One new approach to study genomic function is analysis of the full complement of proteins. The characterization of all the proteins expressed by a genome in a defined cell or tissue has now acquired the connotation of *proteomics*. This is a new field whose name was first used in 1994 at the Sienna, Italy, Two-Dimensional (2-D) Electrophoresis Meeting, and the term *proteomics* first appeared in print in 1995 (318). Most mammalian cells express approximately 10,000 different proteins at any given time. However, the proteome, unlike the genome, undergoes complex changes as proteins are modified by posttranslational modifications such as phosphorylation and glycosylation. The complexity of protein expression underscores the challenges in conducting protein analysis on a large scale. Successful proteomic analysis depends on three groups of techniques (Fig. 11): (1) protein extraction and separation; (2) protein identification and characterization; and (3) protein database construction.

Protein Extraction and Separation

Tissue samples are first treated to extract cellular proteins. This step must solubilize, denature, and reduce cross-linking bonds in order to eliminate protein–protein interactions, and remove nonprotein components such as nucleic acids. After the extraction phase, protein samples are resolved by two-dimensional polyacrylamide gel electrophoresis (2D-PAGE). O'Farrell

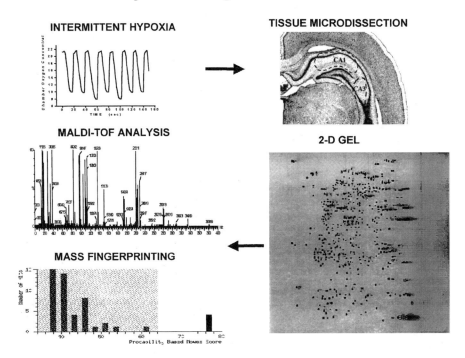

Figure 11 Schematic diagram of a proteomic approach. Rats are exposed to intermittent hypoxia and, at the desired time points, the hippocampus is extracted and microdissected to separate tissues corresponding to the vulnerable CA1 region and the more resistant CA3 region. Tissues are homogenized in appropriate buffers and the amount of protein in the sample is quantified. Equal loads of protein undergo 2D gel electrophoresis to separate the proteins according to their molecular weights and their isoelectric properties. The individual spots corresponding to individual proteins are carefully removed from the gel, and after tryptic digest, are analyzed by MS (MALDI-TOF). The resulting patterns of the measured masses from each spot in the 2D gel are then compared to existing protein databases (peptide fingerprinting). The protein displaying the highest matching probability is retained as the identified protein in the particular spot. Although not always necessary, Western blotting can then be used to further confirm the identity of the detected protein.

and Klose first described modern 2D-PAGE in 1975 and the basic technique has changed little since that time (319,320). Two-dimensional polyacrylamicle gel electrophoresis is the only practical method currently available to resolve complex mixtures of proteins. The first dimension of 2D-PAGE is the isoelectric focusing (IEF) phase. During IEF, proteins are separated in a pH gradient and migrate in the gel until they reach a point where their net charge is zero (the isoelectric point [pI]). The first-dimension IEF gel is then applied to the top of a second gel and electrophoresis is carried out in the presence of sodium dodecyl sulfate (SDS) in the orthogonal direction, such as to separate those proteins that have similar isoelectric properties and align them according to their molecular weights. The second-dimension gels resolve proteins by mass alone, because the protein charges have been dispersed by SDS.

O'Farrell's original 2D-PAGE technique described in 1975 resolved 1000 proteins on a single gel (319). The use of silver staining, complex ampholyte sets, and larger dimension gels now allow resolution of approximately 10,000 proteins in a single gel. Using these methods, complex protein mixtures can be separated and the charge, size, and relative quantity of individual proteins can be measured. However, 2D-PAGE alone does not yield information about the identity, posttranslational changes, or functions of the visualized proteins.

Protein Identification and Characterization

Information from 2D-PAGE gels regarding protein sequence, posttranslational modifications, and functions require analysis by Edman degradative sequencing or mass spectroscopy. For Edman sequencing, proteins are blotted to polyvinylidenedifluoride (PVDF) membranes and identified with a general protein stain. The spots of interest are excised and subjected to Edman analysis to obtain N-terminal sequence data. This approach offers high efficiency, but many proteins have their amino group blocked by posttranslational modifications and cannot be analyzed by Edman techniques. Two types of mass spectroscopy can also be used to analyze proteins separated by the 2D gels. In the peptide mass mapping approach initially described by Henzel et al. (321), the mass spectrum of the eluted protein mixture is acquired and results in a peptide-mass fingerprinting of the protein being studied. This mass spectrum is obtained using matrix-assisted laser desorption/ionization (MALDI), which results in a time-of-flight (TOF) distribution of peptides comprising the mixture. For mass fingerprinting, proteins resolved by 2D-PAGE are subjected to in-gel enzymatic digestion, MALDI-TOF analysis is then used to determine the masses of the cleaved fragments, and the patterns of the measured masses are further matched against the theoretical masses of proteins derived from the available databases. This allows for high-throughput identification of proteins. However, the identification process is based on probability matching. In other words, computerized searches for a given protein will yield names of several candidate proteins and the respective probabilities that they match. The currently available software programs will "electronically cleave" the sequences of known proteins, producing a set of theoretical masses resulting from trypsin cleavage. These candidate, high-probability matching proteins are then ranked according to the probability level, i.e., probability indexing, using annotated protein databases. SWISS-PROT and TrEMBL are examples of annotated protein databases that are accessible through the Internet (http://www.expasy.ch/sprot/) and contain information on more than 225,000 proteins. Depending on the level of probability matching, the definitive identification of the protein may require further confirmation by immunoblotting using specific antibodies.

Although peptide mass fingerprinting can identify a protein in a gel, it cannot provide information about posttranslational modifications or amino acid sequence. The second method for protein identification, which is less applicable for large peptide mixtures, is based on fragmentation of individual peptides to gain sequence information. This is done by electrospray ionization (ESI) directly from the liquid phase, such that the ionized peptides are sprayed into a tandem mass spectrometer that can resolve isolate one peptide species at a time, dissociate it into amino- or carboxy-terminal containing fragments, and the information is then processed for identification using protein or nucleotide databases such as expressed sequence tag (EST) databases. Another recently developed technology, termed MALDI-quadripolar TOF, may offer the advantages of both methods. It combines a MALDI ion source with the highly efficient tandem spectrometric approaches, and theoretically should provide both the high throughput of the peptide mapping and the specificity of peptide sequencing.

Posttranslational modifications of proteins can be identified by metabolic labeling of cells prior to protein extraction or by immunostaining of electroblots of 2D gels. As mentioned, ESI-mass spectrometry (MS) can then be used to identify posttranslational modifications, such that the identification of glycoproteins and phospoproteins is significantly enhanced by MS/MS and collision-induced decay (CID) in ESI-MS. Approximately 20–40% of protein spots from 2D gels are not listed in annotated nonoverlapping protein databases and therefore cannot be identified by peptide mass fingerprinting. In these instances, partial amino acid sequence data are obtained by ESI-MS and comprise a "peptide sequence tag." Although SWISS-PROT and TrEMBL databases contain more than 225,000 entries, human EST databases have more than 1,000,000 entries. Public EST databases provide more than 50% coverage of human genes, with up to 80% coverage in proprietary databases. Therefore, the searching of EST databases significantly extends the ability of proteomic analysis.

Protein Database Construction

Proteomic data must be housed in a flexible database in order to be useful. The goal of proteomic databases is to construct a map of the full complement of proteins that can be searched by several parameters in a given cell or tissue. These parameters include spot location on the gel image, molecular size, isoelectric point, partial sequence data, and mass spectra. Finally, the laboratory database must be linked to annotated protein databases such as TrEMBL and SWISS-PROT. Proteomic analysis of mouse brain was performed and led to the identification of interspecies differences in protein expression between 2 mice species, the C57BL/6 mice and the *Mus pretus* mice (322). Another study was performed on rat brain to establish a two-dimensional database of neonatal rat brain proteins (323).

B. Proteomic Approaches to Intermittent Hypoxia

It is evident from the capabilities of the proteomic approach that the use of high-resolution 2D gels should allow one to identify gene products modulated by hypoxia, to compare them by computer matching with those expressed in normoxia, and to detect posttranslational modifications of these proteins. Most posttranslationally modified products differ from primary gene products in their isoelectric point and/or molecular weight, thus appearing as distinct spots on high-resolution 2D gels. Localization of these distinct protein spots and identification by MS analysis can then be performed. Examples of proteomic analysis of neural tissue are rapidly emerging in the literature. In a study performed on cortical synaptosomes prepared from fetal cortices obtained from pregnant guinea pigs at term and exposed to 60 min of severe hypoxia, 22 proteins were identified by 2D immunoblot analysis, computer-assisted gel analysis, and matching to a 2D reference map of human brain proteins (324). When compared to normoxic fetal cerebral cortices obtained from pregnant guinea pigs at term exposed to normoxia, five of these proteins were found to be associated with hypoxia-induced tyrosine phosphorylation pathways (324).

   This line of work is currently being pursued in our laboratory for the CA1 and CA3 regions of the hippocampus of the rat exposed to either sustained or intermittent hypoxia using the hypoxic profile described above. Of the 19 proteins that increased expression after 6-hr exposures to intermittent hypoxia, three major functional groups were identified: metabolic enzymes, cytoskeletal proteins, and antioxidants (325). The proteomic analysis of the hypoxia-sensitive CA1 region and the more resistant CA3 region after in vivo exposure to mild intermittent hypoxia should allow us to determine whether posttranscriptional modifications occur following hypoxia-induced gene activation, thereby providing new insight into mechanisms underlying regional differences in susceptibility to hypoxia, and elucidating possible strategies of neuronal adaptation to intermittent hypoxia.

IX. Conclusions

Obstructive sleep apnea comprises three major pathophysiological modalities: intermittent nocturnal hypoxia, sleep fragmentation, and abnormal load imposed on the cardiorespiratory system. It is clear from this review of the animal-model-based and cellular research relevant to OSA that there are extensive amounts of data on the cellular and systemic effects of hypoxia, both sustained and intermittent (326). Similarly, a great deal is known about the effects of sleep loss, although the effects of sleep fragmentation mimicking that in OSA have been minimally studied in robust animal models. This major void needs to be filled in order to determine whether, and to what extent, the information gained from various earlier sleep deprivation studies is applicable to the pathophysiological changes in the sleep–wake control, cognitive, and affective functions associated with OSA.

The central and reflex control of the upper muscles is altered in OSA subjects. The wakefulness level of upper airway muscle activity is elevated (327,328; reviewed in Ref. 329), but there have been, so far, no studies of the underlying central mechanisms. It is likely that reflex pathways to upper airway motoneurons become reorganized in response to recurring obstructions and the magnitude of the central wakefulness-related drive to relevant motoneurons is increased. Such changes, if present, should be associated with altered expression of mRNA and proteins that determine the neurochemical control of motoneurons and guide the adaptive changes in their afferent pathways. This is another area that needs more studies in suitable animal models.

Acknowledgments

The authors' research was supported by grants HL-47600, HL-42236, and HL-60287 from the National Institutes of Health (LK); HL-58687 and HL-66312 from the National Institutes of Health, American Cancer Society Research Scholar Grant GMC-101430, and Von Hippel-Lindau Family Alliance Research Grant (MF C-K); HL-65270, HL-63912, HL-66358 from the National Institutes of Health and American Heart Association Grant 0050442N (DG).

References

1. Dinges, D. F., Pack, F., Williams, K., Gillen, K. A., Powell, J. W., Ott, G. E., Aptowicz, C., and Pack, A. I. Cumulative sleepiness, mood disturbance, and psychomotor vigilance performance decrements during a week of sleep restricted to 4–5 hours per night. Sleep 1997; 20:267.
2. Findley, L. J., Suratt, P. M., and Dinges, D. F. Time-on-task decrements in "steer clear" performance of patients with sleep apnea and narcolepsy. Sleep 1999; 22:804–809.
3. Morisson, F., Decary, A., Petit, D., Lavigne, G., Malo, J., and Montplaisir, J. Daytime sleepiness and EEG spectral analysis in apneic patients before and after treatment with continuous positive airway pressure. Chest 2001; 119:45–52.
4. Morgan, B. J., Crabtree, D. C., Puleo, D. S., Badr, M. S., Toiber, F., and Skatrud, J. B. Neurocirculatory consequences of abrupt change in sleep state in humans. J Appl Physiol 1996; 80:1627–1636.
5. Brooks, D., Horner, R. L., Kozar, L. F., Render-Teixeira, C. L., and Phillipson, E. A. Obstructive sleep apnea as a cause of systemic hypertension. J Clin Invest 1997; 99:106–109.
6. Schneider, H., Schaub, C. D., Chen, C. A., Andreoni, K. A., Schwartz, A. R., Smith, P. L., Robotham, J. L., and O'Donnell, C. P. Effects of arousal and sleep state on systemic and pulmonary hemodynamics in obstructive apnea. J Appl Physiol 2000; 88:1084–1092.
7. Peppard, P. E., Young, T., Palta, M., and Skatrud, J. Prospective study of the association between sleep-disordered breathing and hypertension. N Engl J Med 2000; 342:1378–1384.
8. Shahar, E., Whitney, C. W., Redline, S., Lee, E. T., Newman, A. B., Nieto, F. J., O'Connor, G. T., Boland, L. L., Schwartz, J. E., and Samet, J. M. Sleep-disordered breathing and cardiovascular disease: cross-sectional results of the sleep heart health study. Am J Respir Crit Care Med 2001; 163:19–25.
9. Lojander, J., Kajaste, S., Maasilta, P., and Partinen, M. Cognitive function and treatment of obstructive sleep apnea syndrome. J Sleep Res 1999; 8:71–76.
10. Engelman, H. M., Kingshott, R. N., Martin, S. E., and Douglas, N. J. Cognitive function in the sleep apnea/hypopnea syndrome (SAHS). Sleep 2000; 23(suppl 4):S102–S108.
11. Henke, K. G., Grady, J. J., and Kuna, S. T. Effect of nasal continuous positive airway pressure on neuropsychological function in sleep apnea-hypopnea syndrome. A randomized, placebo-controlled trial. Am J Respir Crit Care Med 2001; 163:911–917.
12. Persson, H. E. and Svanborg, E. Sleep deprivation worsens obstructive sleep apnea. Chest 1996; 109:645–650.
13. Petrof, B. J., Pack, A. I., and Kelly, A. M. Pharyngeal myopathy of loaded upper airway in dogs with sleep apnea. J Appl Physiol 1994; 76:1746–1752.
14. Gea, J., Hamid, Q., Czaika, G., Zhu, E., Mohan-Ram, V., Goldspink, G., and Grassino, A. Expression of myosin heavy-chain isoforms in the respiratory

muscles following inspiratory resistive breathing. Am J Respir Crit Care Med 2000; 161:1274–1278.

15. Friberg, D., Ansved, T., Borg, K., Carlsson-Norlander, B., Larsson, H., and Svanborg, E. Histological indications of a progressive snorers disease in the upper airway muscles. Am J Respir Crit Care Med 1998; 157:586–593.

16. Svanborg, E. Upper airway nerve lesions in obstructive sleep apnea. Am J Respir Crit Care Med 2001; 164:187–189.

17. Kimoff, R. J., Sforza, E., Champagne, V., Ofiara, L., and Gendron, D. Upper airway sensation in snoring and obstructive sleep apnea. Am J Respir Crit Care Med 2001; 164:250–255.

18. Sica, A. L., Gootman, P. M., and Ruggiero, D. A. CO_2-induced expression of c-fos in the nucleus of the solitary tract and the area postrema of developing swine. Brain Res 1999; 837:106–116.

19. Berquin, P., Bodineau, L., Gros, F., and Larnicol, N. Brainstem and hypothalamic areas involved in respiratory chemoreflexes: a Fos study in adult rats. Brain Res 2000; 857:30–40.

20. Cirelli, C., Tononi, G., and Ruggiero, D. A. On the functional significance of c-fos induction during the sleep-waking cycle. Sleep 2000; 23:453–469.

21. Kimoff, J. R., Makino, H., Horner, R. L., Kozar, L. F., Lue, F., Slutsky, A. S., and Phillipson, E. A. Canine model of obstructive sleep apnea: model description and preliminary application. J Appl Physiol 1994; 76:1810–1816.

22. Baker, T. L. and Mitchell, G. S. Episodic but not continuous hypoxia elicits long-term facilitation of phrenic motor output in rats. J Physiol (Lond) 2000; 529:215–219.

23. Hamrahi, H., Stephenson, R., Mahamed, S., Liao, K. S., and Horner, R. L. Regulation of sleep-wake states in response to intermittent hypoxic stimuli applied only in sleep. J Appl Physiol 2001; 90:2490–2501.

24. Sica, A. L., Greenberg, H. E., Scharf, S. M., and Ruggiero, D. A. Chronic-intermittent hypoxia induces immediate early gene expression in the midline thalamus and epithalamus. Brain Res 2000; 883:224–228.

25. Sica, A. L., Greenberg, H. E., Scharf, S. M., and Ruggiero, D. A. Immediate-early gene expression in cerebral cortex following exposure to chronic-intermittent hypoxia. Brain Res 2000; 870:204–210.

26. Schaub, C. D., Tankersley, C., Schwartz, A. R., Smith, P. L., Robotham, J. L., and O'Donnell, C. P. Effect of sleep/wake state on arterial blood pressure in genetically identical mice. J Appl Physiol 1998; 85:366–371.

27. Franken, P., Chillet, D., and Tafti, M. The homeostatic regulation of sleep need is under genetic control. J Neurosci 2001; 21:2610–2621.

28. Mathur, R. and Douglas, N. J. Family studies in patients with the sleep apnea-hypopnea syndrome. Ann Intern Med 1995; 122:174–178.

29. Redline, S., Tishler, P. V., Schluchter, M., Aylor, J., Clark, K., and Graham, G. Risk factors for sleep-disordered breathing in children. Associations with obesity, race, and respiratory problems. Am J Respir Crit Care Med 1999; 159:1527–1532.

30. Cakirer, B., Hans, M. G., Graham, G., Aylor, J., Tishler, P. V., and Redline, S. The relationship between craniofacial morphology and obstructive sleep apnea in whites and in African-Americans. Am J Respir Crit Care Med 2001; 163:947–950.

31. Newman, A. B., Nieto, F. J., Guidry, U., Lind, B. K., Redline, S., Pickering, T. G., and Quan, S. F., Sleep Heart Health Study Research Group. Relation of sleep-disordered breathing to cardiovascular disease risk factors: the Sleep Heart Health Study. Am J Epidemiol 2001; 154:50–59.

32. Jacob, H. J. Physiological genetics: application to hypertension research. Clin Exp Pharmacol Physiol 1999; 26:530–535.

33. Kwitek-Black, A. E. and Jacob, H. J. The use of designer rats in the genetic dissection of hypertension. Curr Hypertens Rep 2001; 3:12–18.

34. Heisler, L. K. and Tecott, L. H. A paradoxical locomotor response in serotonin 5-HT$_{2C}$ receptor mutant mice. J Neurosci 2000; 20:1–5.

35. Van Gelder, R., van Zastrow, M. E., Yool, A., Dement, W. C., Barchas, J. D., and Eberwine, J. H. Amplified RNA synthesized from limited quantities of heterogenous cDNA. Proc Natl Acad Sci USA 1990; 87:1663–1667.

36. Eberwine, J., Yeh, H., Miyashiro, K., Cao, Y., Nair, S., Finnell, R., Zettel, M., and Coleman, P. Analysis of gene expression in single live neurons. Proc Natl Acad Sci USA 1992; 89:3010–3014.

37. Wang, E., Miller LDOGA, Liu, E. T., and Marincola, F. M. High-fidelity mRNA amplification for gene profiling. Nat Biotechnol 2000; 18:457–459.

38. Okabe, S., Mackiewicz, M., and Kubin, L. Serotonin receptor mRNA expression in the hypoglossal motor nucleus. Respir Physiol 1997; 110:151–160.

39. Comer, A. M., Yip, S., and Lipski, J. Detection of weakly expressed genes in the rostral ventrolateral medulla of the rat using micropunch and RT-PCR techniques. Clin Exp Pharm Physiol 1997; 24:755–759.

40. Mackiewicz, M., Sollars, P. J., Ogilvie, M. D., and Pack, A. I. Modulation of IL-1β gene expression in the rat CNS during sleep deprivation. Neuroreport 1996; 7:529–533.

41. Horikoshi, T. and Sakakibara, M. Quantification of relative mRNA expression in the rat brain using simple RT-PCR and ethidium bromide staining. J Neurosci 2000; 99:45–51.

42. Thellin, O., Zorzi, W., Lakaye, B., De Borman, B., Coumans, B., Hennen, G., Grisar, T., Igout, A., and Heinen, E. Housekeeping genes as internal standards: use and limits. J Biotechnol 1999; 75:291–295.

43. Schmittgen, T. D. and Zakrajsek, B. A. Effect of experimental treatment on housekeeping gene expression: validation by real-time, quantitative RT-PCR. J Biochem Biophys 2000; 46:69–81.

44. Sucher, N. J. and Deitcher, D. L. PCR patch clamp analysis of single neurons. Neuron 1995; 14:1095–1100.

45. Dixon, A. K., Richardson, P. J., Pinnock, R. D., and Lee, K. Gene-expression analysis at the single-cell level. Trends Pharmacol Sci 2000; 21:65–70.

46. Comer, A. M., Gibbons, H. M., Qi, J., Kawai, Y., Win, J., and Lipski, J. Detection of mRNA species in bulbospinal neurons isolated from the rostral ventrolateral medulla using single-cell RT-PCR. Brain Res Prot 1999; 4:367–377.

47. Phillips, J. K. and Lipski, J. Single-cell RT-PCR as a tool to study gene expression in central and peripheral autonomic neurones. Auton Neurosci 2000; 86:1–12.

48. Plant, T. D., Schirra, C., Katz, E., Uchitel, O. D., and Konnerth, A. Single-cell RT-PCR and functional characterization of Ca^{2+} channels in motoneurons of the rat facial nucleus. J Neurosci 1998; 18:9573–9584.

49. Franz, O., Liss, B., Neu, A., and Roeper, J. Single-cell mRNA expression of *HCN1* correlates with a fast gating phenotype of hyperpolarization-activated cyclic nucleotide-gated ion channels (Ih) in central neurons. Eur J Neurosci 2000; 12:2685–2693.

50. Volgin, D. V., Mackiewicz, M., and Kubin, L. α_{1B} receptors are the main postsynaptic mediators of adrenergic excitation in brainstem motoneurons, a single-cell RT-PCR study. J Chem Neuroanat 2001; 22:157–166.

51. Luo, L., Salunga, R. C., Guo, H., Bittner, A., Joy, K. C., Galindo, J. E., Xiao, H., Rogers, K. E., Wan, J. S., Jackson, M. R., and Erlander, M. G. Gene expression profiles of laser-captured adjacent neuronal subtypes. Nat Med 1999; 5:117–122.

52. Fend, F., Emmert-Buck, M. R., Chuaqui, R., Cole, K., Lee, J., Liotta, L. A., and Raffeld, M. Immuno-LCM: laser capture microdissection of immunostained frozen sections for mRNA analysis. Am J Pathol 1999; 154:61–66.

53. Specht, K., Richter, T., Muller, U., Walch, A., Werner, M., and Hofler, H. Quantitative gene expression analysis in microdissected archival formalin-fixed and paraffin-embedded tumor tissue. Am J Pathol 2001; 158:419–429.

54. Goldsworthy, S. M., Stockton, P. S., Trempus, C. S., Foley, J. F., and Maronpot, R. R. Effects of fixation on RNA extraction and amplification from laser capture microdissected tissue. Mol Carcinog 1999; 25:86–91.

55. Best, C. J., Gillespie, J. W., Englert, C. R., Swalwell, J. I., Pfeifer, J., Krizman, D. B., Petricoin, E. F., Liotta, L. A., and Emmert-Buck, M. R. New approaches to molecular profiling of tissue samples. Anal Cell Pathol 2000; 20:1–6.

56. Martinez, A., Miller, M.-J., Quinn, K., Unsworth, E. J., Ebina, M., and Cuttitta, F. Non-radioactive localization of nucleic acids by direct in situ PCR and in situ RT-PCR in paraffin-embedded sections. Histochem Cytochem 1995; 43:739–747.

57. Mee, A. P., Denton, J., Hoyland, J. A., Davies, M., and Mawer, E. B. Quantification of vitamin D receptor mRNA in tissue sections demonstrates the relative limitations of in situ-reverse transcriptase-polymerase chain reaction. J Pathol 1997; 182:22–28.

58. Wang, H. and Wessendorf, M. W. Mu- and delta-opioid receptor mRNAs are expressed in spinally projecting serotonergic and nonserotonergic neurons of the rostral ventromedial medulla. J Comp Neurol 1999; 404:183–196.

59. Wang, H. and Wessendorf, M. W. Equal proportions of small and large DRG neurons express opioid receptor mRNAs. J Comp Neurol 2001; 429:590–600.

60. Smith, M. D., Parker, A., Wikaningrum, R., and Coleman, M. Combined immunohistochemical labeling and in situ hybridization to colocalize mRNA and protein in tissue sections. Methods Mol Biol 2000; 123:165–175.

61. Pinault, D. A novel single-cell staining procedure performed in vivo under electrophysiological control: morpho-functional features of juxtacellularly labeled thalamic cells and other central neurons with biocytin or Neurobiotin. J Neurosci Methods 1996; 65:113–136.

62. Baro, D. J., Levini, R. M., Kim, M. T., Willms, A. R., Lanning, C. C., Rodriguez, H. E., and Harris-Warrick, R. M. Quantitative single-cell-reverse transcription-PCR demonstrates that A-current magnitude varies as a linear function of *shal* gene expression in identified stomatogastric neurons. J Neurosci 1997; 17:6597–6610.

63. Boudin, H., Sarret, P., Mazella, J., Schonbrunn A., and Beaudet A. Somatostatin-induced regulation of SST_{2A} receptor expression and cell surface availability in central neurons: role of receptor internalization. J Neurosci 2000; 20:5932–5939.

64. Semba, K., Pastorius, J., Wilkinson, M., and Rusak, B. Sleep deprivation-induced *c-fos* and *junB* expression in the rat brain: effects of duration and timing. Behav Brain Res 2001; 120:75–86.

65. Estabrooke, I. V., McCarthy, M. T., Ko, E., Chou, T., Chemelli, R. M., Yanagisawa, M., Saper, C. B., and Scammell, T. E. Fos expression in orexin neurons varies with behavioral state. J Neurosci 2001; 21:1656–1662.

66. Merchant-Nancy, H., Vazquez, J., Aguilar-Roblero, R., and Drucker-Colin, R. C-fos protooncogene changes in relation to REM sleep duration. Brain Res 1992; 579:342–346.

67. Pompeiano, M., Cirelli, C., and Tononi, G. Immediate-early genes in spontaneous wakefulness and sleep: expression of c-*fos* and NGFI-A mRNA and protein. Sleep Res 1994; 3:80–96.

68. Grassi-Zucconi, G., Giuditta, A., Mandile, P., Chen, S., Vescia, S., and Bentivoglio, M. c-fos spontaneous expression during wakefulness is reversed during sleep in neuronal subsets of the rat cortex. J Physiol 1994; 88:91–93.

69. Cirelli, C. and Tononi, G. Differences in gene expression during sleep and wakefulness. Ann Med 1999; 31:117–124.

70. Pompeiano, M., Cirelli, C., and Tononi, G. Effects of sleep deprivation on fos-like immunoreactivity in the rat brain. Arch Ital Biol 1992; 130:325–335.

71. O'Hara, B. F., Young, K. A., Watson, F. L., Heller, H. C., and Kilduff, T. S. Immediate early gene expression in brain during sleep deprivation: pre-liminary observations. Sleep 1993; 16:1–7.

72. Cirelli, C., Pompeiano, M., and Tononi, G. Sleep deprivation and c-*fos* expression in the rat brain. J Sleep Res 1995; 4:92–106.

73. Lin, J. S., Hou, Y., and Jouvet, M. Potential brain neuronal targets for amphetamine-, methylphenidate-, and modafinil-induced wakefulness, evidenced by c-*fos* immunocytochemistry in the cat. Proc Natl Acad Sci USA 1996; 93:14128–14133.

74. Wisor, J. P., Nishino, S., Sora, I., Uhl, G. H., Mignot, E., and Edgar, D. M. Dopaminergic role in stimulant-induced wakefulness. J Neurosci 2001; 21:1787–1794.

75. Scammell, T. E., Estabrooke, I. V., McCarthy, M. T., Chemelli, R. M., Yanagisawa, M., Miller, M. S., and Saper, C. B. Hypothalamic arousal regions are activated during modafinil-induced wakefulness. J Neurosci 2000; 20:8620–8628.

76. Porkka-Heiskanen, T., Smith, S. E., Taira, T., Urban, J. H., Levine, J. E., Turek, F. W., and Stenberg, D. Noradrenergic activity in rat brain during rapid eye movement sleep deprivation and rebound sleep. Am J Physiol 1995; 268:R1456–R1463.

77. Neuner-Jehle, M., Rhyner, T. A., and Borbely, A. A. Sleep deprivation differentially alters the mRNA and protein levels of neurogranin in rat brain. Brain Res 1995; 685:143–153.

78. Toppila, J., Asikainen, M., Alanko, L., Turek, F. W., Stenberg, D., and Porkka-Heiskanen, T. The effect of REM sleep deprivation on somatostatin and growth hormone-releasing hormone gene expression in the rat hypothalamus. J Sleep Res 1996; 5:115–122.

79. Cirelli, C. and Tononi, G. Differential expression of plasticity-related genes in waking and sleep and their regulation by the noradrenergic system. J Neurosci 2000; 20:9187–9194.

80. Maloney, K. J., Mainville, L., and Jones, B. E. Differential c-Fos expression in cholinergic, monoaminergic and GABAergic cell groups of the pontomesencephalic tegmentum after paradoxical sleep deprivation and recovery. J Neurosci 1999; 19:3057–3072.

81. Maloney, K. J., Mainville, L., and Jones, B. E. c-Fos expression in GABAergic, serotonergic, and other neurons of the pontomedullary reticular formation and raphe after paradoxical sleep deprivation and recovery. J Neurosci 2000; 20:4669–4679.

82. Yamuy, J., Sampogna, S., López-Rodríguez, F., Luppi, P.-H., Morales, F. R., and Chase, M. H. Fos and serotonin immunoreactivity in the raphe nuclei of the cat during carbachol-induced active sleep: a double-labeling study. Neuroscience 1995; 67:211–223.

83. Rhyner, T. A., Borbély, A. A., and Mallet, J. Molecular cloning of forebrain mRNAs which are modulated by sleep deprivation. Eur J Neurosci 1990; 2:1063–1073.

84. Cirelli, C. and Tononi, G. Differences in gene expression between sleep and waking as revealed by mRNA differential display. Mol Brain Res 1998; 56:293–305.

85. Cirelli, C. and Tononi, G. Gene expression in the brain across the sleep-waking cycle. Brain Res 2001; 885:303–321.

86. Bobillier, P., Sakai, F., Seguin, S., and Jouvet, M. Deprivation of paradoxical sleep and in vitro cerebral protein synthesis in the rat. Life Sci 1971; 10:1349–1357.

87. Giuditta, A., Rutigliano, B., and Vitale-Neugebauer, A. Influence of synchronized sleep on the biosynthesis of RNA in two nuclear classes isolated from rabbit cerebral cortex. J Neurochem 1980; 35:1259–1266.

88. Panov, A. RNA and protein content of brain stem cells after sleep deprivation. Riv Biol 1982; 75:95–99.

89. Prospero-Garcia, O., Jimenez-Anguiano, A., and Drucker-Colin, R. Chloramphenicol prevents carbachol-induced REM sleep in cats. Neurosci Lett 1993; 154:168–170.

90. Cirelli, C., Pompeiano, M., and Tononi, G. Neuronal gene expression in the waking state: a role for the locus coeruleus. Science 1996; 274:1211–1215.

91. Liquori, C. L., Ricker, K., Moseley, M. L., Jacobsen, J. F., Kress, W., Naylor, S. L., Day, J. W., and Ranum, L. P. Myotonic dystrophy type 2 caused by a CCTG expansion in intron 1 of ZNF9. Science 2001; 293:864–867.

92. Sutcliffe, J. G. Open-system approaches to gene expression in the CNS. J Neurosci 2001; 21:8306–8309.

93. Sherin, J. E., Shiromani, P. J., McCarley, R. W., and Saper, C. B. Activation of ventrolateral preoptic neurons during sleep. Science 1996; 271:216–219.

94. Kilduff, T. S. and Peyron, C. The hypocretin/orexin ligand-receptor system: implications for sleep and sleep disorders. Trends Neurosci 2000; 23:359–365.

95. Willie, J. T., Chemelli, R. M., Sinton, C. M., and Yanagisawa, M. To eat or to sleep? Orexin in the regulation of feeding and wakefulness. Annu Rev Neurosci 2001; 24:429–458.

96. Butcher, K. S. and Cechetto, D. F. Receptors in lateral hypothalamic area involved in insular cortex sympathetic responses. Am J Physiol 1998; 275:H689–H696.

97. Allen, G. V. and Cechetto, D. F. Functional and anatomical organization of cardiovascular pressor and depressor sites in the lateral hypothalamic area: I. descending projections. J Comp Neurol 1992; 315:313–332.

98. Greenberg, H. E., Sica, A. L., Scharf, S. M., and Ruggiero, D. A. Expression of c-fos in the rat brainstem after chronic-intermittent hypoxia. Brain Res 1999; 816:638–645.

99. Ford, B., Holmes, C. J., Manville, L., and Jones, B. E. GABAergic neurons in the rat pontomesencephalic tegmentum: codistribution with cholinergic and other tegmental neurons projecting to the posterior lateral hypothalamus. J Comp Neurol 1995; 363:177–196.

100. Steininger, T. L., Gong, H., McGinty, D., and Szymusiak, R. Subregional organization of preoptic area/anterior hypothalamic projections to arousal-related monoaminergic cell groups. J Comp Neurol 2001; 429:638–653.

101. Peyron, C., Tighe, D. K., van de Pol, A. N., de Lecea, L., Heller, H. C., Sutcliffe, J. G., and Kilduff, T. Neurons containing hypocretin (orexin) project to multiple neuronal systems. J Neurosci 1998; 18:9996–10015.

102. Hervieu, G. L., Cluderay, J. E., Harrison, D. C., Roberts, J. C., and Leslie, R. A. Gene expression and protein distribution of the orexin-1 receptor in the rat brain and spinal cord. Neuroscience 2001; 103:777–797.

103. Fung, S. J., Yamuy, J., Sampogna, S., Morales, F. R., and Chase, M. H. Hypocretin (orexin) input to trigeminal and hypoglossal motoneurons in the cat: a double-labeling immunohistochemical study. Brain Res 2001; 903:257–262.

104. Kubin, L., Davies, R. O., and Pack, A. I. Control of upper airway motoneurons during REM sleep. News Physiol Sci 1998; 13:91–97.

105. Kubin, L., Tojima, H., Davies, R. O., and Pack, A. I. Serotonergic excitatory drive to hypoglossal motoneurons in the decerebrate cat. Neurosci Lett 1992; 139:243–248.

106. Kubin, L., Kimura, H., Tojima, H., Davies, R. O., and Pack, A. I. Suppression of hypoglossal motoneurons during the carbachol-induced atonia of REM sleep is not caused by fast synaptic inhibition. Brain Res 1993; 611:300–312.

107. Kubin, L., Reignier, C., Tojima, H., Taguchi, O., Pack, A. I., and Davies, R. O. Changes in serotonin level in the hypoglossal nucleus region during the carbachol-induced atonia. Brain Res 1994; 645:291–302.

108. Woch, G., Davies, R. O., Pack, A. I., and Kubin, L. Behavior of raphe cells projecting to the dorsomedial medulla during carbachol-induced atonia in the cat. J Physiol (Lond) 1996; 490:745–758.

109. Rekling, J. C., Funk, G. D., Bayliss, D. A., Dong, X-W, and Feldman, J. L. Synaptic control of motoneuronal excitability. Physiol Rev 2000; 80:767–852.

110. Zifa, E. and Fillion, G. 5-Hydroxytryptamine receptors. Pharmacol Rev 1992; 44:401–458.

111. Bylund, D. B., Eikenberg, D. C., Hieble, J. P., Langer, S. Z., Lefkowitz, R. J., Minneman, K. P., Molinoff, P. B., Ruffolo, R. R. Jr, and Trendelenburg, U. International Union of Pharmacology nomenclature of adrenoceptors. Pharmacol Rev 1994; 46:121–136.

112. Zhang, X. Y. and Ehrlich, M. Detection and quantitation of low numbers of chromosomes containing bcl-2 oncogene translocations using semi-nested PCR. Biotechniques 1994; 16:502–507.

113. Léna, C., de Kerchove d'Exaerde, A., Cordero-Erausquin, M., Le Novère, N., del Mar Arroyo-Jimenez, M., and Changeux, J.-P. Diversity and distribution of nicotinic acetylcholine receptors in the *locus ceruleus* neurons. Proc Natl Acad Sci USA 1999; 96:12126–12131.

114. Yan, Z., Vrana, S., Vrana, K., Song W.-J., and Surmeier, D. J. The application of RT-PCR techniques to the analysis of mRNA in tissue and single cells. In: Ariano M. A., ed. Receptor Localization. Laboratory Methods and Procedures. New York: Wiley-Liss, 1998:160–181.

115. Cauli, B., Audinat, E., Lambolez, B., Angulo, M. C., Ropert, N., Tsuzuki, K., Hestrin, S., and Rossier, J. Molecular and physiological diversity of cortical nonpyramidal cells. J Neurosci 1997; 17:3894–3906.

116. Mermelstein, P. G., Song, W. J., Tkatch, T., Yan, Z., and Surmeier, D. J. Inwardly rectifying potassium (IRK) currents are correlated with IRK subunit expression in rat nucleus accumbens medium spiny neurons. J Neurosci 1998; 18:6650–6661.

117. Stefani, A., Chen, Q., Flores-Hernandez, J., Jiao, Y., Reiner, A., and Surmeier, D. J. Physiological and molecular properties of AMPA/Kainate receptors expressed by striatal medium spiny neurons. Dev Neurosci 1998; 20:242–252.

118. Tyagi, S. and Kramer, F. R. Molecular beacons: probes that fluoresce upon hybridization. Nat Biotechnol 1996; 14:303–308.

119. Holland, P. M., Abramson, R. D., Watson, R., and Gelfand, D. H. Detection of specific polymerase chain reaction product by utilizing the 5′-3′ exonuclease activity of *Thermus aquaticus* DNA polymerase. Proc Natl Acad Sci USA 1991; 88:7276–7280.

120. Lee, L. G., Connell, C. R., and Bloch, W. Allelic discrimination by nick-translation PCR with fluorogenic probes. Nucl Acids Res 1993; 21:3761–3766.

121. Medhurst, A. D., Harrison, D. C., Read, S. J., Campbell, C. A., Robbins, M. J., and Pangalos, M. N. The use of TaqMan RT-PCR assays for semiquantitative analysis of gene expression in CNS tissues and disease models. J Neurosci Methods 2000; 98:9–20.

122. Thelwell, N., Millington, S., Solinas, A., Booth, J., and Brown, T. Mode of action and application of Scorpion primers to mutation detection. Nucl Acids Res 2000; 28:3752–3761.

123. Kandimalla, E. R. and Agrawal, S. 'Cyclicons' as hybridization-based fluorescent primer-probes: synthesis, properties and application in real-time PCR. Bioorg Med Chem 2000; 8:1911–1916.

124. Wattjes, M. P., Krauter, J., Heidenreich, O., Ganser, A., and Heil, G. Comparison of nested competitive RT-PCR and real-time RT-PCR for the detection and quantification of AML1/MTG8 fusion transcripts in t(8;21) positive acute myelogenous leukemia. Leukemia 2000; 14:329–335.

125. Volgin, D. V., Saghir, M., and Kubin, L. Developmental changes in the orexin 2 receptor mRNA in hypoglossal motoneurons. Neuroreport 2002; 13:433–436.

126. Kim, D. Y., Kim, S. H., Choi, H. B., Min, C., and Gwag, B. J. High abundance of GluR1 mRNA and reduced Q/R editing of GluR2 mRNA in individual NADPH-diaphorase neurons. Mol Cell Neurosci 2001; 17:1025–1033.

127. Plant, T., Schirra, C., Geraschuk, O., Rossier, J., and Konnerth, A. Molecular determinants of NMDA receptor function in GABAergic neurones of the rat forebrain. J Physiol (Lond) 1997; 499:47–63.

128. Lanneau, C., Viollet, C., Faivre-Bauman, A., Loudes, C., Kordon, C., Epelbaum, J., and Gardette, R. Somatostatin receptor subtypes sst1 and sst2 elicit opposite effects on the response to glutamate of mouse hypothalamic neurones: an electrophysiological and single cell RT-PCR study. Eur J Neurosci 1998; 10:204–212.

129. Volgin, D., Fay, R., and Kubin, L. Postnatal changes in serotonin (5-HT) receptor mRNA and protein expression in hypoglossal (XII) motoneurons (mns). Soc Neurosci Abstr 2001; 27:A696.17.
130. Volgin, D. V. and Kubin, L. Serotonergic 1B, 2A and 2C receptor mRNA expression in upper airway motoneurons in mature rats and during postnatal development. Sleep 2001; 24:A299–A300.
131. Fay, R. and Kubin, L. Pontomedullary distribution of 5-HT$_{2A}$ receptor-like protein in the rat. J Comp Neurol 2000; 418:323–345.
132. Fenik, V., Davies, R. O., and Kubin, L. Adrenergic receptor subtypes mediating excitatory effects in hypoglossal motoneurons. Sleep 1999; 22(suppl):S37.
133. Gozlan, H., El Mestikawy, S., Pichat, L., Glowinski, J., and Hamon, M. Identification of presynaptic serotonin autoreceptors using a new ligand: ^{3}H-PAT. Nature 1983; 305:140–142.
134. Boschert, U., Amara, D. A., Segu, L., and Hen, R. The mouse 5-hydroxytryptamine$_{1B}$ receptor is localized predominantly on axon terminals. Neuroscience 1994; 58:167–182.
135. Umemiya, M. and Berger, A. J. Presynaptic inhibition by serotonin of glycinergic inhibitory synaptic currents in the rat brain stem. J Neurophysiol 1995; 73:1192–1200.
136. Singer, J. H., Bellingham, M. C., and Berger, A. J. Presynaptic inhibition of glutamatergic synaptic transmission to rat motoneurons by serotonin. J Neurophysiol 1996; 76:799–807.
137. Okabe, S. and Kubin, L. Role of 5HT$_1$ receptors in the control of hypoglossal motoneurons in vivo. Sleep 1996; 19:S150–S153.
138. Behan, M. and Brownfield, M. S. Age-related changes in serotonin in the hypoglossal nucleus of rat: implications for sleep-disordered breathing. Neurosci Lett 1999; 267:133–136.
139. Kubin, L., Tojima, H., Reignier, C., Pack, A. I., and Davies, R. O. Interaction of serotonergic excitatory drive to hypoglossal motoneurons with carbachol-induced, REM sleep-like atonia. Sleep 1996; 19:187–195.
140. Veasey, S. C., Fenik, P., Panckeri, K., Pack, A. I., and Hendricks J. C. The effects of trazodone with L-trytophan on sleep-disordered breathing in the English bulldog. Am J Respir Crit Care Med 1999; 160:1659–1667.
141. Carley, D. W., Depoortere, H., and Radulovacki, M. R-zacopride, a 5-HT3 antagonist/5-HT4 agonist, reduces sleep apneas in rats. Pharmacol Biochem Behav 2001; 69:283–289.
142. Jelev, A., Sood, S., Liu, H., Nolan, P., and Horner, R. L. Microdialysis perfusion of 5-HT into hypoglossal motor nucleus differentially modulates genioglossus activity across natural sleep-wake states in rats. J Physiol (Lond) 2001; 532:467–481.
143. Berry, R. B., Yamaura, E. M., Gill, K., and Reist, C. Acute effects of paroxetine on genioglossus activity in obstructive sleep apnea. Sleep 1999; 22:1087–1092.

144. Sunderram, J., Parisi, R. A., and Strobel, R. J. Serotonergic stimulation of the genioglossus and the response to nasal continuous positive airway pressure. Am J Respir Crit Care Med 2000; 162:925–929.

145. Caverely, P. M. A. Blood pressure, breathing, and the carotid body. Lancet 1999; 354:969–970.

146. Lesske, J., Fletcher, E. C., Bao, G., and Unger, T. Hypertension caused by chronic intermittent hypoxia—influence of chemoreceptors and sympathetic nervous system. J Hypertens 1997; 15:1593–1603.

147. Grassi, G. Role of sympathetic nervous system in human hypertension. J Hypertens 1998; 16:1979–1987.

148. Czyżyk-Krzeska, M. F., Bayliss, D. A., Lawson, E. E., and Millhorn, D. E. Regulation of tyrosine hydroxylase gene expression in the rat carotid body by hypoxia. J Neurochem 1992; 58:1538–1546.

149. Czyżyk-Krzeska, M. F., Bayliss, D. A., Lawson, E. E., and Millhorn, D. E. Expression of messenger RNAs for peptides and tyrosine hydroxylase in primary sensory neurons that innervate arterial baroreceptors and chemoreceptors. Neurosci Lett 1991; 129:98–102.

150. Dahlström, A. and Fuxe, K. Evidence for the existence of monoamine containing neurons in the central nervous system. I. Demonstration of monoamines in the cell bodies of brainstem neurons. Acta Physiol Scand 1964; 62:1–55.

151. Erickson, J. T. and Millhorn, D. E. Fos-like protein is induced in neurons of the medulla oblongata after stimulation of the carotid sinus nerve in awake and anesthetized rats. Brain Res 1991; 567:11–24.

152. Soulier, V., Cottet-Emard, J. M., Pequignot, J., Hanchin, F., Peyrin, L., and Pequignot, J.-M. Differential effects of long-term hypoxia on norepinephrine turnover in brain stem cell groups. J Appl Physiol 1992; 73:1810–1814.

153. Schmitt, P., Pequignot, J., Garcia, C., Pujol, J. F., and Pequignot, J.-M. Regional specificity of the long-term regulation of tyrosine hydroxylase in some catecholaminergic rat brainstem areas. I. Influence of long-term hypoxia. Brain Res 1993; 14:53–60.

154. Soulier, V., Dalmaz, Y., Cottet-Emard, J. M., Kitahama, K., and Pequignot, J.-M. Delayed increase of tyrosine hydroxylase in the rat A2 medullary neurons upon long-term hypoxia. Brain Res 1995; 674:188–195.

155. Pepin, J. L., Levy, P., Garcin, A., Feuerstein, C., and Savasta, M. Effects of long-term hypoxia on tyrosine hydroxylase protein content in catecholaminergic rat brainstem areas: a quantitative autoradiographic study. Brain Res 1996; 733:1–8.

156. Roux, J. C., Pequignot, J.-M., Dumas, S., Pascual, O., Ghilini, G., Pequignot, J., Mallet, J., and Denavit-Saubie, M. O₂ sensing after carotid chemodenervation: hypoxic ventilatory responsiveness and upregulation of tyrosine hydroxylase mRNA in brainstem catecholaminergic cells. Eur J Neurosci 2000; 12:3181–3190.

157. Hayashi, Y., Miwa, S., Lee, K., Koshimura, K., Hamahata, K., Hasegawa, H., Fujiwara, M., and Watanabe, Y. Enhancement of in vivo tyrosine

hydroxylation in the rat adrenal gland under hypoxic conditions. J Neurochem 1990; 54:1115–1121.

158. Schmitt, P., Garcia, C., Soulier, V., Pujol, J. F., and Pequinot, J. M. Influence of long term hypoxia on tyrosine hydroxylase in the rat carotid body and adrenal gland. J Auton Nerv Syst 1992; 40:13–20.

159. Czyżyk-Krzeska, M. F., Furnari, B. A., Lawson, E. E., and Millhorn, D. E. Hypoxia increases rate of transcription and stability of tyrosine hydroxylase mRNA in pheochromocytoma (PC12) cells. J Biol Chem 1994; 269:760–764.

160. Gonzalez, C., Kwok, Y., Gibb, J., and Fidone, S. Effects of hypoxia on tyrosine hydroxylase activity in rat carotid body. J Neurochem 1979; 33:713–719.

161. Gonzalez, C., Kwok, Y., Gibb, J., and Fidone, S. Physiological and pharmacological effects on TH activity in rabbit and cat carotid body. Am J Physiol 1981; 240:R38–R43.

162. Fidone, S., Gonzalez, C., and Yoshizaki, K. Effects of low oxygen on the release of dopamine from the rabbit carotid body in vitro. J Physiol (Lond) 1982; 333:93–110.

163. Fishman, M. C., Greene, W. L., and Platika, D. Oxygen chemoreception by carotid body cells in culture. Proc Natl Acad Sci USA 1985; 82:1448–1450.

164. Norris, M. L. and Millhorn, D. E. Hypoxia-induced protein binding to O_2-responsive sequences on the tyrosine hydroxylase gene. J Biol Chem 1995; 270:23774–23779.

165. Czyżyk-Krzeska, M. F., Domiński, Z., Kole, R., and Millhorn, D. E. Hypoxia stimulates binding of a cytoplasmic protein to a pyrimidine rich sequence in the 3'-untranslated region of rat tyrosine hydroxylase mRNA. J Biol Chem 1994; 269:9940–9945.

166. Czyżyk-Krzeska, M. F. and Beresh, J. E. Characterization of the hypoxia inducible protein binding site within the pyrimidine rich tract in the 3' untranslated region of the tyrosine hydroxylase mRNA. J Biol Chem 1996; 271:3293–3299.

167. Paulding, W. R. and Czyżyk-Krzeska, M. F. Regulation of tyrosine hydroxylase mRNA stability by protein-binding, pyrimidine-rich sequence in the 3' untranslated region. J Biol Chem 1999; 274:2532–2538.

168. Mishra, R. R., Adhikary, G., Simonson, M. S., Cherniack, N. S., and Prabhakar, N. R. Role of c-fos in hypoxia-induced AP-1 cis-element activity and tyrosine hydroxylase gene expression. Mol Brain Res 1998; 59:74–83.

169. Feinsilver, S. H., Wong, R., and Rayabin, D. M. Adaptation of neurotransmitter synthesis to chronic hypoxia in cell culture. Biochem Biophys Acta 1997; 928:56–62.

170. Zhu, W. H., Conforti, L., Czyżyk-Krzeska, M. F., and Millhorn, D. E. Membrane depolarization and dopamine secretion in PC12 cells during hypoxia are regulated by an O_2-sensitive K^+ current. Am J Physiol 1996; 271:C658–C665

171. Brown, E. R., Coker, G. T., and O'Malley, K. L. Organization and evolution of the rat tyrosine hydroxylase gene. Biochemistry 1987; 26:5208–5212.

172. Grima, B., Lamouroux, A., Blanot, F., Biguet, N. F., and Mallet, J. Complete coding sequence of rat tyrosine hydroxylase mRNA. Proc Natl Acad Sci USA 1985; 82:617–621.

173. Yoon, S. O. and Chikaraishi, D. M. Tissue specific transcription of the rat tyrosine hydroxylase gene requires synergy between an AP-1 motif and an overlapping E box-containing dyad. Neuron 1992; 9:55–67.

174. Kim, K.-S., Lee, M. K., Carroll, J., and Joh, T. H. Both the basal and inducible transcription of the tyrosine hydroxylase gene are dependent upon a cAMP responsive element. J Biol Chem 1993; 268:15689–15695.

175. Banerjee, S. A., Roffler-Tarlov, S., Szabo, M., Frohman, L., and Chikaraishi, D. M. DNA regulatory sequences of the rat tyrosine hydroxylase gene direct correct catecholaminergic cell-type specificity of a human growth hormone reporter in CNS of transgenic mice causing a dwarf phenotype. Mol Brain Res 1994; 24:89–106.

176. Min, N., Joh, T. H., Jkim, K. S., Peng, C., and Son, J. H. 5′ upstream DNA sequence of the rat tyrosine hydroxylase gene directs high-level and tissue specific expression to catecholaminergic neurons in the central nervous system of transgenic mice. Mol Brain Res 1994; 27:281–289.

177. Wong, S. C., Moffat, M. A., Coker, G. T., Merlie, J. P., and O'Malley, K. L. The 3′ flanking region of the human tyrosine hydroxylase gene directs reporter gene expression in peripheral neuroendocrine tissues. J Neurochem 1995; 65:23–31.

178. Kilbourne, E. J., Nankova, B. B., Lewis, E. J., McMahon, A. N., Osaka, H., Sabban, D. B., and Sabban, E. L. Regulated expression of the tyrosine hydroxylase gene by membrane depolarization. J Biol Chem 1992; 267:7563–7569.

179. Nagamoto-Combs, K., Piech, K. M., Best, J. A., Sun, B., and Tank, A. W. Tyrosine hydroxylase gene promoter activity is regulated by both cyclic AMP-responsive element and AP1 sites following calcium influx. J Biol Chem 1997; 272:6051–6058.

180. Nankova, B., Hiremagalur, B., Menezes, A., Zeman, R., and Sabban, E. Promoter elements and second messenger pathways involved in transcriptional activation of tyrosine hydroxylase by ionomycin. Mol Brain Res 1996; 35:164–172.

181. Tinti, C., Yang, C., Seo, H., Conti, B., Kim, C., Joh, T. H., and Kim, K.-S. Structure/function relationship of the cAMP response element in tyrosine hydroxylase gene transcription. J Biol Chem 1997; 272:19158–19164.

182. Tinti, C., Conti, B., Cubells, J. F., Kim, K.-S., Baker, H., and Joh, T. H. Inducible cAMP early repressor can modulate tyrosine hydroxylase gene expression after stimulation of cAMP synthesis. J Biol Chem 1996; 271:25375–25381.

183. Ghee, M., Baker, H., Miller, J. C., and Ziff, E. B. AP1, CREB and CBP transcription factors differentially regulate the tyrosine hydroxylase gene. Mol Brain Res 1998; 55:101–114.

184. Beitner-Johnson, D. and Millhorn, D. E. Hypoxia induces phosphorylation of the cyclic AMP response element-binding protein by a novel signaling mechanism. J Biol Chem 1998; 273:19834–19839.

185. Lopez-Barneo, J., Pardal, R., and Ortega-Saenz, P. Cellular mechanisms of oxygen sensing. Annu Rev Physiol 2001; 63:259–287.

186. Huang, L. E., Arany, Z., Livingston, D. M., and Bunn, H. F. Activation of hypoxia-inducible transcription factor depends primarily upon redox-sensitive stabilization of its alpha subunit. J Biol Chem 1996; 271:32253–32259.

187. Ciechanover, A. and Schwartz, A. L. The ubiquitin-proteosome pathway: The complexity and myriad functions of proteins death. Proc Natl Acad Sci USA 1998; 95:2727–2730.

188. Karin, M., Liu, Z. G., and Zandi, E. AP-1 function and regulation. Curr Opin Cell Biol 1997; 9:240–246.

189. Abate, C., Patel, L., Rauscher, F. J., and Curran, T. Redox regulation of fos and Jun DNA binding activity in vitro. Science 1990; 249:1157–1161.

190. Xanthoudakis, S., Miao, G., Wang, Y. C., Pan, E., and Curran, T. Redox activation of Fos-Jun DNA binding activity is mediated by a DNA repair enzyme. EMBO J 1992; 11:3323–3335.

191. Xanthoudakis, S. and Curran, T. Identification and characterization of Ref-1, a nuclar protein that facilitates AP-1 DNA binding activity. EMBO J 1992; 11:653–665.

192. Yao, K. S., Xanthoudakis, S., Curran, T., and O'Dwyer, P. J. Activation of AP-1 and of a nuclear redox factor, Ref-1, in the response of HT29 colon cancer cells to hypoxia. Mol Cell Biol 1994; 14:5997–6003.

193. Arias, J., Alberts, A. S., Brindle, P., Claret, F. X., Smeal, T., Karin, M., Feramisco, J., and Montminy, M. Activation of cAMP and mitogen responsive genes relies on a common nuclear factor. Nature 1994; 370:226–229.

194. Hermida Matsumoto, M. L., Chock, P. B., Curran, T., and Yang, D. C. H. Ubiquitinylation of transcription factors c-Jun and c-fos using reconstituted ubiquitinylating enzymes. J Biol Chem 1996; 271:4930–4936.

195. Stancovski, I., Gonen, H., Orian, A., Schwartz, A. L., and Ciechanover, A. Degradation of the protooncogene product c-fos by ubiquitin proteolytic system in vivo and in vitro: identification and characterization of the conjugating enzymes. Mol Cell Biol 1995; 15:7106–7116.

196. Fuchs, S. Y., Xie, B., Adler, V., Fried, V. A., Davis, R. J., and Ronai, Z. C.-Jun NH2 terminal kinases target the ubiquitination of their associated transcription factors. J Biol Chem 1997; 272:32163–32168.

197. Fuchs, S. Y., Fried, V. A., and Ronai, Z. Stress-regulated kinases regulate protein stability. Oncogene 1998; 17:1483–1490.

198. Semenza, G. L. HIF-1: mediator of physiological and pathophysiological responses to hypoxia. J Appl Physiol 2000; 88:1474–1480.

199. Wang, G. L. and Semenza, G. L. Purification and characterization of hypoxia inducible factor 1. J Biol Chem 1995; 27:1230–1237.

200. Arany, Z., Huang, L. E., Eckner, R., Bhattacharya, S., Jiang, C., Goldberg, M. A., Bunn, H. F., and Livingstone, D. M. An essential role for p300/CBP in cellular response to hypoxia. Proc Natl Acad Sci USA 1996; 93:12969–12973.
201. Ebert, B. and Bunn, H. F. Regulation of transcription by hypoxia requires a multiprotein complex that induces hypoxia-inducible factor 1, an adjacent transcription factor, and p300/CREB binding protein. Mol Cell Biol 1998; 18:4089–4096.
202. Kallio, P. J., Okamoto, K., O'Brien S., Carrero, P., Makino, Y., Tanaka, H., and Poellinger, L. Signal transduction in hypoxic cells: inducible nuclear translocation and recruitment of the CBP/p300 coactivator by the hypoxia indcuible factor-1α. EMBO J 1998; 17:6573–6586.
203. O'Rourke, J. F., Tian, Y. M., Ratcliffe, P. J., and Pugh, C. W. Oxygen-regulated and transactivating domains in endothelial PAS protein 1: comparison with hypoxia inducible factor-1α. J Biol Chem 1999; 274:2060–2071.
204. Tian, H., McKnight, S. L., and Russell, D. W. Endothelial PAS domain protein 1 (EPAS1), a transcription factor selectively expressed in endothelial cells. Genes Dev 1997; 11:72–82.
205. Tian, H., Hammer, R. E., Matsumoto, A. M., Russell, D. W., and McKnight, S. L. The hypoxia-responsive transcription factor EPAS1 is essential for catecholamine homeostasis and protection against heart failure during embryonic development. Genes Dev 1998; 12:3320–3324.
206. Wiesener, M. S., Turley, H., Allen, W. E., Wiliam, C., Eckardt, K.-U., Talks, K. L., Wood, S. M., Gatter, K. C., Harris, A. L., Pugh, C. W., Ratcliffe, P. J., and Maxwell, P. H. Induction of endothelial PAS domain protein 1 by hypoxia: characterization and comparison with hypoxia inducible factor 1α. Blood 1998; 92:2260–2268.
207. Gu, Y. Z., Moran, S. M., Hogenesch, J. B., Wartman, L., and Bradfield, C. A. Molecular characterization and chromosomal localization of a third α-class hypoxia inducible factor subunit, HIF3α. Gene Expr 1998; 7:205–213.
208. Huang, L. E., Gu, J., Schau, M., and Bunn, H. F. Regulation of hypoxia-inducible factor 1α is mediated by an O_2-dependent degradation domain via the ubiquitin-proteasome pathway. Proc Natl Acad Sci USA 1998; 95:7987–7992.
209. Kallio, P. J., Wilson, W. J., O'Brien, S., Makino, Y., and Poellinger, L. Regulation of the hypoxia-inducible transcription factor 1 alpha by the ubiquitin-proteasome pathway. J Biol Chem 1999; 274:6519–25.
210. Sutter, C. H., Laughner, E., and Semenza, G. L. Hypoxia-inducible factor 1 alpha protein expression is controlled by oxygen-regulated ubiquitination that is disrupted by deletions and missense mutations. Proc Natl Acad Sci USA 2000; 97:4748–4753.
211. Richard, D., Berra, E., Gothie, E., Roux, D., and Poussegur, J. p42/p44 mitogen activated protein kinases phosphorylate hypoxia-inducible factor 1 (HIF-1) and enhance the transcripitonal activity of HIF-1. J Biol Chem 1999; 274:32631–32637.

212. Conrad, P. W., Freeman, T. L., Beitner-Johnson, D., and Millhorn, D. E. EPAS1 trans-activation during hypoxia requires p42/p44 MAPK. J Biol Chem 1999; 274:33709–33713.
213. Bhattacharya, S., Michels, C. L., Leung, M. K., Arany, Z. P., Kung, A. L., and Livingston, D. M. Functional role of p35srj, a novel p300/CBP binding protein, during transactivation by HIF-1. Genes Dev 1999; 13:64–75.
214. Carrero, P., Okamoto, K., Coulmailleau, P., O'Brien, S., Tanaka, H., and Poellinger, L. Redox-regulated recruitment of the transcriptional co-activators CREB-binding protein and SRC-1 to hypoxia-inducible factor 1α. Mol Cell Biol 2000; 20:402–415.
215. Kvietikova, I., Wenger, R. H., Marti, H. H., and Gassman, M. The transcription factors ATF-1 and CREB-1 bind constitutively to the hypoxia-inducible factor-1 (HIF-1) DNA recognition site. Nucl Acids Res 1995; 23:4542–4550.
216. Iwai, K., Yamanaka, K., Kamura, T., Minato, N., Conaway, R. C., Conaway, J. W., Klausner, D. R., and Pause A. Identification of the von Hippel-Lindau tumor-suppressor protein as part of an active E3 ubiquitin ligase complex. Proc Natl Acad Sci USA 1999; 96:12436–12441.
217. Maxwell, P. H., Wiesener, M. S., Chang, G.-W., Clifford S. C., Vaux E. C., Cockman M. E., Wykoff C. C., Pugh C. W., Maher E. R., and Ratcliffe P. J. The tumor suppressor protein VHL targets hypoxia-inducible factors for oxygen-dependent proteolysis. Nature 1999; 399:271–275.
218. Cockman, M. E., Masson, N., Mole, D. R., Jaakkola, P., Chang, G.-W., Clifford, S. C., Maher, E. R., Pugh, C. W., Ratcliffe, P. J., and Maxwell, P. H. Hypoxia inducible factor-α binding and ubiquitylation by the von Hippel-Lindau tumor suppressor protein. J Biol Chem 2000; 275:25733–25741.
219. Kamura, T., Sato, S., Iwai, K., Czyżyk-Krzeska, M. F., Conaway, R. C., and Conaway, J. W. Activation of HIF 1α ubiquitination by a reconstituted von Hippel-Lindau (VHL) tumor suppressor complex. Proc Natl Acad Sci USA 2000; 97:10430–10435.
220. Ohh, M., Park, C. W., Ivan, M., Hoffman, M. A., Kim, T. Y., Huang, L. E., Pavletich, N., Chau, V., and Kaelin, W. G. Ubiquitination of hypoxia-inducible factor requires direct binding to the domain of the von Hippel-Lindau protein. Nat Cell Biol 2000; 2:423–427.
221. Ivan, M., Kondo, K., Yang, H., Kim, W., Valiando, J., Ohh, M., Salic, A., Asara, J. M., Lane, W. S., and Kaelin, W. G. Jr. HIF alpha targeted for VHL-mediated destruction by proline hydroxylation: implications in oxygen sensing. Science 2001; 292:464–468.
222. Jaakkola, P., Mole, D. R., Tian, Y. M., Wilson, M. I., Gielbert, J., Gaskell, S. J., Kriegsheim, A. V., Hebestreit, H. F., Mukherji, M., Schofield, C. J., Maxwell, P. H., Pugh, C. W., and Ratcliffe, P. J. Targeting of HIF-alpha to the von Hippel-Lindau ubiquitylation complex by regulated prolyl hydroxylation. Science 2001; 292:468–472.
223. Ravi, R., Mookerjee, B., Bhujwalla, Z. M., Sutter, C. H., Artemov, D., Zeng, Q., Dillehay, L. E., Madan, A., Semenza, G. L., and Bedi, A. Regulation of

tumor angiogenesis by p53-induced degradation of hypoxia-inducible factor 1α. Genes Dev 2001: 14:34–44.

224. Giles, R. H., Peters, D. J. M., and Breuning, M. H. Conjunction dysfunction:CBP/p300 in human disease. Trends Gen 1998; 14:5

225. Kamei, Y., Xu, L., Heinzel, T., Torchia, J., Kurokawa, R., Gloss, B., Lin, S. C., Heyman, R. A., Rose, D. W., Glass, C. K., and Rosenfeld, M. G. A CBP integrator complex mediates transcriptional activation and AP-1 inhibition by nuclear receptors. Cell 1996; 85:403–414.

226. Horvai, A. E., Xu, L., Korzus, E., Brard, G., Kalafaus, D., Muellin, T.-M., Rose, D. W., Rosenfeld, M. G., and Glass, C. K. Nuclear integration of JAK/STAT and Ras/Ap-1 signaling by CBP and p300. Proc Natl Acad Sci USA 1997; 94:1074–1079.

227. Maher, E. R. and Kaelin, W. G. Jr. Von Hippel-Lindau disease. Rev Mol Med 1997; 76:381–384.

228. Bender, B. U., Altehofer, C., Januszewicz, A., Gartner, R., Schmidt, H., Hoffmann, M. M., Heidemann, P. H., and Neumann, H. P. H. Functioning thoracic paraganglioma: association with von Hippel-Lindau syndrome. J Clin Endocrinol Metabol 1997; 82:3356–3360.

229. Zanelli, M. and Van Der Walt, J. D. Carotid body paraganglioma in von Hippel-Lindau disease. Histopathology 1996; 29:178–181.

230. Latif, F., Tory, K., Gnarra, J., Yao, M., Duh, F. M., Orcutt, M. L., Stackhouse, T., Kuzmin, I., Modi, W., Geil, L., Schmidt, L., Zhou, F., Li, H., Wei, M. H., Chen, F., Glenn, G., Choyke, P., Walther, M. M., Weng, Y., Duan, D.-S. R., Dean, M., Glavac, D., Richards, F. M., Crossey, P. A., Ferguson-Smith, M. A., Le Paslier, D., Chumakov, I., Cohen, D., Chinault, A. C., Maher, E. R., Linehan, W. M., Zbar, B., and Lerman, M. I. Identification of the von Hippel-Lindau disease tumor suppressor gene. Science 1993; 260:1317–1320.

231. Iliopoulos, O., Kibel, A., Gray, S., and Kaelin, W. G. Jr. Tumour suppression by the human von Hippel-Lindau gene product. Nat Med 1995; 1:822–826.

232. Duan, D. R., Humphrey, J. S., Chen, D. Y., Weng, Y., Sukegawa, J., Lee, S., Gnarra, J. R., Linehan, W. M., and Klausner, R. D. Characterization of the VHL tumor suppressor gene product: localization, complex formation, and the effect of natural inactivating mutations. Proc Natl Acad Sci USA 1995; 92:6459–6463.

233. Kroll, S. L., Paulding, W. R., Schnell, P. O., Barton, M. C., Conaway, J. W., Conaway, R. C., and Czyżyk-Krzeska, M. F. Von Hippel-Lindau protein induces hypoxia-regulated arrest of tyrosine hydroxylase transcript elongation in pheochromocytoma cells. J Biol Chem 1999; 274:30109–30114.

234. Stebbins, C. E., Kaelin, W. G., and Paveletich, N. P. Structure of the VHL-elongin C-elongin B complex: implications for VHL tumor suppressor function. Science 1999; 284:455–461.

235. Kibel, A., Iliopoulos, O., DeCaprio, J. A., and Kaelin, W. G. Binding of the von Hippel-Lindau tumor suppressor protein to elongin B and C. Science 1995; 269:1444–1445.

236. Takagi, Y., Pause, A., Conaway, R. C., and Conaway, J. W. Identification of elongin C sequences required for interaction with the von Hippel-Lindau tumor suppressor protein. J Biol Chem 1997; 272:27444–27449.

237. Pause, A., Lee, S., Worrell, R. A., Chen, D. Y. T., Burgess, W. H., Linehan, W. M., and Klausner, R. D. The von Hippel-Lindau tumor-suppressor gene product forms a stable complex with human CUL-2, a member of the Cdc53 family of proteins. Proc Natl Acad Sci USA 1997; 94:2156–2161.

238. Kamura, T., Koepp, D. M., Conrad, M. N., Skowyra, D., Moreland, R. J., Iliopoulos, O., Lane, W. S., Kaelin, W. G., Elledge, S. J., Conaway, R. C., Harper, J. W., and Conaway, J. W. Rbxl, a component of the VHL tumor suppressor complex and SCF ubiquitin ligase. Science 1999; 284:657–661.

239. Iliopoulos, O., Levy, A. P., Jiang, C., Kaelin, W. G., and Jr Goldberg, M. A. Negative regulation of hypoxia-inducible genes by the von Hippel-Lindau protein. Proc Natl Acad Sci USA 1996; 93:10595–10599.

240. Wizigmann-Voos, S., Breier, G., Risau, W., and Plate, K. H. Up-regulation of vascular endothelial growth factor and its receptors in von Hippel-Lindau disease-associated and sporadic hemangioblastomas. Cancer Res 1995; 55:1358–1364.

241. Los, M., Aarsman, C. J., Terpstra, L., Wittebol-Post, D., Lips, C. J., Blijham, G. H., and Voest, E. E. Elevated ocular levels of vascular endothelial growth factor in patients with von Hippel-Lindau disease. Ann Oncol 1997; 8:1015–1022.

242. Krieg, M., Marti, H. H., and Plate, K. H. Coexpression of erythropoietin and vascular endothelial growth factor in nervous system tumors associated with von Hippel-Lindau tumor suppressor gene loss of function. Blood 1998; 92:3388–3393.

243. Paulding, W. R. and Czyżyk-Krzeska, M. F. Post-transcriptional regulation of gene expression by hypoxia. Adv Exp Med Biol 2000; 475:111–122.

244. Czyżyk-Krzeska, M. F., Paulding, W. R., Beresh, J. E., and Kroll, S. L. Posttranscriptional regulation of tyrosine hydroxylase gene expression by oxygen in PC12 cells. Kidney Int 1997; 51:585–590.

245. Czyżyk-Krzeska, M. F. and Bendixen, A. C. Identification of the poly(C) binding protein in the complex associated with the 3′ untranslated region of erythropoietin mRNA. Blood 1999 93:2111–2120.

246. Dibbens, J. A., Miller, D. L., Damert, A., Risau, W., Vadas, M. A., and Goodall, G. J. Hypoxic regulation of vascular endothelial growth factor mRNA stability requires the cooperation of multiple RNA elements. Mol Biol Cell 1999; 10:907–919.

247. Roehrs, T., Merrion, M., Pedrosi, B., Stepanski, E., Zorick, F., and Roth, T. Neuropsychological function in obstructive sleep apnea syndrome (OSAS) compared to chronic obstructive pulmonary disease. Sleep 1995; 18:382–388.

248. Gozal, D. and Pope, D. W. Objective sleepiness measures in pediatric obstructive sleep apnea. Pediatrics 2001; 108:693–697.

249. Kales, A., Caldwell, A. B., Cadieux, R. J., Vela-Bueno, A., Ruch, L. G., and Mayes, S. D. Severe obstructive sleep apnea: II. Associated psychopathology and psychosocial consequences. J Chronic Dis 1985; 38:427–434.

250. Gozal, D. Sleep-disordered breathing and school performance in children. Pediatrics 1998; 102:616–620.

251. Nelson, T. O., Dunlosky, J., White, D. M., Steinberg, J., Townes, B. D., and Anderson, D. Cognition and metacognition at extreme altitudes on Mount Everest. J Exp Psychol Gen 1990; 119:367–374.

252. Hornbein, T. F. Long term effects of high altitude on brain function. Int J Sports Med 1992; 13:S43–S45.

253. West, J. B. The 1988 Stevenson Memorial lecture. Physiological responses to severe hypoxia in man. Can J Physiol Pharmacol 1989; 67:173–178.

254. Cavaletti, G., Garavaglia, P., Arrigoni, G., and Tredici, G. Persistent memory impairment after high altitude climbing. Int J Sports Med 1990; 11:176–178.

255. Dudkin, K. N., Kruchinin, V. K. Chueva, I. V., and Samoilov, M. O. The effect of brain hypoxia on cognitive processes and the neuronal correlates in monkeys. Dokl Akad Nauk 1993; 333:543–555.

256. Chleide, E., Bruhwyler, J., and Mercier, M. Effect of chronic hypoxic treatment on the retention of fixed interval responding. Physiol Behav 1991; 49:465–470.

257. Saletu, B., Gronberger, J., Anderer, P., Linzmayer, L., and Koenig, P. On the cerebro-protective effects of caroverine, a calcium channel blocker and antiglutamatergic drug: double-blind, placebo-controlled, EEG mapping and psychometric studies under hypoxia. Br J Clin Pharmacol 1996; 41:89–99.

258. Davis, H. P., Tribuna, J., Pulsinelli, W. A., and Volpe, B. T. Reference and working memory of rats following hippocampal damage induced by transient forebrain ischemia. Physiol Behav 1986; 37:387–392.

259. Hagan, J. J. and Beaughard, M. The effects of forebrain ischemia on spatial learning. Behav Brain Res 1990; 14:161–160.

260. Shukitt-Hale, B., Stillman, M. J., Welch, D. I., Levy, A., Devine, J. A., and Lieberman, H. R. Hypobaric hypoxia impairs spatial memory in an elevation-dependent fashion. Behav Neural Biol 1994; 62:244–252.

261. Nelson, A., Sowinski, P., and Hodges, H. Differential effects of global ischemia on delayed matching-to-position tasks in the water maze and Skinner Box. Neurobiol Learn Mem 1997; 67:228–247.

262. Timiras, P. S. Hypoxia and the CNS: maturation and adaptation at high altitude. Int J Biometeorol 1977; 21:147–156.

263. Chavez, J. C., Pichiule, P., Boero, J., and Arregui, A. Reduced mitochondrial respiration in mouse cerebral cortex during chronic hypoxia. Neurosci Lett 1995; 193:169–172.

264. Arregui, A. and Barer, G. R. Chronic hypoxia in rats: alterations of striato-nigral angiotensin converting enzyme, GABA, and glutamic acid decarboxylase. J Neurochem 1980; 34:740–743.

265. Arregui, A., Barer, G. R., and Emson, P. C. Neurochemical studies in the hypoxic brain: substance P, met-enkephalin, GABA and angiotensin converting enzyme. Life Sci 1981; 28:2925–2929.

266. Arregui, A., Hollingsworth, Z., Penney, J. B., and Young, A. B. Autoradiographic evidence for increased dopamine uptake sites in striatum of hypoxic mice. Neurosci Lett 1994; 167:195–197.

267. Pichiule, P., Chavez, J. C., Boero, J., and Arregui, A. Chronic hypoxia induces modification of the N-methyl-D-aspartate receptor in rat brain. Neurosci Lett 1996; 218:83–86.

268. Samuel, W., Masliah, E., Brush, D. E., Garcia-Munoz, M., Patino, P., Young, S. J., and Groves, P. M. Lesions in the dentate hilum and CA2/CA3 regions of the rat hippocampus produce cognitive deficits that correlate with site-specific glial activation. Neurobiol Learn Mem 1997; 68:103–116.

269. Muller, R. U., Stead, M., and Pach, J. The hippocampus as a cognitive graph. J Gen Physiol 1996; 107:663–694.

270. Kadar, T., Dachir, S., Shukkitt-Hale, B., and Levy, A. Sub-regional hippocampal vulnerability in various animal models leading to cognitive disfunction. Neural Transm 1998; 105:987–1004.

271. Bernaudin, M., Nouvelot, A., MacKenzie, E. T., and Petit, E. Selective neuronal vulnerability and specific glial reactions in hippocampal and neocortical organotypic cultures submitted to ischemia. Exp Neurol 1998; 150:30–39.

272. Davolio, C. and Greenamire, J. T. Selective vulnerability of the CA1 region of hippocampus to the indirect excitotoxic effects of malonic acid. Neurosci Lett 1995; 192:29–32.

273. Wilde, G. J., Pringle, A. K., Wright, P., and Iannotti, F. Differential vulnerability of the CA1 and CA3 subfields of the hippocampus to superoxide and hydroxyl radicals in vitro. J Neurochem 1997; 69:883–886.

274. Strasser, U. and Fisher, G. Protection from neuronal damage induced by combined oxygen and glucose deprivation in organotypic hippocampal cultures by glutamate receptor antagonists. Brain Res 1995; 687:167–174.

275. Pringle, A. K., Iannotti, F., Wilde, G. J. C., Chad, J. E., Seeley, P. J., and Sundstorm, L. E. Neuroprotection by both NMDA and non-NMDA receptor antagonists in in vitro ischemia. Brain Res 1997; 755:36–46.

276. Chow, E. and Haddad, G. G. Differential effects of anoxia and glutamate on cultured neocortical neurons. Exp Neurol 1998; 150:52–59.

277. Ohmori, T., Hirashima, Y., Kurimoto, M., Endo, S., and Takaku, A. In vitro hypoxia of cortical and hippocampal CA1 neurons: glutamate, nitric oxide, and platelet activating factor participate in the mechanism of selective neuronal death in CA1 neurons. Brain Res 1996; 743:109–115.

278. Matson, M. P. and Katter, S. B. Development and selective neurodegeneration in cell cultures from different hippocampal regions. Brain Res 1989; 490:110–125.

279. Nabetani, M. and Okada, Y. Developmental and regional differences in the vulnerability of rat hippocampal slices to brief and prolonged periods of hypoxia. Dev Neurosci 1994; 16:301–306.

280. Kreisman, N. R. and LaManna, J. C. Rapid and slow swelling during hypoxia in the CA1 region of rat hippocampal slices. J Neurophysiol 1999; 82:320–329.

281. Kreisman, N. R., Soliman, S., and Gozal, D. Regional differences in hypoxic depolarization and swelling in hippocampal slices. J Neurophysiol 2000; 83:1031–1038.

282. Kawasaki, K., Traynelis, S. F., and Dingledine, R. Different responses of CA1 and CA3 regions to hypoxia in rat hippocampal slice. J Neurophysiol 1990; 63:385–394.

283. Wang, H. D., Fukuda, T., Suzuki, T., Hashimoto, K., Liou, S. Y., Momoi, T., Kosaka, T., Yamamoto, K., and Nakanishi, H. Differential effects of Bcl-2 overexpression on hippocampal CA1 neurons and dentate granule cells following hypoxic ischemia in adult mice. J Neurosci Res 1999; 57:1–12.

284. Tsujimoto, Y., Gorham, J., Cossmann, J., Jaffe, E., and Croce, C. The t(14; 18) chromosome translocations involved in B-cell neoplasms results from mistakes in VDJ joining. Science 1985; 229:1300–1303.

285. Korsmeyer, S. J. Bcl-2: an antidote to programmed cell death. Cancer Surv 1992; 15:105–118.

286. Kane, D., Sarafian, T., Anton, R., Hahn, H., Gralla, E., Selvestone, V., Ord, T., and Bredesen, D. Bcl-2 inhibition of neural death: decreased generation of reactive oxygen species. Science 1993; 262:1274–1277.

287. Zhong, L., Sarafian, T., Kane, D. J., Charles, A. C., Mah, S. P., Edwards, R. H., and Bredesen, D. Bcl-2 inhibits death of central neural cells induced by multiple agents. Proc Natl Acad Sci USA 1993; 90:4533–4537.

288. Behl, C., Hovey, L. I., Krajewski, S., Schubert, D., and Reed, J. Bcl-2 prevents killing of neuronal cells by glutamate but not amyloid beta protein. Biochem Biophys Res Commun 1993; 197:949–956.

289. Banasiak, K. J., Cronin, T., and Haddad, G. G. bcl-2 prolongs neuronal survival during hypoxia-induced apoptosis. Mol Brain Res 1999; 72:214–225.

290. An, W. G., Kanekal, M., Simon, M. C., Maltepe, E., Blagosklonny, M. V., and Neckers, L. M. Stabilization of wild-type p53 by hypoxia-inducible factor 1 α. Nature 1998; 392:405–408.

291. Baker, S. J., Fearon, E. R., Nigro, J. M., Hamilton, S. R., Preisinger, A. C., Jessup, J. M., van Tuinen, P., Ledbetter, D. H., Barker, D. F., and Nakamura, Y. Chromosome 17 deletions and p53 gene mutations in colorectal carcinomas. Science 1989; 44:217–221.

292. Zhan, Q., Carrier, F., and Fornace, A. J. Induction of cellular p53 activity by DNA-damaging agents and growth arrest. Mol Cell Biol 1993; 13:4242–4250.

293. Kastan, M. B., Zhan, Q., El-Deiry, W. S., Carrier, F., Jacks, T., Walsh, W. V., Plunkett, B. S., Vogelstein, B., and Fornace, A. J. A mammalian cell cycle checkpoint pathway utilizing p53 and GADD45 is defective in ataxia-telangiectasia. Cell 1992; 13:587–597.

294. Lowe, S. W., Schmitt, E. M., Smith, S. W., and Osborne, B. A., Jacks, T. p53 is required for radiation induced apoptosis in mouse thymocytes. Nature 1993; 362:847–849.

295. Banasiak, K. J. and Haddad, G. G. Hypoxia-induced apoptosis: effect of hypoxic severity and role of p53 in neuronal cell death. Brain Res 1998; 797:295–304.

296. Weil, J. V. Sleep at high altitude. Clin Chest Med 1985; 6:615–621.

297. Coote, J. H., Stone, B. M., and Tsang, G. Sleep of Andean high altitude natives. Eur J Appl Physiol Occup Physiol 1992; 64:178–181.

298. Gozal, D., Daniel, J. M., and Dohanich, G. P. Behavioral and anatomical correlates of chronic episodic hypoxia during sleep in the rat. J Neurosci 2001; 21:2442–2450.

299. Albin, R. L. and Greenamyre, J. T. Alternative excitotoxic hypotheses. Neurology 1992; 42:733–738.

300. Hoffman, D. J., McGowan, J. E., Marro, P. J., Mishra, O. P., and Delivoria-Papadopoulos, M. Hypoxia-induced modification of the N-methyl-D-aspartate receptor in the brain of the newborn piglet. Neurosci Lett 1994; 167:156–160.

301. Beal, M. F. Aging, energy, and oxidative stress in neurodegenerative diseases. Ann Neurol 1995; 38:357–366.

302. Alberghina, M., Ragusa, N., and Giuffrida, A. Changes of nucleic acid and protein synthesis in hypertrophied guinea-pig heart during intermittent hypoxia. Ital J Biochem 1981; 30:229–241.

303. Serra, I., Alberghina, M., Viola, M., and Giuffrida, A. M. Effect of hypoxia on nucleic acid and protein synthesis in different brain regions. Neurochem Res 1981; 6:595–605.

304. Lee, P. J., Jiang, B.-H., Chin, B. Y., Iyer, N. V., Alam, J., Semenza, G. L., and Choi, A. M. K. Hypoxia-inducible factor-1 mediates transcriptional activation of the heme oxygenase-1 gene in response to hypoxia. J Biol Chem 1997; 272:5375–5381.

305. Tamm, M., Bihl, M., Eickelberg, O., Stulz, P., Perruchoud, A. P., and Roth, M. Hypoxia-induced interleukin-6 and interleukin-8 production is mediated by platelet-activating factor and platelet-derived growth factor in primary human lung cells. Am J Resp Cell Mol Biol 1998; 19:653–661.

306. Bossenmeyer, C., Chihab, R., Muller, S., Schroeder, H., and Daval, J. L. Hypoxia/reoxygenation induces apoptosis through biphasic induction of protein synthesis in cultured rat brain neurons. Brain Res 1998; 787:107–116.

307. Chihab, R., Ferry, C., Koziel, V., Monin, P., and Daval, J.-L. Sequential activation of activator protein-1-related transcription factors and JNK protein kinases may contribute to apoptotic death induced by transient hypoxia in developing brain neurons. Mol Brain Res 1998; 63:105–120.

308. Gozal, D. and Gozal, E. Episodic hypoxia potentiates the late hypoxic ventilatory response in the developing rat: putative role of neuronal nitric oxide synthase. Am J Physiol 1999; 276:R17–R22.

309. Gozal, D., Xue, Y. D., and Simakajornboon, N. Hypoxia induces c-fos protein expression in NMDA but not AMPA glutamate receptor labeled neurons within the nucleus tractus solitarii of the conscious rat. Neurosci Lett 1999; 262:93–96.

310. Prabhakar, N. R., Pieramici, S. F., Premkumar, D. R. D., Kumar, G. K., and Kalaria, R. N. Activation of nitric oxide synthase gene expression by hypoxia in central and peripheral neurons. Mol Brain Res 1996; 43:341–346.

311. Conforti, L., Kobayashi, S., Beitner-Johnson, D., Conrad, P. W., Freeman, T., and Millhorn, D. E. Regulation of gene expression and secretory functions in oxygen-sensing pheochromocytoma cells. Respir Physiol 1999; 115:249–260.

312. Kobayashi, S., Zimmermann, H., and Millhorn, D. E. Chronic hypoxia enhances adenosine release in rat PC12 cells by altering adenosine metabolism and membrane transport. J Neurochem 2000; 74:621–632.

313. Beitner-Johnson, D., Seta, K., Yuan, Y., Kim, H., Rust, R. T., Conrad, P. W., Kobayashi, S., and Millhorn, D. E. Identification of hypoxia-responsive genes in a dopaminergic cell line by subtractive cDNA libraries and microarray analysis. Parkins Rel Dis 2001; 7:273–281.

314. Sinor, A. D., Irvin, S. M., Cobbs, C. S., Chen, J., Graham, S. H., and Greenberg, D. A. Hypoxic induction of vascular endothelial growth factor (VEGF) protein in astroglial cultures. Brain Res 1998; 812:289–291.

315. Ikeda, E., Achen, M. G., Breier, G., and Risau, W. Hypoxia-induced transcriptional activation and increased mRNA stability of vascular endothelial growth factor in C6 glioma cells. J Biol Chem 1995; 270:19761–19766.

316. Preedy, V. R., Smith, D. M., and Sugden, P. H. The effects of 6 hours of hypoxia on protein synthesis in rat tissues in vivo and in vitro. Biochem J 1985; 228:179–185.

317. Gage, A. T. and Stanton, P. K. Hypoxia triggers neuroprotective alterations in hippocampal gene expression via a heme-containing sensor. Brain Res 1996; 719:172–178.

318. Soskic, V., Gorlach, M., Poznanovic, S., Boehmer, F. D., and Godovac-Zimmerman, J. Functional proteomic analysis of signal transduction pathways of the platelet derived growth factor β receptor. Biochemistry 1999; 38:1757–1764.

319. O'Farrell, P. H. High resolution two-dimensional electrophoresis of proteins. J Biol Chem 250: 1975; 4007–4021.

320. Klose, J. Protein mapping by combined isoelectric focusing and electrophoresis of mouse tissues. A novel approach to testing for induced point mutations in mammals. Humangenetik 1975; 26:231–243.

321. Henzel, W. J., Billeci, T. M., Stults, J. T., and Wong, S. Identifying proteins from two-dimensional gels by molecular mass searching of peptide fragments in protein sequence databases. Proc Natl Acad Sci USA 1993; 90:5011–5015.

322. Gauss, C., Kalkum, M., Lowe, M., Lehrach, H., and Klose, J. Analysis of the mouse proteome. (I) Brain proteins: separation by two-dimensional electro-

phoresis and identification by mass spectrometry and genetic variation. Electrophoresis 1999; 20:575–600.

323. Fountoulakis, M., Schuller, E., Hardmeier, R., Berndt, P., and Lubec, G. Rat brain proteins: two-dimensional protein database and variations in the expression levels. Electrophoresis 1999; 20:3572–3579.

324. Buonocore, G., Liberatori, S., Bini, L., Mishra, O. P., Delivoria-Papadopoulos M., Pallini V., and Bracci, R. Hypoxic response of synaptosomal proteins in term guinea pig fetuses. J Neurochem 1999; 73:2139–2148.

325. Gozal, E., Klein, J. B., Pierce, W. M., Cai, J., Scherzer, J. A., Sachleben, L. R., and Gozal, D. Proteomic analysis of CA1 and CA3 regions of hippocampus following 6 hours of intermittent hypoxia. Soc Neurosci Abstr 2000; 26:A655.12.

326. Prabhakar, N. R. Oxygen sensing during intermittent hypoxia: cellular and molecular mechanisms. J Appl Physiol 2001; 90:1986–1994.

327. Mezzanotte, W. S., Tangel, D. J., and White, D. P. Waking genioglossal electromyogram in sleep apnea patients versus normal controls (a neuromuscular compensatory mechanism). J Clin Invest 1992; 89:1571–1579.

328. Hendricks, J. C., Petrof, B. J., Panckeri, K., and Pack, A. I. Upper airway dilating muscle hyperactivity during non-rapid eye movement sleep in English bulldogs. Am Rev Respir Dis 1993; 148:185–194.

329. Kubin, L. and Davies, R. O. Mechanisms of upper airway hypotonia. In: Pack AI., ed. Sleep Apnea. Pathogenesis, Diagnosis and Treatment. New York: Marcel Dekker, 2002:99–154.

Part Three

EXPERIMENTAL SLEEP-RELATED BREATHING DISORDERS

6

Cardiovascular Effects of Intermittent Hypoxia in the Rat

EUGENE C. FLETCHER

University of Louisville School of Medicine
Louisville, Kentucky, U.S.A.

I. Introduction

Previous publications indicate that sleep apnea syndrome is found in 30–35% of patients with clinical systemic hypertension (1–4). There is a growing consensus among sleep disorders investigators that obstructive sleep apnea is a risk factor for systemic hypertension independent of obesity or age. Acute apnea is accompanied by several autonomic responses including marked increase in blood pressure, tachycardia–bradycardia, elevation of intracranial pressure, and other hemodynamic and neurologic changes (5). Closely repetitive apneas show not only an acute blood pressure rise with each apnea, but also a gradual rise in baseline blood pressure that is extended well beyond termination of the apneas (6). This suggests that repetitive apneas could lead to a form of secondary systemic hypertension. Snoring and repetitive sleep apnea may be major etiologic contributors to the pool of patients with essential hypertension, and particularly in cases of difficult to manage or refractory hypertension.

Hypothetically, repetitive apnea may lead to sustained diurnal systemic hypertension in patients with sleep apnea. Several laboratories

183

are now using rodent models of episodic hypoxia over a period of weeks or months to test the hypothesis that hypoxia leads to chronic sustained blood pressure elevation. This chapter will discuss the *episodic hypoxia rat* preparation. Rats are exposed to recurrent short periods of episodic or intermittent hypoxia for 8 hr/day over a 35-day period to induce sustained elevation of daytime blood pressure. It should be noted that episodic hypoxia may be applied in many different forms, ranging from hypoxic cycles (as in our model) every 30 sec to hypoxia episodes lasting 2 min to 2 hr. These cycles may be applied continuously over days or weeks, or for variable periods (e.g., 8 hr) during the day, simulating the recurrent episodic hypoxia of sleep apnea. Currently, 70% of hypertension research is carried out in rodents because of the many similarities of blood pressure and cardiovascular response between these animals and humans. Because of the short life span of rodents, many of the models of chronic renal and endocrine hypertension paralleling human clinical disease can be studied in greater depth in rodents than is possible in humans.

II. The Chronic Episodic Hypoxia Model

Acute hypoxia leads to stimulation of the peripheral chemoreceptors, which in turn directly increases sympathetic outflow via two peripheral neuro-transmitters. *Epinephrine* is excreted into adrenal venous blood during hypoxia, stimulating sympatho-renal discharge to counter the stress of oxygen deficit (7,8). *Norepinephrine* is a ganglionic neurotransmitter of the peripheral sympathetic nervous system as well as the adrenal medulla. The adrenal medulla and the peripheral sympathetic nervous system act together during hypoxia to preserve homeostasis by increasing cardiac output, and redistributing blood flow to optimize oxygen delivery to vital tissues. We designed and constructed 25 chambers where rodents could be exposed to rapid swings in ambient oxygen concentration (FIO_2) which induced changes in oxygen saturation (SaO_2) similar to that seen in humans with sleep apnea (Fig. 1). The animals are housed in individual cylindrical Plexiglas chambers (length 28 cm, diameter 10 cm, volume 2.4 L) with snug-fitting lids. Using a timed solenoid valve, nitrogen (100%) is distributed to each chamber for 12 sec at a flow that is adjusted to reduce the FIO_2 to 3–5% for approximately 3–6 sec. This is followed by infusion of compressed air over 15–18 sec to an FIO_2 of 20.9%. The cycle is repeated twice per minute during the day for 6–8 hr on 30–40 consecutive days. Multiple serial arterial blood samples as well as continuous arterial catheter oximetry monitoring during episodic hypoxia have shown the average nadir level of SaO_2 in this system to be 70% (range 60–80%) (Fig. 2). At the same time as nitrogen is being

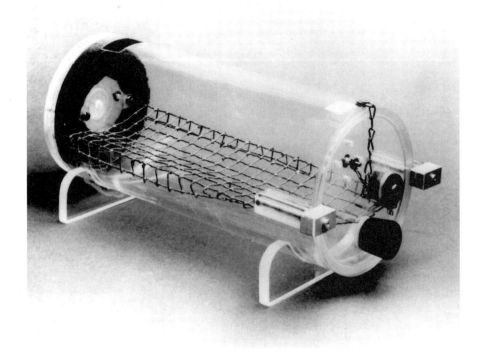

Figure 1 Normobaric chamber which would contain a single rat, where infusion of N_2 lowers FIO_2 creating transient hypoxia or asphyxia. Infusion of N_2 lasts about 12 sec (with a range of 6–14 sec) followed by compressed air for the balance of each 30-sec cycle.

distributed to hypoxic chambers, compressed air at approximately the same liter flow can be distributed to sham cages simulating the same noise and air disturbance. A dampening device at the intake end of the chamber is used to dissipate the airstream so that no direct gas jets disturb the animal. The system can be manipulated to combine nitrogen with varying concentrations of CO_2 such that any blood gas change associated with apnea can be simulated (hypo-, hyper-, eucapnea) and can be administered chronically. The rat is active nocturnally and sleeps during the day. Thus, the 8-hr episodic hypoxia exposure period is during the usual sleep cycle of the rat. Behaviorally, the rats continue to sleep during the day throughout the 35-day cycle.

Our first publication describing this model demonstrated that repetitive episodic hypoxia patterned after that seen in sleep apnea results

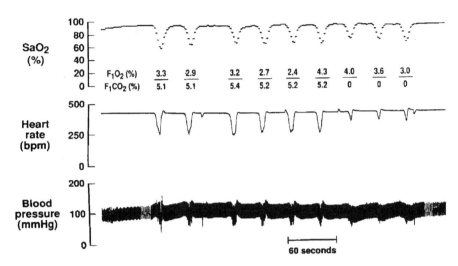

Figure 2 Example of continuous oxyhemoglobin saturation change (SaO$_2$) (top channel), continuous heart rate (middle channel), and blood pressure (bottom channel) in a single rat undergoing acute episodic hypoxia challenge (FIO$_2$ = % indicated in numerator) with and without added CO$_2$ (FICO$_2$ = % indicated in denominator). Before the seventh desaturation, the added CO$_2$ was stopped, with rapid return to hypocapnic hypoxia, reducing the bradycardia and blood pressure response. The continuous SaO$_2$ was measured with an indwelling fiberoptic catheter placed in the carotid artery of a rat.

in persistent mean arterial blood pressure elevation (9). Six Sprague Dawley rats were subjected to intermittent hypoxia, 8 hr per day for 35 days while six controls were exposed only to episodic exchanges of compressed air. At the end of study, diurnal tail cuff systolic blood pressures were 21 mmHg higher in hypoxia-exposed animals than in six sham and four unhandled controls ($p < 0.05$). A similar study was performed using Wistar Thomae rats measuring blood pressure intra-arterially. Some rats were removed from episodic hypoxia at 20, 30, and 35 days. There was a progressive increase in mean arterial pressure among the three groups. The 35-day Wistar rat episodic hypoxia group showed a 13.7 mmHg increase in mean arterial pressure, whereas sham (compressed air) and unhandled controls showed no change in mean arterial pressure (9).

III. The Sympathetic Nervous System in Chronic Episodic Hypoxia

We hypothesized that episodic hypoxia stimulated carotid chemoreceptors, which in turn increased sympathetic activity. The first of a pair of studies examined the role of chemoreceptors in producing the diurnal blood pressure increase in the episodic hypoxia rat (10,11). Carotid body denervation was performed on two groups of male Wistar rats by severing both carotid sinus nerves (10). A sham-operated, nondenervated group exposed to episodic hypoxia displayed a 13 mmHg increase in mean arterial pressure, whereas carotid body denervated rats exposed to episodic hypoxia showed no change in blood pressure. Unhandled sham-operated and unhandled carotid body denervated rats showed no significant change in blood pressure from baseline.

Next, we examined the role of the peripheral sympathetic nervous system in the episodic hypoxia rat (11). Chemical sympathectomy was performed using a drug (6-OH dopamine) that accumulates only at norepinephrine uptake sites, destroying nerve synapses of the peripheral sympathetic nervous system. Two intraperitoneal injections of 6-OH dopamine were given 20 days apart in two groups of male Wistar Thomae rats: one was subjected to episodic hypoxia and one remained unhandled (11). A third group received only vehicle but was subjected to episodic hypoxia. The latter group showed a 7.7 mmHg increase (post 40 days) in mean arterial pressure above baseline whereas the 6-OH dopamine-injected, episodic hypoxia and unhandled controls showed no change in mean arterial pressure. Measurement of catecholamines in cardiac muscle homogenate confirmed sympathetic denervation in 6-OH dopamine animals. The results imply that the sympathetic nervous system plays a major role in the sustained blood pressure increase in the episodic hypoxia rat.

Confirming that the sympathetic nervous system is substantially involved in the *chronic* blood pressure response to episodic hypoxia, we performed a series of acute studies to examine the relationship between hypoxia, sympathetic nervous system activity, and acute blood pressure changes (12). One thing that this study examined was whether episodic eucapnic hypoxia was a more potent stimulus to *acute* blood pressure elevation than was episodic hypocapnic hypoxia. Another question was the role of the sympathetic and parasympathetic nervous systems in the heart rate and blood pressure response to episodic hypoxia. Prazosin (α_1-adrenergic blocker), yohimbine (α_2-adrenergic blocker), and atropine were used to block sympathetic and parasympathetic responses. Eucapnic hypoxia caused a three-fold greater elevation in systolic blood pressure and greater bradycardia than hypocapnic hypoxia. Prazosin, but not

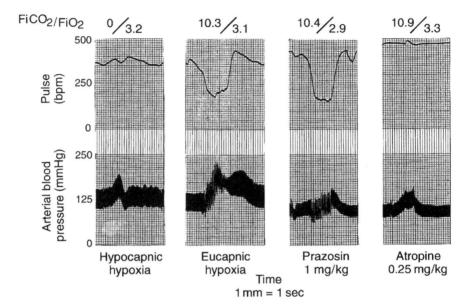

Figure 3   Continuous pulse (upper channel) and blood pressure (lower channel) from a single rat exposed to hypocapnic hypoxia, eucapnic hypoxia, prazosin with eucapnic hypoxia, and prazosin with atropine and eucapnic hypoxia. Eucapnic hypoxia produced a greater pressor response than hypocapnic hypoxia with more profound bradycardia. Prazosin blocks much of the pressor response, doing little to the bradycardia. Atropine completely eliminated the bradycardia, doing little to the pressor response. $FICO_2\%$ for each episodic hypoxia episode appears in the numerator (top) and FIO_2 appears in the denominator. (From Ref. 12.)

yohimbine, blunted the blood pressure response and atropine blocked the hypoxia-associated bradycardia (Fig. 3). Direct recording of splanchnic nerve activity in the awake, unrestrained rat confirmed that adding CO_2 to episodic hypoxia caused a profound increase in sympathetic nervous system activity (not shown). This study confirmed that in the *acute setting*, eucapnic hypoxia is a more potent stimulus to blood pressure elevation than hypocapnic hypoxia.

Because the usual blood gas change of apnea is mildly increased CO_2, and the blood pressure change of *acute* apnea is markedly enhanced by hypercapnia, we hypothesized that the chronic blood pressure response to hypercapnic hypoxia might cause a greater sustained rise in blood pressure than hypocapnia hypoxia (13). Numerous arterial blood gas samples were drawn in 33 rats under varying conditions of $FICO_2$, to establish blood gas changes that occur in the same chambers under chronic gas exposure. In the *chronic* experiment, unhandled, sham-air controls, hypocapnic hypoxia (no added CO_2), eucapnic hypoxia (7–10% F_{ICO_2}), and hypercarbic hypoxia (11–14% F_{ICO_2}) groups were studied. Mean arterial pressure was measured in conscious animals at baseline and after 35 days under their respective study conditions. Neither episodic eucapnic nor hypercarbic hypoxia had any additional effect upon changes in chronic diurnal blood pressure compared to hypocapnic hypoxia. These results suggest that the sympathetic nervous system or other neurohumoral systems contributing to *chronic* diurnal blood pressure elevation are maximally stimulated by hypoxia.

It is well known that arousal from sleep, or startle in the awake animal/human, causes sympathetic discharge and other cardiovascular changes similar to those seen with hypoxia. Several studies suggest that arousal and sleep disruption could be important factors in acute and chronic blood pressure changes with apnea (14,15). We were interested in testing whether the chronic effect of repetitive arousal could induce the same chronic blood pressure changes as episodic hypoxia in our model. We exposed 12-week-old ($N = 10$) Sprague Dawley rats in individual chambers to recurrent buzzer noise (500 Hz, 100 dB) 6 out of every 30 sec, 8 hr/day for 35 days (16). Nine sham rats housed in identical cages were not exposed to noise. An infrared beam positioned at the end of each cage quantified motion by registering the number of times the rat broke the beam per 8-hr "sleep" period. Mean arterial pressure was invasively measured in unrestrained conscious animals at baseline and at the end of 35 days of their respective conditions. All animals showed a significant *acute* blood pressure response to noise that diminished after 30–60 min of noise exposure. Acoustic stimulated rats showed higher movement activity throughout the day than did the nonstimulated rats, but there was no difference in mean arterial pressure in either group before and after the respective 35-day experimental conditions.

Establishing that the sympathetic nervous system plays a direct role in the chronic blood pressure response to episodic hypoxia, we undertook a study to further dissect how the various components of the sympathetic nervous system interacted (17). We were interested in the specific roles of the renal artery sympathetics and the adrenal medulla in the chronic blood pressure increase. Male Sprague Dawley rats had either adrenal medullectomy or bilateral renal artery denervation, or an abdominal incision only (sham surgery). Demedullated rats, sham-operated rats, and renal denervated rats were subjected to episodic hypoxia as described above for 35 days. Control groups were subjected either to compressed air or were left unhandled. Both adrenal demedullation and separately, renal artery denervation, eliminated the chronic diurnal systemic blood pressure increase in response to episodic hypoxia, whereas sham-operated controls continued to show no elevation. Plasma and renal tissue catecholamines at the end the experiment confirmed successful adrenal demedullation or renal denervation in the respective groups. In the sham-operated, hypoxia-exposed rats, renal tissue norepinephrine was elevated five times baseline at the end of the hypoxia period.

The results of this study suggest that adrenal-secreted, circulating epinephrine may be an important regulator of blood pressure in the setting of chronic episodic hypoxia (17). There are several ways that combined action of adrenal epinephrine and renal artery sympathetic nerves may both bring about diurnal blood pressure elevation. One is that circulating epinephrine binds to presynaptic sympathetic nervous system receptors, enhancing norepinephrine release across the neural junction, facilitating neurogenic vasoconstriction as described by Floras et al. (18,19). It is postulated that the secretion of renin may persist in the face of renal artery denervation because of the existence of an extrarenal renin-producing site that is stimulated by circulating adrenal epinephrine (20,21).

IV. The Renin Angiotensin System in Chronic Episodic Hypoxia

Sympathetic nerves may regulate plasma renin activity, affecting chronic blood pressure level through the renin-angiotensin system. On the basis of the results of the renal denervation experiment, we examined plasma renin activity in 24 Sprague Dawley rats after 35 days of episodic hypoxia (22). Half of the group was treated with losartan (an angiotensin 1 [AT_1] receptor blocker) 15 mg/kg/day by gastric gavage and half were treated with vehicle only. The groups were divided as follows: five rats remained unhandled to establish plasma renin activity normals for our methods and another five unhandled rats received losartan; seven rats were exposed to episodic hypoxia without losartan and seven were exposed to episodic hypoxia with losartan. Both at the beginning and at the end of the experiment, arterial blood was rapidly withdrawn from quiet, resting rats for later measurement of angiotensin II and plasma renin activity. In the episodic hypoxia vehicle and the episodic hypoxia losartan-treated rats, blood pressure was monitored at room air rest (unrestrained) using implanted telemetry sensors (Data Sciences, St. Paul, MN) at baseline and every seventh day throughout a 35-day period. In the remaining rats, blood pressure was measured at baseline and day 36 only, by indwelling arterial catheter (Fig. 4).

Episodic hypoxia was associated with a 12 mmHg increase in mean arterial pressure (Fig. 4, BPs) and a three-fold rise in plasma renin activity as

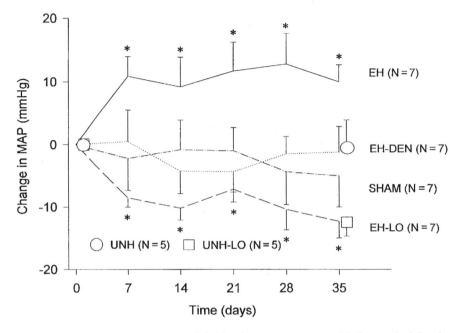

Figure 4 Change in mean arterial blood pressure over a 35-day period in six groups of rats exposed to experimental or control conditions. Only the episodic hypoxia (EH) rats showed significant elevation of BP above baseline. Both losartan-treated groups (EH-LO, UNH-LO) showed a significant fall in BP by day 35 of treatment. The open circle and square represent the UNH and UNH-LO groups, respectively. Blood pressure and heart rate were measured by indwelling arterial catheter in these two groups as opposed to telemetry in the other groups, thus making data available only on days before and after the 35-day exposure. EH, episodic hypoxia; EH-DEN, episodic hypoxia with bilateral renal artery denervation; SHAM, sham operated, exposed to episodic compressed air; EH-LO, episodic hypoxia with losartan; UNH, unhandled; UNH-LO, unhandled rats given losartan. (*) Indicates a significant change from baseline at $p < 0.05$ or greater. (From Ref. 22.)

compared to no increase in blood pressure or plasma renin activity in the unhandled controls (Fig. 5). Unhandled losartan-treated animals showed a fall in mean arterial pressure over 35 days. Losartan effectively blocked the blood pressure response to episodic hypoxia. The results show that plasma renin activity *increases* in response to episodic hypoxia and that an AT_1 antagonist prevents the rise in blood pressure. As would be expected in any study with AT_1 blockade, losartan caused a small fall in mean arterial pressure in the unhandled and episodic hypoxia rats along with a large

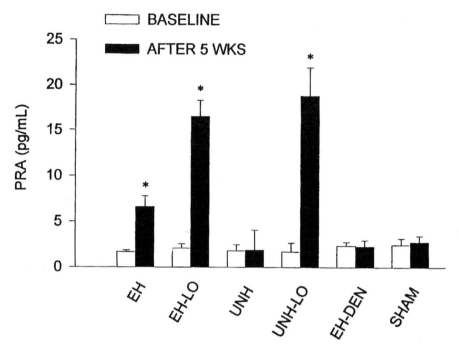

Figure 5 Plasma renin activity at baseline and 35 days in all study and control groups. Plasma renin activity in episodic hypoxia exposed group was elevated about three times baseline, whereas there was no change in plasma renin activity in the EH-DEN, SHAM, or UNH groups. Both groups treated with losartan (EH-LO and UNH-LO) showed marked increases in plasma renin activity, as would be expected with AT_1 blockade alone. (*) Indicates a significant change from baseline at $p < 0.05$ or greater. (From Ref. 22.)

increase in plasma renin activity in all treated animals (Fig. 5). These data indicate that chronic blood pressure elevation from episodic hypoxia is at least in part regulated through the renin–angiotensin system.

These two studies suggest that chronic blood pressure elevation in episodic hypoxia is regulated by increased sympathetic activity induced by chemoreceptor stimulation, acting through renal nerve sympathetics to increase plasma renin and perhaps renal tissue renin–angiotensin system activity. We further analyzed the relationship between episodic hypoxia and the effect of renal sympathetics on sustained blood pressure elevation by challenging the rat with conflicting stimuli (23). On the one hand, episodic hypoxia should chronically increase renal nerve activity, whereas a high-salt diet expanding intravascular volume should suppress renal nerve activity and the systemic renin–angiotensin system. Separate groups of male Sprague Dawley rats were fed high-salt (8%), ad-lib salt, or low-salt (0.1%) diets for 7 weeks: 2 weeks wash-in for baseline blood pressure measurement and 5 weeks of experimental conditions. Beginning after 2 weeks of diet, rats in each salt group were subjected to episodic hypoxia, whereas controls remained unhandled under normoxic conditions.

Mean arterial pressure remained at basal levels in all nonepisodic hypoxia controls as well as high-salt diet–episodic hypoxia exposed rats. The ad-lib and low-salt episodic hypoxia rats showed an increase in mean arterial pressure from 106 and 104 mmHg at baseline to 112 and 113 mmHg, respectively ($p < 0.05$). Whole kidney renin mRNA was suppressed in high-salt controls and episodic hypoxia rats, whereas kidney AT_1 receptor mRNA showed opposite changes. Suppression of the renin–angiotensin system with a high-salt diet blocked the increase in mean arterial pressure in episodic hypoxia challenged rats, in part by suppression of local tissue renin levels. This implies that the systemic volume stimulus from a high-salt diet appears to supercede (block) the episodic hypoxia-induced sympathetic signal transmitted via the renal nerves to increase renal sympathetic output. It was surprising that the effects of low salt and episodic hypoxia on blood pressure and kidney renin mRNA were not additive, but this may reflect the tendency for renin mRNA to return to baseline levels after 20 days in low-salt animals (24). These data suggest that although the effect of episodic hypoxia upon the kidney via renal sympathetics may in part contribute to systemic blood pressure elevation, the local tissue renin angiotensin system may play a primary role. Upregulation of the tissue angiotensin system appears necessary for the chronic blood pressure changes that occur from episodic hypoxia.

V. Vascular Tone in Chronic Episodic Hypoxia

Although increased sympathetic activity is evident in hypertension resulting from chronic episodic hypoxia, the method by which sympathetic activity is translated into increased blood pressure is unknown. One method could be increased vascular tone persisting beyond the period of episodic hypoxia. To examine vascular tone in 35-day episodic hypoxia exposed rats, we used in vivo video microscopy to examine arteriolar reactivity in the cremaster muscle (25). Video microscoscopy is used to measure blood vessel diameter changes in response to various vasoactive amines. Cremaster muscles of post-35-day episodic hypoxia and control rats were exposed to varying doses of norepinephrine, acetylcholine, and endothelin-1. In an additional experiment, chronic episodic hypoxia and control rats were given one dose of a nitric oxide synthase (eNOS) inhibitor: N^g-nitro-L-arginine methyl ester (L-NAME). We also examined eNOS mRNA levels from the kidneys of episodic hypoxia-stimulated and control rats. Telemetry-monitored episodic hypoxia rats showed a 16 mmHg increase in mean arterial pressure over 35 days, whereas control rats (unhandled, no episodic hypoxia) showed no change. The responses to norepinephrine and endothelin were similar for both groups. Acetylcholine vasodilation of arterioles in episodic hypoxia rats was significantly attenuated when compared to that of nonhypoxia controls (Fig. 6). The degree of vasoconstriction in response to blockade of the nitric oxide system by (L-NAME) was significantly less (83% of baseline diameter with L-NAME) for arterioles of episodic hypoxia rats compared to that for controls (61% of baseline diameter), implying lower basal resting nitric oxide release in the episodic hypoxia rats. Whole kidney mRNA eNOS levels were not different between groups. These indicate that chronic elevation of blood pressure associated with episodic hypoxia involves increased peripheral resistance from decreased basal release or production of nitric oxide.

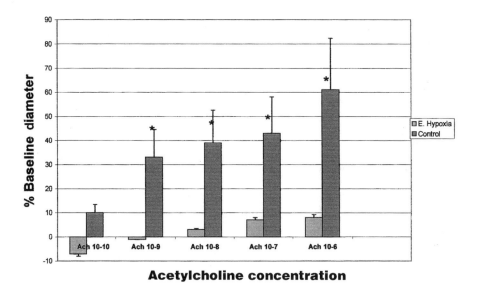

Figure 6 Dose response curve for acetylcholine starting with vessels approximately 50% constricted with norepinephrine 10^{-7}. Horizontal axis shows increasing dose of acetylcholine administered every 5 min, and vertical axis is mean diameter as a percent of baseline or "percent relaxation." (*) Indicates that values for acetylcholine vary from controls by $p < 0.05$ for concentrations 10^{-8} to 10^{-6}. (From Ref. 25.)

VI. Conclusions

Summarizing the studies to date in this model, our data create the following scenario regarding chronic recurrent episodic hypoxia and diurnal blood pressure. Acute and chronic hypoxia recurrently stimulate the peripheral chemoreceptors, probably through increased alpha receptor activity (12). This is verified by observations of acutely increased splanchnic nerve sympathetic activity, and blood pressure and heart rate change in response to episodic hypoxia. Diurnal (chronic or nonstimulated) increased blood pressure changes are blocked by chemical sympathectomy (11). It appears that both the adrenal gland, via circulating epinephrine, and renal sympathetics participate in the chronic diurnal blood pressure elevation (17). These two end organs of sympathetic activity may act synergistically in the setting of episodic hypoxia by adrenal release of epinephrine with potentiation of sympathetic nervous system transmission and/or by facilitating the release of renin through alpha receptors in the kidney or from nonrenal sites (20,21). Supporting this is demonstration of increased renin–angiotensin system activation in episodic hypoxia as well as inhibition of the blood pressure response to episodic hypoxia by AT_1 receptor blockers (22). Finally, it appears that this sympathetic overactivity is somehow translated into chronically increased arteriolar vascular tone as a result of decreased NO activity or responsiveness (25). The exact mechanism for this remains unknown, and there is always the possibility that there is a direct effect of episodic hypoxia on the vascular endothelium.

Evidence for a link between systemic hypertension and sleep apnea, and possibly atherosclerotic events (acute myocardial occlusion, stroke) in middle and older age males is strong. The slow time course and delayed diagnosis of sleep apnea and hypertension clearly limit our ability to examine such possibilities in humans until specific mechanisms of diurnal hypertension are worked out. It is extremely important to develop animal preparations which can mimic some manifestations of obstructive sleep apnea over a reasonable time period, allowing study of likely scenarios in the relationship between obstructive sleep apnea and hypertension, stroke, myocardial infarction, and early cardiovascular death. The flexibility of the episodic hypoxia rat allows manipulation of stress factors, strain, or species, and control of exposure periods. It also allows many invasive functional and anatomic studies not possible in humans, producing a better understanding of endocrine, neural, and renal mechanisms operating to elevate blood pressure. Similar mechanisms of blood pressure control and analogous diurnal and sleeping blood pressure patterns between man and rat lend further validity to the episodic hypoxia rat preparation. Such knowledge may enhance management of hypertension in patients with sleep-disordered breathing.

References

1. Lavie, P., Ben-Yosef, R., and Rubin, A. E. Prevalence of sleep apnea syndrome among patients with essential hypertension. Am J Cardiol 1985; 55:1019–1022.
2. Kales, A., Cadieux, R. J., Shaw, L. C., Vela-Bueno, A., Bixler, E. O., Schneck, D. W., Locke, T. W., and Soldatos, C. R. Sleep apnoea in a hypertensive population. Lancet 1984; ii:1005–1008.
3. Fletcher, E. C., DeBenke, R. D., Lovoi, M. S., and Gorin, A. B. Undiagnosed sleep apnea in patients with essential hypertension. Ann Int Med 1985; 103:190–195.
4. Williams, A. J., Houston, D., Finberg, S., Lam, C., Kinney, J. L., and Santiago, S. Sleep apnoea syndromes and essential hypertension. Am J Cardio 1985; 55:1019–1022.
5. O'Donnell, C. P., Ayuse, T., King, E. D., Schwartz, A. R., Smith, P. L., and Robotham, J. L. Airway obstruction during sleep increases blood pressure without arousal. J Appl Physiol 1996; 80:773–781.
6. Shepard, J. W., Jr. Gas exchange and hemodynamics during sleep. Med Clin North Am 1985; 69:1243–1263.
7. Korner, P. I. and White, S. W. Circulatory control in hypoxia by the sympathetic nerves and adrenal medulla. J Physiol 1966; 184:272–290.
8. Johnson, T. S., Young, J. B., and Landsberg, L. Sympathoadrenal response to acute and chronic hypoxia in the rat. J Clin Invest 1983; 71:1263–1272.
9. Fletcher, E. C., Lesske, J., Qian, W., Miller, C. C., and Unger, T. Repetitive, episodic hypoxia causes diurnal elevation of systemic blood pressure in rats. Hypertension 1992; 19:555–561.
10. Fletcher, E. C., Lesske, J., Behm, R., Miller, C. C., and Unger, T. Carotid chemoreceptors, systemic blood pressure, and chronic episodic hypoxia mimicking sleep apnea. J Appl Physiol 1992; 72:1978–1984.
11. Fletcher, E. C., Lesske, J., Culman, J., Miller, C. C., and Unger, T. Sympathetic denervation blocks blood pressure elevation in episodic hypoxia. Hypertension 1992; 20:612–619.
12. Bao, G. and Fletcher, E. C. Mechanism of acute blood pressure elevation during episodic hypercapnic hypoxia in rats simulating sleep apnea. J Appl Physiol 1997; 82(4):1071–1078.
13. Fletcher, E. C., Bao, G., and Miller, C. C. Effect of recurrent episodic hypocapnic, eucapnic, and hypercapic hypoxia on systemic blood pressure. J Appl Physiol 1995; 78(4):1516–1521.
14. Ringler, J., Basner, R. C., Shannon, R., Schwartzstein, R., Manning, H., Weinberger, S. E., and Weiss, J. W. Hypoxemia alone does not explain blood pressure elevations after obstructive apneas. J Appl Physiol 1990; 69(6):2143–2148.
15. Ringler, J. E., Garpestad, R. C., Basner, R. C., and Weiss, J. W. Systemic blood pressure elevation after airway occlusion during NREM sleep. Am J Respir Crit Care Med 1994; 150:1062–1066.

16. Bao, G., Metreveli, N., and Fletcher, E. C. Acute and chronic blood pressure response to recurrent acoustic arousal in rats. Am J Hypertens 1999; 12:504–510.

17. Bao, G., Metreveli, N., Li, R., Taylor, A., and Fletcher, E. C. Blood pressure response to chronic episodic hypoxia: role of the sympathetic nervous system. J Appl Physiol 1997; 83(1):95–101.

18. Floras, J. S., Aylward, P. E., Victor, R. G., Mark, A. L., and Abboud, F. M. Epinephrine facilitates neurogenic vasoconstriction in humans. J Clin Invest 1988; 81:1265–1274.

19. Floras, J. S., Aylward, P. E., Mark, A. L., and Abboud, F. M. Adrenalin facilitates neurogenic vasoconstriction in borderline hypertensive subjects. J Hypertens 1990; 8:443–448.

20. Blair, M. L., Hisa, H., Sladek, C. D., Radke, K. J., and Gengo, F. M. Dual adrenergic control of renin during non-hypotensive hemorrhage in conscious dogs. Am J Physiol 1991; 260:E910–E919.

21. Blair, M. L. and Gengo, F. M. β-adrenergic control of renin in sodium-deprived conscious dogs: renal versus extrarrenal location. Can J Physiol Pharmacol 1995; 73:1198–1202.

22. Fletcher, E. C., Bao, G., and Li, R. Renin activity and blood pressure in response to chronic episodic hypoxia. Hypertension 1999; 34:309–314.

23. Fletcher, E., Orolinova, N., and Bader, M. Mean arterial pressure change in response to chronic episodic hypoxia: the effect of salt loading. Am Rev Respir Crit Care Med 2001; 163(5):A36.

24. Holmer, S., Eckardt, K. U., LeHir, M., Schricker, K., Riegger, G., and Kurtz, A. Influence of dietary NaCl intake on renin gene expression in the kidneys and adrenal glands of rats. Pflügers Arch 1993; 425:62–67.

25. Tahawi, Z., Orolinova, N., Joshua, G., Bader, M., and Fletcher, E. C. Altered vascular reactivity in arterioles of chronic intermittent hypoxic rats. J Appl Physiology 2001; 90(5):207–213.

7

A Chronic Canine Model of Obstructive Sleep Apnea

R. JOHN KIMOFF

McGill University Health Centre
Montreal, Quebec, Canada

I. Introduction

Obstructive sleep apnea (OSA) is a prevalent disorder that is characterized by repeated episodes of upper airway obstruction during sleep (1–3). Upper airway closure results in reduction or cessation of breathing, leading to progressive hypoxemia and hypercapnia and increasing inspiratory efforts against the occluded airway. These stimuli ultimately provoke arousal from sleep, which leads to restoration of upper airway patency and resumption of breathing. An increasing body of clinical and epidemiological literature indicates that the sleep fragmentation and recurrent hypoxemia associated with OSA lead to a host of important neuropsychological, cardiovascular, respiratory control, and other disturbances, which in turn result in substantial morbidity and mortality (3–5). However, the investigation of the mechanisms by which these complications are produced has been hampered by the methodologic restrictions inherent to investigations involving humans, and by the fact that once the human condition comes to clinical attention, it has typically been present for some time. It is therefore difficult to determine which abnormalities represent a primary

199

factor contributing to the disorder, a secondary complication of it, or an indirectly associated comorbidity.

In view of these considerations, we undertook (in the laboratory of Eliot Phillipson at the University of Toronto) to develop a large-animal model of OSA designed specifically to study the consequences of repeated upper airway obstruction during sleep. The general concept was to use adult animals whose normal physiology could be well characterized in the laboratory, subject the animals to repeated airway occlusion throughout sleep while evaluating physiologic changes over time, and then withdraw the animals from the system and assess further physiologic changes during recovery. The main objectives were to determine the effects of airway occlusion on sleep architecture and on respiratory control and cardiovascular function during wakefulness. We also aimed to evaluate the relative contributions of sleep fragmentation and hypoxemia in mediating the changes observed during the production of repeated airway obstruction.

The studies using this model (6–14) have been conducted at the University of Toronto and in my laboratory at McGill University. We have been privileged to work with a highly capable group of collaborators, who are responsible for much of the data presented in this chapter. Their many contributions are acknowledged in the references cited throughout the text, as well as at the end of the chapter. The scope of this chapter will describe the design of the chronic canine model of OSA and the modifications that have been made to it during the course of our studies. The findings during long-term application of the model will then be discussed, including the changes in sleep architecture, respiratory control, arousal responsiveness, and cardiovascular function, including blood pressure, baroreceptor sensitivity, and ventricular function.

II. Model Description

Adult dogs trained to sleep in the laboratory are prepared with a permanent side-hole tracheostomy and then undergo implantation of a subcutaneous telemetry-amplifier device (Data Sciences, Akron, OH) (Fig. 1). Two different models of telemetry unit have been used: initially one with two bipolar bioelectric channels for electroenclphalogram (EEG) and nuchal electromyogram (EMG), and subsequently a unit with an additional channel for monitoring of blood pressure, consisting of a pressure transducer connected to a fluid-filled catheter implanted in the profunda femoris artery (11,12). The telemetry output of EEG, EMG, and blood pressure is transmitted continuously to a series of receivers placed around the perimeter of the animal's cage, which are interconnected via a

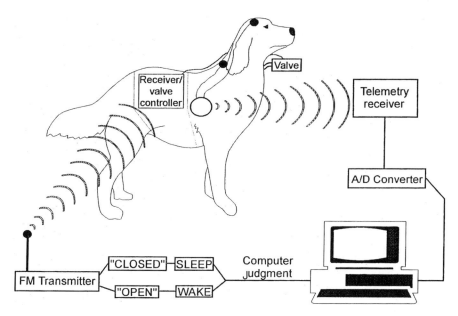

Figure 1 Schematic of OSA model.

multiplexer. The multiplexer selects the strongest signals, i.e., from the receiver closest to the dog. The blood pressure signal is then sent to a personal computer running a commercial data acquisition system for processing of cardiovascular variables (Dataquest IV, Data Sciences). The EEG and EMG signals are sent from the multiplexer to a second personal computer running custom software designed by our group to continuously analyze EEG and EMG via an algorithm described below. The program analyzes the data in 6-sec segments or epochs and identifies wakefulness (W), nonrapid eye movement (NREM) or rapid eye movement (REM) sleep as the preponderant state for each epoch. Thus, a judgment concerning sleep–wake state is produced every 6 sec. After a predetermined number of consecutive epochs of sleep, the computer generates an analog signal that is transmitted to a receiver–controller unit housed in a jacket on the dog's back. This unit controls a silent Plexiglas occlusion valve at the end of the tracheostomy tube, which when activated by the computer, produces airway occlusion. The occlusion is maintained until arousal occurs, which is identified as one epoch of wakefulness. Thus whenever sleep occurs, the airway is obstructed and an apnea ensues, which in turn is relieved when arousal occurs. This sequence of events therefore closely mimics the events that are typical of human OSA. A representative tracing depicting the model in operation is shown in Figure 2.

Advantages of this system include the fact that the animal is freely mobile within its cage, and the equipment can function completely independently. The model can therefore be applied on a continuous basis over many weeks to produce apnea whenever the animal falls asleep. By varying the number of consecutive epochs of sleep required before airway occlusion, the severity of OSA can be varied. During the experiments described below, the model has typically been set to produce a mild degree of OSA (apnea–hypopnea index [AHI] = 15–20 apneas/hr of sleep) for the

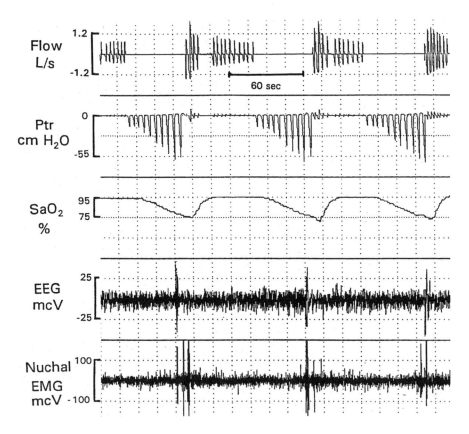

Figure 2 Representative tracing of airway occlusion system during independant operation. Note the repeated occurrence of apnea with resultant hypoxemia and increasing respiratory efforts against the occluded airway, terminating when arousal occurs and the airway occlusion is released.

first 2–4 weeks, and then a severe degree of OSA (AHI 50–60) for the remainder of the intervention period. Another major strength of the model is that each animal serves as its own control. Thus, changes in physiologic variables compared with baseline values which develop during application of the airway occlusion system can be directly attributed to the OSA intervention. Furthermore, as will be described below, the model system can be modified to assess the specific effects of isolated sleep fragmentation or hypoxemia and assess the relative contributions of these factors to the changes observed during repeated airway occlusion.

A. Sleep Analysis Algorithm

The appropriate operation of the model is dependent upon accurate identification of sleep–wake state on a continuous basis. A major step in designing the model was to develop a computerized system for this purpose. The software and hardware were designed in the laboratory, and have been extensively validated by comparison with human scoring of continuous EEG records.

The algorithm for sleep–wake state identification is as follows: The EEG and EMG signals from the multiplexer are filtered (EEG: 1–50 Hz, EMG: 10–100 Hz) and sampled at 300 Hz. The software analyzes 5 sec of data for 1 sec every 6 sec and produces a judgment of sleep versus wake. The EEG frequency is analyzed using the interval histogram technique (6,9,15) to determine the percent of the signal in each of six bandwidths: δ_2 (0.5–2 Hz), δ_1 (2–4 Hz), θ (4–7.5 Hz), α (7.5–13.5 Hz), β_1 (13.5–20 Hz), and β_2 (20–30 Hz). The β_2/δ_1 ratio and the amplitude of the EEG and (moving-averaged) EMG are also determined. The first decision step in the analysis algorithm (6,9) is between NREM versus wake/REM, which is based on EEG frequency. For each animal, a specific upper-limit value β_2/δ_1 ratio during NREM sleep is identified by manual EEG analysis during baseline testing. Thus, epochs with β_2/δ_1 values below the threshold value are identified as NREM sleep. A maximum amplitude cutoff for EEG has been incorporated to compensate for high-amplitude movement artifact deflections, which can be misinterpreted as slow-wave activity and lead to false identification of NREM sleep during W (9). The next decision step in the algorithm is W versus REM, which is judged on the basis of EMG amplitude. During baseline testing, a threshold value for EMG amplitude is identified that reliably distinguishes W from REM sleep and entered in the algorithm for that animal. This system has been shown to reliably detect wake versus sleep during both short- (6) and long-term application of the model (8–10).

B. General Experimental Protocol

The general approach to application of the model to date has been as follows: Following recovery from the preparatory surgery, an animal undergoes baseline measurements over a period of several weeks. These include determination of sleep architecture during overnight operation of the sleep analysis system and measurement of cardiorespiratory variables of interest during quiet wakefulness and sleep during daytime recording sessions. The animal is then placed on the airway occlusion system, with the apparatus being applied continuously 24 hr per day, 7 days per week. Thus, whenever the animal falls asleep, repeated airway occlusions are produced. The exception to this is a period of 4–5 hr each day when the animal is removed from the apparatus to permit cleaning and maintenance of the model equipment, as well as the performance of experimental studies during wakefulness or sleep. During periods when the animal is removed from the model apparatus and other experiments are not being conducted, it is kept under direct observation and prevented from sleeping by verbal or tactile stimulation by the laboratory staff. The model intervention is carried on continuously for a minimum of 8 weeks in most cases, and has been applied for as long as 17 weeks. Following the OSA intervention period, the animal is withdrawn from the model apparatus and once again allowed to sleep without induced airway occlusion. Monitoring of the physiologic variables of interest is then conducted during at least the first 4 weeks of recovery.

The success of long-term application of this model has in general been excellent (8–10,12,14). There have been minor problems of inflammatory reaction to the implanted telemetry equipment which have responded to local treatment, occasional electrode loss or loss of battery power with a need for reimplantation, and occasional malfunction of the airway occlusion valve, such that it fails to close in response to the computer signal. Failure of valve closure can be identified during the routine morning inspection of the epoch-by-epoch record of the previous night's sleep and respiratory events produced by the model software. Several failsafe mechanisms have been incorporated in the occlusion valve to avoid malfunction in the closed position.

C. Model Modification for Acoustic-Induced Sleep Fragmentation

We have also produced a modification of the model to determine the long-term effects of sleep fragmentation without airway occlusion (8,12). The airway occlusion apparatus is replaced by a loudspeaker-amplifier unit such that the computer output which normally generates airway occlusion instead produces an acoustic tone (ramp frequency of 17–30 kHz, with increasing intensity delivered over 10–30 sec), which arouses the dog. This system produces repeated arousals during sleep at a similar frequency to that produced by the original airway occlusion system, but without respiratory disturbance (8). The application of this modification of the model is described further below.

III. Effects of the OSA Model on Sleep Architecture

The effects of long-term OSA on sleep architecture were formally assessed by Horner et al. (9) in 4 animals. The computer records (1930–0730 hr) for 4 consecutive nights were analyzed for sleep–wake state during the baseline pre-OSA period, during the OSA intervention period beginning at an average of 85 days into the intervention, and for a variable number of nights during the recovery phase after withdrawal of the airway occlusion system. The model produced severe OSA with an average AHI of 59 apneas/hr of sleep (range 54–68) during the latter part of the intervention period. We observed a mild reduction in sleep efficiency (number of epochs of sleep/ total number of epochs) from baseline to OSA, likely due to the sleep-disruptive effect of repeated airway occlusion, and then a marked and statistically significant increase in nocturnal sleep efficiency during the recovery period (9). The mild reduction in nocturnal sleep efficiency during the OSA period contrasted with the marked increase in sleepiness observed during daytime hours when the animals were removed from the occlusion system. As the OSA intervention progressed, considerable effort was required on the part of the laboratory staff to ensure that the animals did not fall asleep without the model system in place.

During the OSA period there was a tendency for the amount of NREM sleep during the night to decrease (from 21% to 17% of epochs) and recover to baseline (21% of epochs) afterward, but these changes did not achieve statistical significance. The major finding with respect to sleep state was a marked increase in REM sleep during recovery from OSA (25% of epochs, compared with 15% of epochs during OSA). This was reminiscent of the abundant REM sleep often observed during acute application of nasal continuous positive airway pressure (CPAP) for human OSA (9,16), which has classically been considered to represent a "rebound" because of REM deprivation associated with OSA. However, the striking finding in our animals was that the amount of REM sleep during the baseline pre-OSA recording (15%) was identical to that during the OSA period. Thus, REM was not decreased by OSA, yet despite this, there was a marked increase in REM during recovery from OSA. This suggests that the repeated disruption of REM (as opposed to a simple reduction in REM duration) may lead to an increased drive to REM sleep which then manifests as a rebound following relief of apnea. Alternatively, there could have been a decreased duration of REM early during OSA that was subsequently restored by compensatory mechanisms during the OSA period, with the REM rebound representing short-term persistence of this compensation. Further studies will be required to more clearly elucidate the mechanisms and neural substrates involved. However, these observations with our model represent a unique new insight into the changes in sleep architecture associated with OSA, and illustrate the advantages of a system in which OSA is produced de novo in a previously normal animal.

IV. Changes in Ventilatory Control During Application of the OSA Model

There has been considerable variability in the findings of studies on ventilatory control and chemoreceptor responsiveness in human OSA (3,17–19). It has been difficult to determine whether observed abnormalities represent sequelae of sleep-disordered breathing or a primary underlying defect of control that may predispose to OSA. The use of our model has provided new insights into these issues. We formally assessed the effects of OSA on ventilatory control (10) in 5 dogs subjected to the airway occlusion version of the model for an average of 15 weeks (range 12–17 weeks). The degree of OSA was again severe for the majority of the intervention period with a mean AHI = 57.5 $\pm$ 4.5 events/hr. No significant changes in oxygen saturation (SaO$_2$) during quiet breathing were observed during either wakefulness or sleep. There were minor but statistically significant changes observed in the pattern of resting ventilation during wakefulness for the OSA compared with the preintervention control period, with a shift to a slightly deeper, slower respiratory pattern due to an increase in both Ti (1.2 $\pm$ 0.1 sec [OSA] versus 1.0 $\pm$ 0.1 [CL]) and Te (2.6 $\pm$ 0.3 sec [OSA] versus 2.1 $\pm$ 0.2 [CL]), and in tidal volume (0.31 $\pm$ 0.20 L [OSA] versus 0.28 $\pm$ 0.02 [CL]), with a slight overall reduction in minute ventilation. Despite the reduction in minute ventilation, P$_{ET}$CO$_2$ decreased slightly (37.0 $\pm$ 1.3 mmHg [OSA] versus 38.1 $\pm$ 1.6 [CL]), likely due to reduced dead space ventilation associated with the increased tidal volume.

Similar changes in breathing pattern were observed for unobstructed breathing during both NREM and REM sleep, although the change in rate was offset by the increased tidal volume such that minute ventilation did not change significantly. Values for all variables during the recovery period tended to return to baseline. Thus, long-term application of the model for up to 4 months led to minor changes in resting breathing, but did not result in significant hypoventilation during wakefulness or sleep. Also of note, the variability for respiratory timing variables was not greater during either wakefulness or sleep for the OSA period, and there was no evidence of periodic breathing during unobstructed breathing associated with the OSA intervention.

The effects of induced OSA on ventilatory responses to hypoxia and hypercapnia were also assessed during wakefulness and sleep, using standard rebreathing techniques (10). The most striking finding was a significant decrease in the ventilatory response to hypoxia during wakefulness at the end of the OSA period. This was characterized by both a shift to the right and reduction in slope of the ventilation versus SaO_2 curve (Fig. 3). A reduction in hypoxic ventilatory responses was also observed for NREM and REM sleep, characterized as a right-ward shift in the curve, without a significant change in slope (Fig. 3). The reduction in minute ventilation was due exclusively to a reduction in the breathing frequency response, which in turn was due to a prolongation of Te. Significant reductions in breathing frequency were seen at all levels of SaO_2 recorded for each of W, NREM, and REM sleep during the OSA intervention period. During the recovery phase, the hypoxic ventilatory responses returned to baseline values during W, and tended to overshoot and increase slightly compared with baseline values during NREM and REM sleep (10).

Hypercapnic ventilatory responses showed a different pattern of change from hypoxic responses during the OSA period. The ventilation versus PCO_2 curve was shifted slightly to the left, i.e., ventilation was mildly

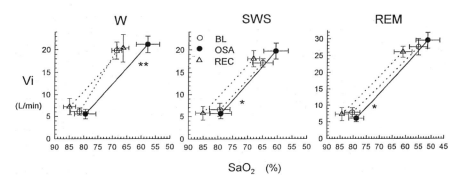

Figure 3 Hypoxic ventilatory responses during wakefulness, slow-wave NREM (SWS) and REM sleep at baseline (open circles), during OSA (closed circles) and recovery (triangles). *$p < 0.05$ for OSA versus baseline and recovery for shift of the curve; **$p < 0.05$ versus baseline and recovery for both a decrease in slope and shift of the curve. (From Ref. 10.)

increased at all levels of P_{CO_2}, without a change in slope during both W and NREM sleep, whereas responses showed no significant change during REM. The increase in ventilation was predominantly due to an increase respiratory frequency response to hypercapnia, particularly during NREM sleep. During the recovery phase, ventilatory responses reverted to baseline (10).

Thus, application of the OSA model led to a selective attenuation of the ventilatory response to hypoxia, whereas there was a mild increase in CO_2 sensitivity. The precise mechanisms underlying these changes remain to be elucidated. It seems unlikely that sleep fragmentation would be the sole mechanism, given the divergent changes in hypoxic and hypercapnic responses. However, differential effects of sleep fragmentation cannot be discounted (19), and this issue could be further evaluated using the acoustic-induced sleep fragmentation system. The change in hypoxic responsiveness may represent an adaptive response elicited by repeated exposure to hypoxemia (10). The increase in central (CO_2) chemosensitivity suggests that reduced hypoxic responsiveness is most likely mediated through adaptations in carotid body sensitivity to hypoxia. Alternatively, given that blood pressure increases in these animals (see Sec. VI.A.), it may be that the pressor response to hypoxia also increases and the reduced ventilatory response is related to an inhibitory effect of blood pressure on breathing.

The relatively minor changes in resting ventilation and chemoreceptor responsiveness resulting from the airway occlusion intervention are in keeping with the clinical observation that human OSA patients without other major cardiorespiratory illness do not demonstrate major respiratory control abnormalities during wakefulness. Our findings suggest, however, that diminished hypoxic ventilatory responsiveness may be an early factor leading to the development of hypoventilation during wakefulness when this does occur. Most studies indicate that lung function abnormalities are an important predisposing factor in the development of awake hypoventilation in severe OSA (17,18). The detailed mechanisms by which repeated airway occlusion during sleep interacts with chemoreceptor function and abnormal respiratory system mechanics to lead to sustained hypoventilation could be investigated in future studies applying simulated respiratory loads to the unoccluded tracheostomy tube of the OSA model.

V. Changes in Arousal Responses to Respiratory Stimuli During Application of the OSA Model

Numerous studies have provided indirect evidence of impaired arousal responses to respiratory stimuli in human OSA (19–22). Such an impairment has been hypothesized to contribute to apnea lengthening, and thereby a progression of OSA severity over time. However, direct evidence that this occurs has been lacking. During the course of the ventilatory control studies just described, the arousal thresholds to hypoxia and hypercapnia were determined for both NREM and REM sleep at baseline, during OSA and after recovery (10). The SaO_2 at arousal from NREM sleep decreased significantly during OSA (mean arousal $SaO_2 = 60.6 \pm 4.2\%$ [OSA] versus $65.0 \pm 3.5\%$ [baseline]) and tended to decrease for REM as well (mean arousal $SaO_2 = 55.0 \pm 3.5\%$ [OSA] versus $51.4 \pm 4.7\%$ [baseline]). The values during recovery increased slightly above baseline values (10). In contrast, the mean values for PCO_2 at arousal showed no change across the three study periods during NREM sleep, and showed a slight but nonsignificant increase during REM in the OSA period. Thus, in our model, OSA produced a specific impairment in the arousal response to hypoxia. Although this change parallels the change in hypoxic ventilatory response, there were increases in both the minute ventilation and tidal volume at arousal during hypoxic rebreathing in the OSA period, suggesting that arousal responses to a variety of stimuli, including carotid body and mechanoreceptor stimuli, may become impaired in OSA (19–22).

We also systematically assessed the changes in arousal responses to airway occlusion during application of the OSA model. Brooks et al. (8) reported findings in 4 animals subjected initially to the airway occlusion model, and then following 6 months of recovery, to the acoustic-induced sleep fragmentation model. Application of the airway occlusion model resulted in a progressive lengthening of apnea duration (Fig. 4), increased respiratory effort at arousal, and decreased SaO_2 at arousal for both NREM and REM sleep, which rapidly recovered following withdrawal from the apnea model. The values for apnea duration and other respiratory variables tended to plateau after approximately 4 weeks of severe OSA, but increased progressively up to 10 weeks in some animals. When these same animals were subjected to repeated acoustic-induced sleep fragmentation, with a similar severity of sleep disruption to that during the airway occlusion intervention, it was found that arousal responses to acutely induced airway occlusion during sleep became blunted to a similar degree to that during the nocturnal airway occlusion intervention.

This study therefore directly demonstrates that impaired arousal responses to respiratory stimuli develop over time in OSA and lead to a progression of apnea duration and worsening of nocturnal O_2 desaturation. These findings extend the observations of other previous short-term studies using other animal models (23–25) and provide new information on the evolution over many weeks of changes in arousal responsiveness. The findings also provide clear evidence that the sleep fragmentation associated with OSA plays a major role both in the short- and long-term (Fig. 4)

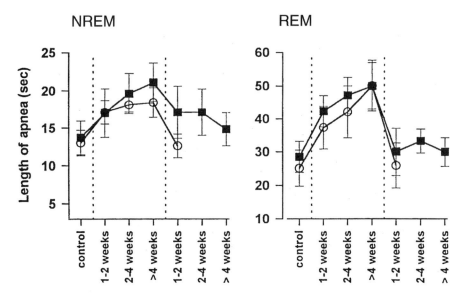

Figure 4 Changes in mean time to arousal in response to induced airway occlusion during OSA (filled squares) and sleep fragmentation (open circles). Data to the left of the first dotted line are for the baseline period, data between the two dotted lines are for the intervention period, and data to the right of the second dotted line are for recovery. (From Ref. 8.)

changes in arousal responses to respiratory stimuli. Future studies with the model could provide further insight into the detailed mechanisms involved in both the initial deterioration in arousal responses and the maintenance of these responses during the plateau phase.

VI. Changes in Cardiovascular Function During Application of the OSA Model

A. Hypertension

There is currently considerable accumulated evidence linking human OSA to cardiovascular disease (4,12–14,26,27). One of the strongest associations in this regard is between OSA and hypertension. However, this association has been controversial, because although hypertension is prevalent among OSA patients, there are potential confounding variables such as obesity that could account for this relationship. Recent large cohort studies have provided statistical evidence that OSA is an independant risk factor for hypertension (26). However this biostatistical association does not prove causality.

We have used the OSA model to (1) determine whether OSA per se leads to sustained hypertension during wakefulness, and (2) evaluate the relative contributions of repeated airway occlusion versus isolated sleep fragmentation in producing changes in blood pressure. Brooks et al. (12) studied 4 animals at baseline, during 1–3 months of OSA and then during 1 month of recovery. At least 6 months after termination of the OSA protocol, the animals were then subjected to 1–2 months of acoustic-induced sleep fragmentation as described above.

The findings are depicted in Figure 5. Both repeated airway occlusion and acoustic-induced sleep fragmentation were associated with nocturnal increases in blood pressure, which resolved rapidly as of the first night following withdrawal from the model system. However, repeated airway occlusion during sleep led to a sustained increase in blood pressure during the daytime, whereas this did not occur with acoustic-induced sleep fragmentation. The increase in daytime blood pressure with OSA was observed in all 4 animals and ranged from 6 to 27 mmHg (mean peak increase $= 15.7 \pm 4.3$ mmHg). Following withdrawal of the airway occlusion system, the blood pressure fell to baseline levels over a 1- to 3-week period.

These findings represent the first direct evidence that repeated episodes of upper airway obstruction during sleep can lead to sustained increases in

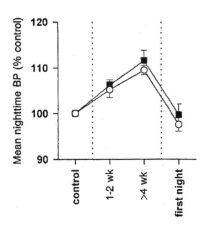 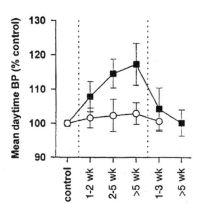

Figure 5 Mean nocturnal (left panel) and daytime (right panel) arterial blood pressure during OSA (filled squares) and sleep fragmentation (open circles) shown in the same format as in Figure 4. Note that both acoustic-induced sleep fragmentation and OSA increased blood pressure at night, whereas sustained hypertension during the daytime occurred only with repeated airway occlusions during sleep. (From Ref. 12.)

blood pressure during the daytime. Furthermore, these changes were reversible following relief of OSA, suggesting that treatment of human OSA may have an important role in the management of hypertension, and thereby contribute to a reduction in cardiovascular risk. The absence of an increase in daytime blood pressure with isolated sleep fragmentation indicates that the respiratory disturbance is of primary importance in mediating the changes in blood pressure associated with OSA.

B. Model Modification for Airway Occlusion Without Hypoxemia

Further experiments are currently underway to examine the interaction of the respiratory disturbance with blood pressure. One major question is whether the changes in blood pressure are more closely linked to the mechanical events associated with airway occlusion or to repeated hypoxemia. To address this, a modification of the airway occlusion system has been produced in which oxygen is delivered to the tracheostomy tube distal to the site of airway occlusion. In this way, apnea episodes with increasing effort against the occluded airway are produced, but in the context of a marked attenuation in associated O_2 desaturation. Data on daytime blood pressure from one animal studied with this system are shown in Figure 6. This animal demonstrated an increase in daytime blood pressure during application of the conventional OSA model, and then a return of blood pressure to baseline following recovery from OSA. When the same animal was subjected to repeated airway occlusion with O_2 supplementation, an increase in daytime blood pressure was not observed over a similar intervention period. Although further experiments are required to confirm these observations in a group of animals, these findings suggest that nocturnal hypoxemia is of key importance in producing the changes in blood pressure associated with OSA. These findings are consistent with observations in other animal models involving either intermittent hypoxia or acute airway occlusion during sleep (28–30) (see also Chap. 6, this volume). Taken together, these observations suggest that nocturnal hypoxemia is a key element in the development of sustained daytime hypertension associated with OSA.

C. Baroreceptor Function

To further evaluate the mechanisms responsible for the blood pressure elevation associated with OSA, Brooks et al. (13) studied baroreceptor function during application of the OSA model (13). The baroreceptor reflex, assessed as the change in heart rate in response to a step change in blood pressure, was determined in 3 dogs at baseline, during 1–3 months of OSA

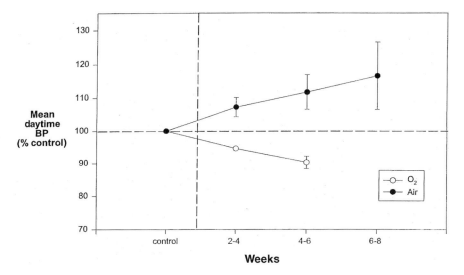

Figure 6 Mean daytime arterial blood pressure at baseline and the end of the intervention period for one animal that underwent standard airway occlusions during sleep (open circles) and then following recovery, underwent airway occlusions with supplemental oxygen (closed circles). *$p < 0.05$ for blood pressure values during OSA versus baseline.

and then during recovery. The changes in R-R interval were assessed during infusion of phenylephrine to increase blood pressure and nitroprusside to lower blood pressure (over a total range of systolic blood pressure of 100–120 mmHg). During the OSA intervention period these animals demonstrated an increase in daytime blood pressure as described above, but no change in resting heart rate. The R-R interval versus systolic blood pressure curve generated during induced changes in blood pressure demonstrated a shift to the right but no change in the slope of the relationship in each of the 3 animals during the OSA intervention period. Thus, the setpoint of baroreceptor function was shifted to a higher level, but the sensitivity of the baroreceptors was not changed. Although the change in baroreceptor sensitivity reported in some forms of essential hypertension was therefore not observed, the increased set point suggests that the baroreceptors could be acting at least indirectly to maintain hypertension. Further studies with the model clearly have the potential to provide insight into the detailed mechanisms of altered baroreceptor function as well as other neural, humoral, or endothelial factors that contribute to sustained hypertension during wakefulness in OSA.

D. Left Ventricular Function

Another area of considerable current interest is the interaction between sleep-disordered breathing and cardiac function (14,27,30). Several lines of evidence suggest that OSA can contribute significantly to ventricular dysfunction and worsen congestive heart failure (27,31). However, prior to our studies with the model, it was unclear whether OSA can impair ventricular function in a previously normal heart.

To evaluate this, Parker et al. (14) studied the acute effects of airway occlusion on ventricular function in 3 dogs after 25–96 days on the OSA model. During daytime sleep recordings, the animals were prepared with a multielectrode impedance catheter positioned in the left ventricle. Using a validated algorithm, measurements from the electrode array on the impedance catheter were used to determine left ventricular (LV) volume. Intraventricular pressure was also available from another port on the cathether and tracheal pressure was used as a measure of intrathoracic pressure during airway occlusions. Left ventricular transmural pressure was then calculated as the difference between intraventricular pressure and tracheal pressure. A representative tracing of events during an airway occlusion are shown in Figure 7. When the data were analyzed for changes associated with consecutive cardiac cycles during an obstructed respiratory effort, in comparison with cycles just prior to the effort, there was a significant increase in LV transmural pressure (i.e., afterload), an increase in LV end-systolic volume, and a trend to decreased end-diastolic volume, with a resultant significant fall in stroke volume. When all cardiac cycles during apneas were compared with pre- and postapneic cycles, the pattern of increased transmural pressure and end-systolic volume was confirmed, with the LV ejection during events falling from $48 \pm 7\%$ (preocclusion) to $43 \pm 7\%$ (post-occlusion). Thus, airway occlusion during sleep led to an acute increase in LV afterload, and a reduction in LV systolic function.

The chronic effects of repeated airway occlusion during sleep were also evaluated. Four animals were studied with two-dimensional echocardiography after 1–3 months of OSA, and the findings were compared with control values. Left ventricular mass tended to increase, but this did not achieve statistical significance. There was a statistically significant increase in LV end-systolic volume from $20 \pm 4\,mL$ (control) to $27 \pm 6\,mL$ (OSA) with a nonsignificant trend for LV end-diastolic to increase as well ($47 \pm 6\,mL$ [control] versus $55 \pm 10\,mL$ [OSA]). Of considerable interest was the significant decrease in LV ejection fraction during wakefulness from $58 \pm 3\%$ under control conditions to $51 \pm 3\%$ at the end of the OSA intervention period.

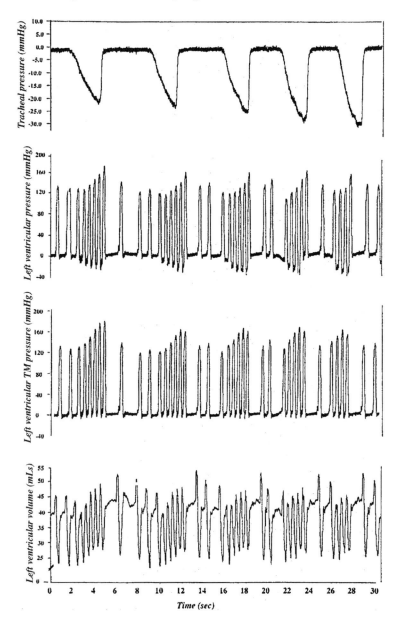

Figure 7 Recordings of tracheal and cardiac pressures and left ventricular volume during obstructed inspiratory efforts against a closed airway. Note the marked increase in LV transmural systolic pressure and volume during the obstructed inspiratory efforts. (From Ref. 14.)

Thus, repeated airway occlusion during sleep led acutely to increased LV afterload and ventricular dilation, and chronic exposure to obstructive apneas produced LV systolic dysfunction during wakefulness. These observations therefore provide strong evidence for a direct link between OSA and cardiac dysfunction. Although our findings on hypertension indicate that hypoxemia is an important factor in producing vascular changes associated with OSA, the acute data on ventricular function strongly suggest that mechanical events during apneas play an important role in the development of chronic ventricular dysfunction. Thus, our model has considerable potential for further studies to elucidate the mechanisms responsible for these interactions, and in this particular context may offer important advantages over small-animal models of intermittent hypoxia, for which inducing upper airway occlusion during sleep is not feasible.

VII. Perspective in Relation to Other Experimental Models

The long-term application of our OSA model has provided important new insights into the effects of repeated airway occlusion during sleep on sleep architecture, respiratory control, arousal responsiveness, and cardiovascular function. Although progress has been made, there is clearly a host of key experimental questions that remain to be addressed, and that could be addressed in future studies using this model. However, as we look forward it is important to consider the strengths and limitations of our model in relation to the other available experimental systems described in this book.

Our model has been criticized because it does not account for one major factor in the pathophysiology of human OSA: the upper airway. In designing our system, we considered numerous possible approaches to producing airway occlusion, including methods that would involve the upper airway. However, a key requirement was feasibility of long-term application, and on the basis of extensive preparatory work, we concluded this would not be possible in a previously normal animal using any approach other than tracheostomy tube occlusion. Furthermore, our first priority in designing the model was to evaluate the consequences of chronic OSA, which our approach of inducing OSA in a previously normal animal that serves as its own control has clearly enabled us to do. Thus, animal models of spontaneously occurring upper airway obstruction during sleep, such as the English bulldog (see Chap. 11) or obese pig model are clearly more appropriate to investigate mechanisms of upper airway collapse during sleep, but with respect to assessing the consequences of OSA suffer the limitations discussed at the beginning of this chapter inherent to animals (and humans) with pre-existing OSA. It should also be noted that although we have not yet conducted such studies, our model does not preclude acute experiments to assess changes in upper airway function during the model intervention.

Another potential disadvantage of our model is that in comparison with small-animal models, e.g., of intermittent hypoxia in rodents, the chronic canine model is very labor intensive and associated with a considerably greater cost per animal (see Chap. 6, this volume). It is clear that the small-animal approach is more appropriate for certain types of investigations, such as those requiring large numbers of animals or technologies that are not currently feasible in large animals, such as the production of genetic knockout strains. However, the use of large animals in our model presents certain advantages. For example, it is currently not feasible to produce mechanical airway obstruction in a spontaneously sleeping rodent. Although intermittent hypoxia is a major factor leading to cardiovascular complications, our findings on ventricular function, as well as those in studies on human congestive heart failure cited above, indicate that mechanical events during apneas play an important role in the development of ventricular dysfunction. Thus, some aspects of cardio-respiratory interactions in OSA will clearly be more appropriately addressed using a long-term model that permits the mechanical events of human OSA to be reproduced.

In conclusion, there is no one ideal model for the study of sleep-disordered breathing. The chronic canine model of OSA we have developed presents both advantages and disadvantages in relation to other experimental systems. However it seems clear that some issues will be best addressed in future studies using a large-animal model in which OSA can be produced de novo in a previously healthy animal. We are therefore confident that our model will continue to provide important new insights into the mechansisms underlying the complications of sleep-disordered breathing, and will also stimulate complementary studies using other model systems.

Acknowledgments

The studies described in this chapter represent a major undertaking by a large group of dedicated investigators. Eliot Phillipson, in whose laboratory much of this work was done, has been the inspiration and guiding force for the investigations using this model. Richard Horner played a major role in all of this work, and Dina Brooks made an enormous contribution to the cardiovascular studies. It is impossible here to specifically mention the numerous contributions of our coinvestigators, but these are all very gratefully acknowledged. The invaluable contribution of our technical staff is also deeply appreciated, in particular that of Vicki Champagne at McGill and most notably Louise Kozar at the University of Toronto.

These studies have been supported by operating grants from the Medical Research Council of Canada, the Canadian Institutes of Health Research, and the Quebec Lung Association. Dr. Kimoff is a clinical research scholar of the Fonds de la Recherche en Santé du Québec.

References

1. Young, T., Palta, M., Dempsey, J., Skatrud, J., Weber, S., and Badr, S. The occurrence of sleep-disordered breathing among middle-aged adults. N Engl J Med 1993; 328:1230–1235.

2. Phillipson, E. A. Sleep apnea—a major public health problem. N Engl J Med 1993; 328:1271–1273.

3. Cistulli, P. A. and Sullivan, C. E. Pathophysiology of sleep apnea. In: Saunders, N. A. and Sullivan, C. E., eds. Sleep and Breathing. 2nd ed. New York: Marcel Dekker, 1994:405–448.

4. Parish, J. M. and Shepard, J. W. Jr. Cardiovascular effects of sleep disorders. Chest 1990; 97:1220–1226.

5. He, J., Kryger, M. H., Zorick, F. J., Conway, W., and Roth, T. Mortality and apnea index in obstructive sleep apnea. Experience in 385 male patients. Chest 1988; 94:9–14.

6. Kimoff, R. J., Makino, H., Horner, R. L., Kozar, L. F., Lue, F., Slutsky, A. S., and Phillipson, E. A. Canine model of obstructive sleep apnea: model description and preliminary application. J Appl Physiol 1994; 76:1810–1817.

7. Pack, A. Canine model of obstructive sleep apnea. J Appl Physiol 1994; 76:1409–1410.

8. Brooks, D., Horner, R. L., Kimoff, R. J., Kozar, L. F., Render-Teixeira, C. L., and Phillipson, E. A. Effect of obstructive sleep apnea versus sleep fragmentation on responses to airway occlusion. Am J Respir Crit Care Med 1997; 155:1609–1617.

9. Horner, R. L., Brooks, D., Kozar, L. F., Leung, E., Hamrahi, H., Render-Teixeira, C. L., Makino, H., Kimoff, R. J., and Phillipson, E. A. Sleep architecture in a canine model of obstructive sleep apnea. Sleep 1998; 21:847–858.

10. Kimoff, R. J., Brooks, D., Horner, R. L., Kozar, L. F., Render-Teixeira, C. L., Champagne, V., Mayer, P. and Phillipson, E. A. Ventilatory and arousal responses to hypoxia and hypercapnia in a canine model of obstructive sleep apnea. Am J Respir Crit Care Med 1997; 156:886–894.

11. Brooks, D., Horner, R. L., Kozar, L. F., Waddell, T. K., Render, C. L., and Phillipson, E. A. Validation of a telemetry system for long-term measurement of blood pressure. J Appl Physiol 1996; 81:1012–1018.

12. Brooks, D., Horner, R. L., Kozar, L. F., Render-Teixeira, C. L., and Phillipson, E. A. Obstructive sleep apnea as a cause of systemic hypertension. Evidence from a canine model. J Clin Invest 1997; 99:106–109.
13. Brooks, D., Horner, R. L., Floras, J. S., Kozar, L. F., Render-Teixeira, C. L., and Phillipson, E. A. Baroreflex control of heart rate in a canine model of obstructive sleep apnea. Am J Respir Crit Care Med 1999; 159:1293–1297.
14. Parker, J. D., Brooks, D., Kozar, L. F., Render-Teixeira, C. L., Horner, R. L., Douglas, B. T., and Phillipson, E. A. Acute and chronic effects of airway obstruction on canine left ventricular performance. Am J Respir Crit Care Med 1999; 160:1888–1896.
15. Kuwahara, H., Higashi, H., Mizuki, Y., Matsunari, S., Tanaka, M., and Inanaga, K. Automatic real-time analysis of human sleep stages by an interval histogram method. Electroencephalogr Clin Neurophysiol 1988; 70:220–229.
16. Issa, F. G. and Sullivan, C. E. The immediate effects of nasal continuous positive airway pressure treatment on sleep pattern in patients with obstructive sleep apnea syndrome. Electroencephalogr Clin Neurophysiol Suppl 1986; 63:10–17.
17. Bradley, T. D., Rutherford, R., Lue, F., Moldofsky, H., Grossman, R. F., Zamel, N., and Phillipson, E. A. Role of diffuse airway obstruction in the hypercapnia of obstructive sleep apnea. Am Rev Respir Dis 1986; 134:920–924.
18. Chan, C. S., Grunstein, R. R., Bye, P. T., Woolcock, A. J., and Sullivan, C. E. Obstructive sleep apnea with severe chronic airflow limitation. Comparison of hypercapnic and eucapnic patients. Am Rev Respir Dis 1989; 140:1274–1278.
19. Kimoff, R. J. Sleep fragmentation in obstructive sleep apnea. Sleep 1996; 19:S61–S66.
20. Kimoff, R. J., Cheong, T. H., Olha, A. E., Charbonneau, M., Levy, R. D., Cosio, M. G., Gottfried, S. B. Mechanisms of apnea termination in obstructive sleep apnea. Role of chemoreceptor and mechanoreceptor stimuli. Am J Respir Crit Care Med 1994; 149:707–714.
21. Montserrat, J. M., Kosmas, E. N., Cosio, M. G., and Kimoff, R. J. Mechanism of apnea lengthening across the night in obstructive sleep apnea. Am J Respir Crit Care Med 1996; 154:988–993.
22. Cala, S. J., Sliwinski, P., Cosio, M. G., and Kimoff, R. J. Effect of topical upper airway anesthesia on apnea duration through the night in obstructive sleep apnea. J Appl Physiol 1996; 81:2618–2626.
23. Fewell, J. E. The effect of short-term sleep fragmentation produced by intense auditory stimuli on the arousal response to upper airway obstruction in lambs. J Dev Physiol 1987; 9:409–417.
24. Fewell, J. E., Williams, B. J., Szabo, J. S., and Taylor, B. J. Influence of repeated upper airway obstruction on the arousal and cardiopulmonary response to upper airway obstruction in lambs. Pediatr Res 1988; 23:191–195.
25. O'Donnell, C. P., King, E. D., Schwartz, A. R., Smith, P. L., and Robotham, J. L. Effect of sleep deprivation on responses to airway obstruction in the sleeping dog. J Appl Physiol 1994; 77:1811–1818.

26. Hla, K. M., Young, T. B., Bidwell, T., Palta, M., Skatrud, J. B., and Dempsey, J. Sleep apnea and hypertension. A population-based study. Ann Intern Med 1994; 120:382–388.
27. Bradley, T. D. and Floras, J. S. Pathophysiologic and therapeutic implications of sleep apnea in congestive heart failure. J Card Fail 1996; 2:223–240.
28. Fletcher, E. C., Lesske, J., Qian, W., Miller, C. C. III, and Unger, T. Repetitive, episodic hypoxia causes diurnal elevation of blood pressure in rats. Hypertension 1992; 19:555–561.
29. O'Donnell, C. P., King, E. D., Schwartz, A. R., Robotham, J. L., and Smith, P. L. Relationship between blood pressure and airway obstruction during sleep in the dog. J Appl Physiol 1994; 77:1819–1828.
30. Scharf, S. M. Cardiovascular effects of airways obstruction. Lung 1991; 169:1–23.
31. Malone, S., Liu, P. P., Holloway, R., Rutherford, R., Xie, A., and Bradley, T. D. Obstructive sleep apnoea in patients with dilated cardiomyopathy: effects of continuous positive airway pressure. Lancet 1991; 338:1480–1484.

Part Four

**NATURALLY OCCURRING SLEEP-RELATED
BREATHING DISORDERS**

8

The Preterm Lamb
A Unique Animal Model of Neonatal Respiratory Instability

JEAN-PAUL PRAUD and
JULIE ARSENAULT   **SYLVAIN RENOLLEAU**

University of Sherbrooke   Armand-Trousseau Children's Hospital
Sherbrooke, Quebec, Canada   Paris, France

I. Introduction

One of the major concerns for newborn infants as they adapt to extrauterine life is respiratory control immaturity, which is responsible for respiratory instability. Characterized by short apneas (3–20 sec) and episodes of periodic breathing, these manifestations are usually without consequences in term newborns, even when present for long periods of time. This situation is very different in preterm infants however, in whom respiratory system immaturity can lead to prolonged and repetitive apneas, and can thereby have disastrous effects on gas exchange.

Apnea of prematurity is defined as "a pause in breathing of greater than 20 sec or one of less than 20 sec and associated with cyanosis, marked pallor, hypotonia or bradycardia" (1), with no known etiology except prematurity. Overall, 50% of all preterm newborns will present apneas of prematurity; this number reaches 90% for those weighing less than 1000 g. Many basic questions about apneas of prematurity are as of yet unresolved, including their pathophysiology, the involvement of upper airways, and the various determinants of hypoxia and bradycardia following only some of the apneas. Furthermore, management of apneas of prematurity still poses daily problems for neonatologists. Indeed, usual treatment modalities such as respiratory stimulants and noninvasive ventilatory support (i.e., nasal/pharyngeal continuous positive airway pressure or intermittent positive pressure ventilation) are not always effective, and tracheal intubation for mechanical ventilation often needs to be implemented (2). Untreated apneas of prematurity carry major risks, including immediate, life-threatening effects on gas exchange, and/or lifelong neurological sequelae because of repeated cerebral hypoxia (3,4). Apneas of prematurity are thus frequently responsible for prolongation of initial hospitalization in neonatal intensive care units (5). Furthermore, continuous cardiorespiratory monitoring is at times prescribed because of fear of severe apneas after hospital discharge, at the expense of significant parental anxiety (6), and follow-up by a specialized team on call 24 hr a day (7). With the survival of increasingly more immature newborns and the use of surfactant to treat respiratory distress syndrome, apneas of prematurity are now the most worrisome respiratory problem in neonatal intensive care units (8).

The understanding of neonatal respiratory instability and testing of new treatments for apneas of prematurity have been hampered by the obvious difficulty in performing research on preterm infants and the lack of a suitable animal model. This chapter describes our recent development of a unique animal model of neonatal respiratory instability, the preterm lamb. The first results obtained in this model, including those related to laryngeal dynamics during apneas and periodic breathing, are also reported.

II. Historical Perspective: The Need for an Animal Model of Neonatal Respiratory Instability

Apart from human newborn infants, there are very few studies on respiration in unanesthetized, spontaneously breathing preterm mammals. Two studies examined the laryngeal chemoreflex in preterm lambs born at 135 days gestational age (full term 147 days) (9,10). Two other studies examined the ventilatory responses to hypercapnia and hypoxia in preterm lambs born at 135 days gestational age (11), and the ventilatory response to hypercapnia in premature monkeys born at 143–151 days gestational age (0.85–0.9 of term) (12). In addition, a few preterm lambs were added in a study on apneas in full-term lambs, with the mention that spontaneous apneas were more frequent in preterm than in full-term lambs (13). Finally, a series of studies were conducted in the very immature newborn opossum (14). Furthermore, although polysomnographic recordings have been performed in full-term, nonhuman infants of several different species, such as dogs (15) and sheep (16), there are, to our knowledge, no previous reports of prolonged recordings of sleep stages and cardiorespiratory variables in preterm, nonhuman infants. Moreover, polysomnographic recordings performed in full-term, nonhuman infants have apparently not allowed recording of a sufficient number of spontaneous apneas or episodes of periodic breathing to warrant systematic study.

Our research program is aimed at determining the characteristics of perinatal control of breathing. Clinical relevance includes a better understanding and management of apneas of prematurity, and of the effects of premature birth on postnatal maturation of respiratory control as potentially related to a higher risk of sudden infant death syndrome (SIDS). Using the full-term lamb, we (and others) have examined maturation of the chemical control of breathing (17–21), maturation of the vagal control of breathing (especially originating from bronchopulmonary C fiber endings) (22,23) and the importance of laryngeal dynamics during both ventilation and induced central apneas (24–27). Our initial attempts to perform prolonged polysomnographic recordings in the laboratory were hampered by the observation of only very few spontaneous apneas in full-term lambs. In an attempt to overcome this problem, we designed polysomnographic recording equipment using radiotelemetry transmission (28), which allowed us to study free-moving, nonsedated lambs in their usual environment, i.e., in their pen and with their mother. This proved to be partially successful because we were able to record seemingly more normal cycles of wakefulness, nonrapid eye movement (NREM) and rapid eye movement (REM) sleep (unpublished results). However, the full-term lambs still displayed rare spontaneous apneas and no periodic breathing episodes. Those results prompted us to turn to the study of preterm lambs.

III. Personal Experience in Preterm Sheep Deliveries
A. Gestation, Delivery, and Immediate Postnatal Care

Nonpregnant ewes were first selected by our local provider using two fetal ultrasound examinations at 50-day intervals. Following estrus induction with vaginal sponges containing 60 mg of medroxyprogesterone acetate, mating was then allowed during 48 hr to ensure accuracy of postconceptional age (± 24 hr). A third ultrasound examination was performed 50 days later to confirm pregnancy, and gestation was continued without any other intervention until transfer from the farm to our animal quarters, between 125 and 129 days postconceptional age.

Beginning at 130 days postconceptional age (48 hr before delivery induction), antenatal lung maturation was accelerated by administration of betamethasone and thyrotropin-releasing hormone (TRH) to the pregnant ewe. A single dose of 0.5 mg/kg betamethasone was injected intramuscularly. Four doses of 400 µg TRH were given by slow intravenous injection at 48, 36, 24, and 12 hr before induction of delivery. Twelve hours before induction of delivery, a prostaglandin (PGE_2) gel was placed intravaginally to accelerate cervical dilation. On the day of delivery (132 days gestational age), a continuous infusion of oxytocin was given intravenously to the ewe to activate preterm labor. The infusion was started at a rate of 6 mUI/min and subsequently increased every 10 min up to a maximum of 60 mUI/min. Labor evolution was monitored by means of regular physical examination. Lambs were born vaginally without assistance except in cases of abnormal presentation.

Immediately after delivery, the first procedure consisted of an intratracheal injection of 8 mL calf surfactant (Survanta®, Abbott Laboratories Ltd., Montreal, Canada) percutaneously, with the intention of performing the injection prior to the lamb's first breath. The lamb was then dried with warmed towels, weighed, and transferred to an incubator for initial clinical examination and standard neonatal care. Continuous monitoring of oxygenation using a transcutaneous oxygen saturation (SpO_2) probe (Nonin 8500, Nonin Medical Inc., Plymouth, MN) attached at the base of the shaved tail was initiated together with rectal temperature monitoring (Mon-a-Therm, Mallinkrodt, Pointe Claire, PQ, Canada). Glycemia was also regularly checked on venous blood samples (BM test, Boehringer Ingelheim Ltd., Burlington, ON, Canada). The lamb was returned to its mother as soon as possible, i.e., when temperature was stabilized over 39°C, SpO_2 was maintained at 95% without tachypnea (respiratory rate > 60/min) in room-air breathing, and glycemia was over 2.5 mmol/L. In case of hypothermia (<38.5°C) and/or hypoglycemia (<2.3 mmol/L) because of insufficient spontaneous feedings, the lamb was kept in an incubator and fed with mother's milk by discontinuous gastric feeding. In case of respiratory distress syndrome, the lamb was also kept in an incubator and standard care presently in use in our institution for human newborns was initiated.

While normal temperature and glycemia were maintained, oxygen was first given by nasal cannulae as needed for maintaining $SpO_2 > 90\%$ and an arterial line was inserted for blood gas monitoring. In case of overt retractions or severe blood gas abnormalities despite nasal O_2 ($PaO_2 <$ 60 torr and/or arterial pH < 7.25), endotracheal ventilatory support was implemented. A time-cycled, pressure-limited, constant-flow neonatal ventilator (Bourns BP 200) was used, with initial settings of 60% F_iO_2, 20 cm H_2O peak inspiratory pressure, 4 cm H_2O positive end-expiratory pressure (PEEP), 60/mn respiratory rate, and 0.3 sec inspiratory time.

Continuous sedation was ensured by intravenous infusion of 0.1 mg/kg/hr midazolam (Versed, Hoffmann-La Roche, Mississauga, ON, Canada) and 5 mg/kg/hr ketamine hydrochloride (Ketaset, Ayerst, Montreal, PQ, Canada). Paralysis was ensured by infusing 1 mg/kg/hr iv pancuronium. Surfactant replacement (Survanta) was given when deemed necessary, up to two doses. Finally, intravenous fluids, consisting of 10% dextrose with 12 mg/kg/hr calcium gluconate, were continuously infused at a rate of 80 mL/kg for the first 24 hr. For intractable respiratory insufficiency, ventilatory support was stopped and the lamb was euthanized with 50 mg/kg iv pentobarbital.

B. Success Rate

Forty-six lambs were born from a total of 28 deliveries performed in our laboratory to date. Thirteen ewes gave birth to one lamb, 12 ewes gave birth to 2 lambs, 2 ewes gave birth to 3 lambs, and 1 ewe gave birth to 4 lambs. Twenty-five preterm lambs survived the first 48 hr of life, including the quadruplet lambs. Six unattended deliveries (7 lambs) occurred unexpectedly during the night following PGE_2 gel application, prior to oxytocin infusion; 4 of those 7 lambs died. Nine lambs died in the first 24 hr from intractable respiratory distress syndrome. Three lambs were discovered dead 24 hr after birth with multiple rib fractures, and lung or liver lacerations due to repetitive traumatisms inflicted by their mothers. One lamb was discovered dead 48 hr after birth, presumably from apnea/bradycardia, after a negative autopsy. Four lambs had to receive nasal oxygen and continuous positive airway pressure (CPAP) for more than 4 hr (max 48 hr), and 1 lamb survived after being ventilated during 48 hr. Overall, 17 lambs from 28 deliveries were sequentially studied up to 6 weeks postnatal age. Of note, our success rate improved greatly since the addition of prophylactic surfactant at birth, because we were able to study at least 1 preterm lamb from each of the 7 last deliveries (132 days gestational age).

IV. Studies of Respiration in Preterm Lambs
A. Breathing Pattern and Laryngeal Dynamics
Chronic Instrumentation

Our initial study in 7 preterm lambs examined basal respiratory pattern and laryngeal dynamics during breathing and apneas. Preterm lambs were chronically instrumented during aseptic surgery under general anesthesia on their second or third day of life. Details of the procedure can be found in a recent publication (29). Chronic instrumentation consisted of electrodes for electroencephalogram and eye movement recording, bipolar wire intramuscular electrodes for recording electromyogram [EMG] of a glottal constrictor muscle (the thyroarytenoid muscle) and the diaphragm, thoracic subcutaneous electrodes for electrocardiogram recording, and a nasal thermocouple for recognizing apneas and periodic breathing. All leads were subcutaneously tunneled to exit from the back of the lamb, where they were connected to a telemetry transmitter before each recording. Early postoperative care included observation in an incubator and continuous monitoring of rectal temperature and SpO_2. The postoperative period was marked by numerous, prolonged apneas with severe desaturations which were managed by one intravenous injection of 10 mg/kg caffeine to which a doxapram infusion (1–2 mg/kg/hr) frequently had to be added for a few hours. After complete recovery, lambs were housed with their mother in our animal quarters before recordings were initiated not sooner than 48 hr after surgery.

Larynx and Ventilation

Experiments consisting of polysomnographic recordings during 3–8 hr were repeated on average six times in each lamb up to a postconceptional age of 147 days corresponding to full-term birth. Overall, recording time totaled 126 hr in 7 lambs, including 29 hr of REM sleep. Apart from apneas, postinspiratory thyroarytenoid muscle EMG was present in 50–60% of breaths during wakefulness and NREM sleep, mainly when respiratory rate was at its lowest. Notably, this percentage did not decrease with age within the study period, contrary to results for term lambs, in which it is known to decrease after the first week (16). Persistence of postinspiratory thyroarytenoid muscle EMG suggested the need for maintaining a high end-expiratory lung volume, presumably through vagal afferent activity originating from the slowly adapting bronchopulmonary stretch receptors (16). A strong Hering-Breuer reflex is present accordingly in preterm lambs during the first weeks of life (J.-P. Praud, unpublished results). Moreover, postinspiratory thyroarytenoid muscle EMG was observed in only 10% of breaths during REM sleep, in agreement with the decrease in functional residual capacity previously reported in preterm human infants during this stage (30).

Larynx During Apneas and Periodic Breathing

Characteristics of apneas are reported in Table 1 in relation to states of consciousness. Overall, 2088 apneas longer than 3 sec were observed, with a mean apnea index of 15 apneas/hr. According to the classical definition of central apneas (no airflow and no respiratory efforts), 2020 apneas were central, 68 were mixed, and no obstructive apneas were observed. However, 89.5% of central apneas were characterized by continuous thyroarytenoid muscle EMG throughout the apnea, with probable complete glottal closure as suggested by the simultaneous, consistent disappearance of cardiac artifact on the airflow trace as soon as thyroarytenoid muscle EMG was present (Fig. 1). Accordingly, complete glottal closure was also observed endoscopically during spontaneous apneas in preterm infants (31), and we have previously reported identical endoscopic observations during induced central apneas in full-term lambs (27). A total of 57 episodes of periodic breathing corresponding to 5 hr of recordings were observed (Table 2). Virtually all apneas (98.5%) observed during episodes of periodic breathing were characterized by continuous thyroarytenoid muscle EMG, even during REM sleep (97.5%) (Fig. 2). Moreover, the presence of continuous thyroarytenoid muscle EMG throughout apneas was associated with

Table 1 Characteristics of Apneas in 7 Preterm Lambs Born at 130 Days Postconceptional Age

	REM	NREM	Wakefulness	Sum
Total recording duration	29 hr 21 min	50 hr 14 min	46 hr 40 min	126 hr 15 min
Total number of apneas	339	1203	546	2088
Number of central apneas	297	1187	536	2020
Central apnea index (hr^{-1})	10 ± 13.5	23.5 ± 47.2	11.2 ± 31.9	15 ± 34.2
n-TA: total (central apnea)	22 (20)	24 (23)	20 (20)	66 (63)
nC-TA: total (central apnea)	69 (47)	74 (72)	34 (30)	177 (149)
C-TA: total (central apnea)	248 (226)	1105 (1096)	492 (486)	1845 (1808)
C-TA (% apneas)	73.2	91.9	90.1	88.4

n-TA = number of apneas with no thyroarytenoid muscle EMG, with number of central apneas in parentheses; nC-TA = noncontinuous TA EMG during apneas; C-TA = continuous TA EMG during apneas; C-TA (% apneas) = percentage of apneas with continuous TA EMG. Values are expressed as means ± standard deviation.
Source: Ref. 29.

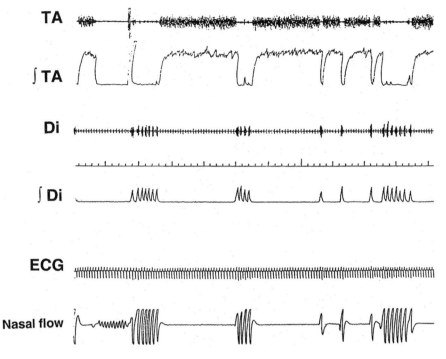

Figure 1 Active glottal closure during spontaneous apneas in a preterm lamb (postconceptional age = 139 days). TA, raw thyroarytenoid muscle electromyogram (EMG); ∫TA, moving time averaged TA EMG; Di, raw diaphragmatic EMG; ∫Di, moving time averaged Di EMG; ECG, electrocardiogram. Disappearance of ECG artifact (see first apnea) on nasal flow tracing indicates that presence of TA EMG during apneas corresponds to total upper airway (glottal) closure. (From Ref. 29. Copyright American Lung Association.)

maintenance of apneic lung volume in an inspiratory position (inspiratory breath-holding) (Fig. 3). Again, repetitive complete glottal closure was equally observed endoscopically during apneas within periodic breathing in an infant (32). Although control of this active glottal closure during neonatal apneas is currently unknown, phylogenetic and ontogenetic links are readily apparent. From a phylogenetic standpoint, the basic respiratory pattern in vertebrates corresponds to alternating pulmonary ventilation and inspiratory breath-holding with the glottis closed and the gas exchanger full of air (33). Maintenance of a high lung volume during apneas appears to be beneficial by favoring continuation of gas exchange in the absence of ventilatory movements. This is especially relevant in the preterm newborn in

Table 2 Characteristics of Periodic Breathing Episodes in 7 Preterm Lambs Born at 130 Days Postconceptional Age

	REM	NREM	Wakefulness	Sum
Number of episodes	3	37	17	57
Total duration	10 min	3 hr 33 min	1 hr 13 min	4 hr 55 min
Duration by PB episode	3 min 18 sec ± 2 min	5 min 45 sec ± 4 min	4 min 17 sec ± 4 min	5 min 11 sec ± 4 min
Percent time spent in PB	0.6%	7.1%	2.6%	3.9%
Number of oscillations				
Total by PB episode	49 (16.3 ± 9.1)	1106 (29.9 ± 18.5)	393 (23.1 ± 22.6)	1548 (27.2 ± 19.6)
Number of apneas				
Total by PB episode	39 (13 ± 10.6)	755 (20.4 ± 16.4)	287 (16.9 ± 19.1)	1081 (19 ± 16.9)
Mean duration of apneas	6.4 ± 1.4 sec	6.1 ± 1.4 sec	5.8 ± 1.1 sec	6.1 ± 1.3 sec
C-TA (% apneas)	38 (97.4)	740 (98)	286 (99.6)	1064 (98.4)

PB = periodic breathing; C-TA = number and percentage of apneas with continuous TA.
Source: Ref. 29.

which lung volume tends to decrease dramatically as soon as inspiratory muscle contractions cease, because of the presence of a highly compliant chest wall with low lung compliance (34). From an ontogenetic standpoint, periods with diaphragmatic "inspiratory" contractions—fetal breathing movements—are separated by prolonged periods with the glottis closed and absence of diaphragmatic contraction in the fetus in utero (35). Respiratory instability with active glottal closure during apneas observed in preterm lambs could well represent persistence of the fetal pattern of respiration. Prenatal lung growth has been clearly shown to be dependent on the increase in tracheal pressure brought about by active glottal closure during periods without fetal breathing movements (36). An intriguing hypothesis is that repetitive inspiratory breath-holdings during prolonged episodes of

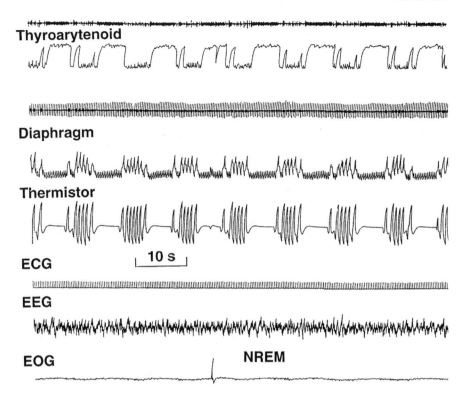

Thyroarytenoid

Diaphragm

Thermistor

ECG   ⌊ **10 s** ⌋

EEG

EOG   **NREM**

Figure 2 Active glottal closure during apneas within a 35-min epoch of periodic breathing in a preterm lamb (postconceptional age = 148 days) during NREM sleep. Raw and moving time-averaged EMG are reported for thyroarytenoid muscle and diaphragm. Thermistor, nasal flow; ECG, electrocardiogram; EEG, electroencephalogram; EOG, eye movements. (From Ref. 29. Copyright American Lung Association.)

periodic breathing in the immature newborn mammal also enhance postnatal lung growth.

B. Ventilatory Responses to Respiratory Stimuli

We are currently examining the postnatal development of ventilatory responses to respiratory stimuli in preterm lambs versus full-term lambs. Experiments under way aim at examining postnatal maturation of the central and peripheral chemoreceptor function and of the responses to stimulation of bronchopulmonary vagal receptors from 24 hr to 6 weeks postnatally. Although many experiments have yet to be completed, unique

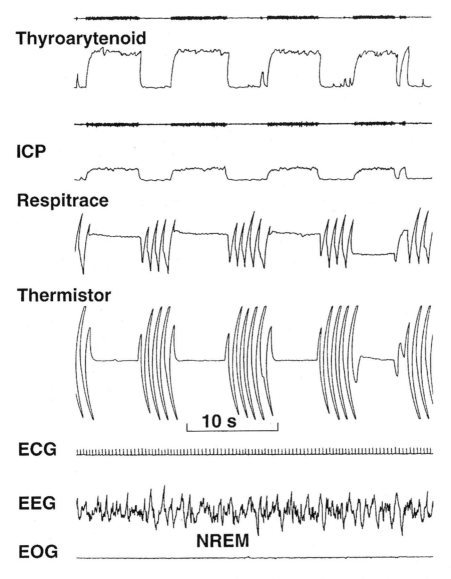

Figure 3 Maintenance of apneic lung volume above previous end-expiratory lung volume with active glottal closure. ICP, raw and moving time-averaged EMG of the inferior pharyngeal constrictor; Respitrace, sum signal of the respiratory inductive plethysmograph; Thermistor, nasal flow; ECG, electrocardiogram; EEG, electro-encephalogram; EOG, eye movements. (From Ref. 29. Copyright American Lung Association.)

preliminary results have already shown that bronchopulmonary C fibers are functional at birth in preterm lambs. This is of special relevance because our previous studies on pulmonary edema in lambs have shown that bronchopulmonary C fibers appear to be necessary for the presence of active expiratory laryngeal closure (22), an important defense mechanism in the preterm human newborn with respiratory distress syndrome. This phenomenon is well known by neonatologists as the expiratory grunting of the newborn. Of particular note, bronchopulmonary C fibers were claimed to be nonfunctional at birth until only recently (22,23,37), even in the full-term newborn mammal.

Further experiments will focus on postnatal maturation of the responses to laryngeal stimulation, and of the arousal response to various stimuli in NREM versus REM sleep. Cardiac responses will also be examined in all of the above conditions. Such extensive characterization of cardiorespiratory physiology in our animal model is required in preparation for future studies on neonatal apneas and periodic breathing, including new management strategies. Moreover, it is hoped that results from these experiments will provide new light in our attempt to better understand the clinical observation that preterm infants are at a higher risk of dying from SIDS (38), and that the risk period for this syndrome is different in the preterm infant compared to that of the full-term infant (39).

V. Relevance of the Preterm Lamb Model

The choice of the sheep as a model of neonatal respiratory instability may appear to be questionable, especially to the reader unfamiliar with the study of perinatal physiological functions. Indeed, the more advanced neurological maturation of the newborn sheep when compared to the human infant could be considered a major drawback. However, the sheep has been and still is one of the most frequently used animal models of perinatal respiratory physiology. Numerous studies on fetal breathing movements, respiratory adaptation at birth, and postnatal maturation of respiratory control have been performed in sheep, especially since the pioneering work of Dawes et al. on fetal breathing movements (40). Initially, experimental use of lambs mostly stemmed for practical and/or technical advantages: sheep are readily available worldwide, and artificial induction of ovulation provides lambs year round. Because of its size and small number of newborns per litter, the fetal lamb in utero is the model of choice for studying fetal physiology and in designing/testing fetal surgical techniques readily applicable to the human fetus. In addition, the identical size of the newborn lamb and human infant is appealing for neonatal surgeons and neonatologists, allowing them to use familiar techniques and instrumentation during neonatal care, surgical procedures, and physiological measurements. Moreover, robustness and calmness of the lamb, e.g., in comparison to the piglet, makes a real difference for performing repetitive and/or prolonged studies without sedation. Aside from practical/technical issues, scientific relevance of studying newborn lambs has been repeatedly shown. Indeed, despite a more advanced neurological maturation than that of the human infant, results from numerous studies in the fetal lamb in utero and the full-term newborn lamb have clearly provided invaluable new knowledge, directly translatable to the human infant. The body of results obtained in both the fetal and term lamb also offers particular advantages in terms of understanding normal maturation of physiological functions from prenatal to postnatal life. In this context, the preterm lamb is a tremendous addition to this armamentarium, and offers a unique opportunity to perform studies in abnormal conditions mimicking the preterm human infant with clear respiratory instability. Our first results showing that spontaneous apneas and periodic breathing are frequent and observed during all states of consciousness confirm the relevance of our ovine model. This is further confirmed by the observations that regular periodic breathing predominates in NREM sleep (8), more severe apneas occur in the hours following surgery, and caffeine and doxapram are efficacious. These observations are all well-known characteristics of respiratory instability observed in human preterm newborns.

VI. Conclusions

The preterm lamb is an exciting model of spontaneous respiratory instability, which should enable us to provide answers to numerous questions relevant to neonatal breathing. Aside from physiological studies on breathing pattern and maturation of cardiorespiratory control, the pathophysiology of neonatal apneas is currently being examined. Several questions about the characteristics of postoperative apneas in the preterm infant, the effects of respiratory syncytial virus infection on control of breathing and respiratory instability, the pathophysiology of apneas during feeding, and the postnatal maturation of the laryngeal chemoreflex can be readily addressed. Furthermore, the preterm lamb is a model of choice for a thorough examination of the effects of several treatment options for apneas of prematurity. These treatments include administration of various candidate drugs such as TRH, antagonists of prostanoid receptors, or antagonists of adenosine A_1 receptors; inhalation of low CO_2 concentrations, or mechanical treatment such as nasal CPAP and nasal inspiratory positive pressure ventilation.

Refinement in the acceleration of antenatal lung surfactant maturation and in management of surfactant insufficiency at birth should offer additional possibilities to study even younger immature lambs, allowing researchers to extend the capabilities of the preterm lamb model.

Acknowledgments

The authors wish to acknowledge the expert technical assistance of Bruno Gagné throughout the experiments performed in full-term and preterm lambs. The authors also acknowledge generous donations of Survanta by Abbott Laboratories and Relefact® by Hoechst-Marion-Roussel Inc. These studies were supported by grants from the Canadian Institutes for Health Research (Grants MT 7137 and MT 15571), the Quebec Lung Association, and the University of Sherbrooke.

References

1. National Institutes of Health Consensus Development Panel on Infantile Apnea and Home Monitoring. Consensus Statement. Pediatrics 1987; 79:292–299.
2. Bathia, J. Current options in the management of apnea of prematurity. Clin Pediatr 2000; 39:327–336.
3. Perlman, J. and Volpe, J. Episodes of apnea and bradycardia in the preterm newborn: impact on the cerebral circulation. Pediatrics 1985; 76:333–338.
4. Livera, L. N., Spencer, S. A., Thorniley, M. S., Wickramasinghe, Y. A., and Rolte, P. Effects of hypoxaemia and bradycardia on neonatal cerebral haemodynamics. Arch Dis Child 1991; 66:376–380.
5. Darnall, R. A., Kattwinkel, J., Nattie, C., and Robinson, M. Margin of safety for discharge after apnea in preterm infants. Pediatrics 1997; 100:795–801.
6. Williams, P. D., Press, A., and Williams, A. R. Fatigue in mothers of infants discharged to the home on apnea monitors. Appl Nurs Res 1999; 12:69–77.
7. Côté, A., Hum, C., Brouillette, R. T., and Themens, M. Frequency and timing of recurrent events in infants using home cardiorespiratory monitors. J Pediatr 1998; 132:783–789.
8. Rigatto, H. Breathing and sleep in preterm infants. In: Loughlin, G. M., Carroll, J. L., and Marcus, C. L., eds. Sleep and Breathing in Children: A Developmental Approach. Lung Biology in Health and Disease. Vol 147. New York: Marcel Dekker, 2000:495–523.

9. Marchal, F., Corke, B. C., and Sundell, H. Reflex apnea from laryngeal chemo-stimulation in the sleeping premature newborn lamb. Pediatr Res 1982;16:621–627.

10. Grogaard, J., Kreuger, E., Lindstrom, D., and Sundell, H. Effects of carotid body maturation and terbutaline on the laryngeal chemoreflex in newborn lambs. Pediatr Res 1986; 20:724–729.

11. Davey, M. G., Moss, T. J., McCrabb, G. J., and Harding, R. Prematurity alters hypoxic and hypercapnic ventilatory responses in developing lambs. Respir Physiol 1996; 105:57–67.

12. Guthrie, R. D., Standaert, T. A., Hodson, W. A., and Woodrum, D. E. Sleep and maturation of eucapnic ventilation and CO_2 sensitivity in the premature primate. J Appl Physiol 1980; 48:347–354.

13. Henderson-Smart, D. J. and Read, D. J. C. Depression of intercostal and abdominal muscle activity and vulnerability to asphyxia during active sleep in the newborn. In: Guilleminault, C. and Dement, W. C., eds. Sleep Apnea Syndromes. New York: Alan R Liss, 1978:93–117.

14. Farber, J. P. Development of pulmonary reflexes and pattern of breathing in the Virginia opossum. Respir Physiol 1972; 14:278–286.

15. England, S. J. Laryngeal muscle and diaphragmatic activities in conscious dog pups. Respir Physiol 1985; 60:95–108.

16. Harding, R. The upper respiratory tract in perinatal life. In: Johnston, B. M. and Gluckman, P. D., eds. Respiratory Control and Lung Development in the Fetus and Newborn. Ithaca, New York: Perinatology Press, 1986:332–376.

17. Canet, E., Praud, J. P., Laberge, J. M., Blanchard, P. W., and Bureau, M. A. Apnea threshold and breathing rhythmicity in newborn lambs. J Appl Physiol 1993; 74:3013–3019.

18. Delacourt, C., Canet, E., Praud, J. P., and Bureau, M. A. Influence of vagal afferences on diphasic ventilatory response to hypoxia in newborn lambs. Respir Physiol 1995; 99:29–39.

19. Canet, E., Kianicka, I., and Praud, J. P. Postnatal maturation of peripheral chemoreceptor ventilatory response to O_2 and CO_2 in newborn lambs. J Appl Physiol 1996; 80:1928–1933.

20. Canet, E., Praud, J. P., and Bureau, M. A. Periodic breathing induced on demand in the awake newborn lamb. J Appl Physiol 1997; 82:607–612.

21. Praud, J. P., Kianicka, I., Diaz, V., Chevalier, J. Y., and Thisdale, Y. Abolition of breathing rhythmicity in lambs by extracorporeal CO_2 unloading in the immediate postnatal period. Respir Physiol 1997; 110:1–8.

22. Diaz, V., Dorion, D., Renolleau, S., Létourneau, P., Kianicka, I., and Praud, J. P. Laryngeal dynamics during pulmonary edema in capsaicin-desensitized lambs. J Appl Physiol 1999; 86:1570–1577.

23. Diaz, V., Arsenault, J., and Praud, J. P. Consequences of capsaicin treatment on pulmonary vagal reflexes and chemoreceptor activity in lambs. J Appl Physiol 2000; 89:1709–1718.

24. Kianicka, I., Leroux, J. F., and Praud, J. P. Thyroarytenoid muscle activity during hypocapnic central apneas in awake non-sedated lambs. J Appl Physiol 1994; 76:1262–1268.

25. Praud, J. P., Kianicka, I., Leroux, J. F., and Dalle, D. Laryngeal response to hypoxia in awake lambs during the first postnatal days. Pediatr Res 1995; 37:482–488.

26. Praud, J. P., Kianicka, I., Leroux, J. F., and Dalle, D. Prolonged active glottis closure after barbiturate-induced fatal respiratory arrest in lambs. Respir Physiol 1996; 104:221–229.

27. Lemaire, D., Létourneau, P., Dorion, D., and Praud, J. P. Complete glottic closure during central apnea in lambs. J Otolaryngol 1999; 28:13–19.

28. Létourneau, P., Dumont, S., Kianicka, I., Diaz, V., Dorion, D., Drolet, R., and Praud, J. P. Radiotelemetry system for apnea study in lambs. Respir Physiol 1999; 116:85–93.

29. Renolleau, S., Létourneau, P., Niyonsenga, T., and Praud, J. P. Thyroarytenoid muscle electrical activity during spontaneous apneas in preterm lambs. Am J Respir Crit Care Med 1999; 159:1396–1404.

30. Henderson-Smart, D. J. and Read, D. J. Reduced lung volume during behavioral active sleep in the newborn. J Appl Physiol 1979; 46:1081–1085.

31. Ruggins, N. R. and Milner, A. D. Site of upper airway obstruction in preterm infants with problematical apnoea. Arch Dis Child 1991; 66:787–792.

32. Ruggins, N. R. and Milner, A. D. Site of upper airway obstruction in infants following an acute life-threatening event. Pediatrics 1993; 91:595–601.

33. Shelton, G. and Boutilier, R. G. Apnea in amphibians and reptiles. J Exp Biol 1982; 100:245–273.

34. Bryan, A. C. and Wohl, M. E. Respiratory mechanics in children. In: Fishman, A. P., ed. Handbook of Physiology. Section 3, Vol. III, Part 1. Bethesda, M.D.: American Physiological Society, 1986:179–191.

35. Kianicka, I., Diaz, V., Dorion, D., and Praud, J. P. Coordination between glottic adductor muscle and diaphragm EMG activity in the fetal lamb in utero. J Appl Physiol 1998; 84:1560–1565.

36. Harding, R. and Hooper, S. B. Regulation of lung expansion and lung growth before birth. J Appl Physiol 1996; 81:209–224.

37. Nault, M. A., Vincent, S. G., and Fisher, J. T. Mechanisms of capsaicin and lactic acid-induced bronchoconstriction in the newborn dog. J Physiol 1999; 515:567–578.

38. Hodgman, J. E. Apnea of prematurity and risk of SIDS. Pediatrics 1998; 102:969–971.

39. Malloy, M. H. and Hoffman, H. F. Prematurity, sudden infant death syndrome, and age of death. Pediatrics 1995; 96:464–471.

40. Dawes, G. S. Fœtal and Neonatal Physiology. A Comparative Study of the Changes at Birth. Chicago: Year Book Medical Publishers, 1968.

9

Neonatal Models and Ventilatory Behavior

KINGMAN P. STROHL

Case Western Reserve University
and Louis Stokes Cleveland VA Medical Center
Cleveland, Ohio, U.S.A.

I. Introduction

Ventilatory behavior in the neonate is the combined result of innate factors including genetic predisposition and neural capacity, and of experiential factors that facilitate adaptation to the immediate postnatal (PN) environment (1–6). Neonatal acquisition of behavior exhibits features of learning and memory (7–11) and direction of neural development by external cues (2,12,13). Structural and functional flexibility are an essential feature of development, maintenance, and expression of neural circuitry (14).

Insight into the systems that determine ventilatory behavior can be gained by perturbations during certain critical periods of development. If perturbations produce altered behavior beyond that of the initiating event, then the systems exhibit flexibility beyond that of genetic determination (3,15–17). If such acquired behavior leads to illness, there may also be a way to decondition the behavior or design appropriate studies to define and prevent the initial adverse conditions operating to produce adult human illness.

The goals of this review are to present the logic and significance of animal studies, and those in the rat in particular, in the neonatal period that are relevant to disorders of ventilation and respiration. One focus will be on the potential for state (active sleep [AS] in particular) to be a crucial element determining ventilatory behavior in the adult.

II. Neonatal Animal Models

In our laboratory, the rat is considered to be a good model organism on the basis of its historical record of neuroanatomical and neurophysiological studies, and the size of its brain nuclei, which compared to the mouse, permit separate and combined interventions to be controlled and examined efficiently using such methods as microdialysis and extracellular recordings. The rat also offers the opportunity to study the effect of genetic background, because there are reproducible differences among strains relating to adult nonrespiratory and respiratory physiology (18–20). Although the mouse is more generally available for genetic studies, there will be soon a complete rat genome database that will permit gene identification and genetic engineering in the rat. It is our belief that studies in the rat can be designed to complement those in the mouse, and that findings in both rats and mice might give clues to the design of studies and interventions relevant to human disease.

The ventilatory behavior of the neonate is the product of intrauterine development and experience. There is precedent in studies of nonrespiratory systems that take advantage of the ability to intervene in utero and subsequently assess PN behavior, including such complex events as adversive conditioning (21). Related to this is the ability to examine mammals at earlier developmental periods than in the human, because PN day 1 in the rat corresponds roughly to a 30-week postgestational human. Animals like the rat are large enough that interventions can be performed in the perinatal and/or neonatal period that target selected neural structures (22,23). In model organisms the life span of the animal permits study of adult animals with interventions to reverse abnormal behavior (17) or to observe spontaneous deconditioning over time (24). Studies in model organisms are also preferable to examining the "proof of principle" before proceeding to human studies, including those that involve the potential effects of drug abuse (25).

One may design studies or observe behaviors in rats with stimuli that may accompany everyday events relevant to the human condition. Interventions can manipulate touching, auditory tones, and hypoxia with breath-holding or feeding. For instance, differences in maternal licking and grooming will result in synaptic changes in the hippocampus and differences in cognitive development (26,27) in the rat. These observations are potentially relevant to understanding how environmental factors influence the development of cardiovascular and stress responses in humans (28–32).

Another experimental approach is to study the effects of neonatal exposure to medications that alter the central nervous system (CNS). Commonly used drugs prescribed for hypertension in nursing mothers or during pregnancy (e.g., clonidine) or used as over-the-counter sleeping aids (e.g., scopolamine) have been shown to change developmental expression of neurotransmitters when given to the rat neonate. One potential area of study is the effects of drugs given for behavioral problems in adolescents (33): Medications taken by women in their childbearing years may produce unanticipated effects on the unborn child. Both the mechanisms of acquisition of this altered behavior and its countermeasures are best addressed in animal models such as the rat.

Alternative model organisms for the study of the acquisition of ventilatory behavior include larger animals (e.g., dogs, cats, and pigs) and lower organisms such as snails (25). Life-span issues preclude study of larger animals, and the lack of a formal breathing mechanism in lower organisms is problematic. These alternative model organism approaches, however, have an appropriate place (34). For instance, the study of the genetic architecture of a protein system or gene expression response may be more efficient in the lower organism where the reduced anatomy combined with knowledge of the entire genome can disclose structural and functional consequences of interventions potentially relevant to the mammalian system.

In summary, the neonatal rat may serve as a model in which controlled interventions, highly selective neuroactive agents, genetic manipulation, and neurophysiologic monitoring can dissect the complexity of mammalian neural development.

III. The Perinatal Period and Active Sleep

In the first PN week of the rat (post-natal day (PD) 1–7 corresponds roughly to a 30 to 31-week gestation in the human) there is rapid growth and integration of CNS sensory and motor pathways (1,35–37). This is a critical period in which sensory input is known to direct neural structure and function in the visual, auditory, and olfactory systems (38–42). This literature suggests that sensory neural networks "learn" in this period, setting up responses that persist throughout growth and influence the adult phenotype.

The mode and strength of stimuli direct specific anatomic connections and the development of behavioral characteristics for adaptation to the immediate PN environment. Notably, these characteristics continue to be functionally operative into adulthood (8,43) in the absence of the original sensory challenge (1). These behaviors are less easily created or acquired in the older animal and in some instances there may not be reacquisition or restoration of normal structure once it is altered by neonatal interventions (35,44). These studies underscore the brain's capacity for plasticity in neural structure, biochemistry, and function (45). An ability to rapidly change behavior appears to assist genetic heterogeneity as a mechanism for evolutionary success (4).

In mammals, the rapid neural development and acquisition of behavior in the early PN period takes place against the background of intense and prolonged AS (44,46,47). Active sleep is characterized neurophysiologically by constant neuronal firing in the region of the pons also known to influence respiratory behavior during prenatal life in lambs (48,49). During PN life, particularly during the first few days of life, the pons is involved in critical regulatory functions including sleep, and is functionally operational before the maturation of other brain areas known to be associated in the adult with sleep, including the suprachiasmatic nucleus (SCN) and hippocampal areas (50), or areas associated with the coordination of motor behavior, such as the cerebellum (51). Active sleep at this age (the first 21 days of life) may provide the brain with intense endogenous sensory information (52–54). The neurochemical equivalent would be presynaptic depolarization that would promote postsynaptic differentiation and growth (8,12,55).

Rats and human neonates spend 70–80% of the time in AS; the remainder of time is spent in wakefulness (feeding and active movements), indeterminate sleep, or slow-wave sleep (SWS) (56). Then, AS rapidly reduces into smaller segments of time. By 3–4 weeks in the rat and 5–6 months in the human, only 20–30% of time is spent in AS; the remainder of time is equally spent in SWS or wakefulness (56,57). In the adult, AS occurs intermittently in 10–15% of sleep time, and total sleep only occupies one-third of the day (37). How this fractionation of state is created is unknown; one theory suggests that the states of SWS and perhaps wakefulness (self-awareness) are derived from a primordial state of AS in the perinatal and neonatal period (58).

Although the precise function of AS is unknown, there is evidence that fetal/neonatal AS (rapid eye movement [REM]-like state in neonates) has an important role in neuronal growth (45,59), synaptic plasticity (54,60), learning and unlearning (52,61,62), genetic "readout" and individual differences (56,63), the maintenance of cortical networks (54,64), and thermoregulation (65). In the neonatal period, interruption of sleep by behavioral arousal methods (66) or by pharmacological blockade of AS (5) results in alterations in adult behavior. Some of the identified altered behaviors include hyperactivity, hyperanxiety, attentional distractibility, sleep disturbances, and reduced sexual behavior, alone and in concert with changes in adult neuroanatomy (reduction in size of the cortex and brainstem), and biochemistry (especially changes in adrenergic responses to stress) (46). Evidence for the specificity of sleep as the critical state is derived from studies where AS is selectively inhibited by behavioral interventions or comparison of similar classes of drugs with profiles that either inhibit or do not inhibit AS (66,67). A selectivity for critical period is derived from the observations that these same interventions in the adult or neonatal rat after the second PN week do not have long-lasting effects on either structure or function (46).

Such models are relevant to the human condition. As a result of findings in rats, which suggested that clonidine given in the neonatal period altered behavior (46), Huisjes et al. (68) designed a study that compared children (mean age 6.3 years) of mothers with gestational hypertension who were treated with clonidine to children born to gestational hypertensive mothers who were treated with bed rest and/or diuretics. Results showed no abnormalities in clinical neurological examination or differences in school performance; however, there were some differences that appeared to be dose dependent in reports of hyperactivity and sleep disturbances, including night awakenings, restlessness, nightmares, night terrors, and somnambulism. There was no screening for disorders of sleep; however, many of these behaviors are associated with sleep-disordered breathing (69–71).

In summary, a state called AS is fully operative at birth, and is of major importance in the PN maturation of neural structures and functions needed by the neonate for adaptation to its extrauterine environment. Furthermore, interventions directed at the animal during AS can produce measurable effects on subsequent behavior.

IV. Neonatal Modulation of Adult Behavior

Opportunities for entrainment, encoding, and conditioning of sensory stimuli are especially enriched in the neonatal period (1,43,72). Both transfer between sensory modes (intermodal) and amodal transfer of responses occur, presumably because of the variations in the timing of different developing systems (1). At a cellular level, there is increasing dendritic spine formation and glial cell proliferation, and therefore, a greater chance of learning an inhibitory behavior; but after 21 days (the normal weaning period in rats) there is a decrease in spine formation with a decreased chance of learning associations that would be paired with and lead to inhibitory responses (73–77). Although experiential effects on cell growth and proliferation can be produced throughout the entire life span of rats, cellular effects produced by sensory deprivation, distortion, and/or enrichment are more sharply restricted to those presented during the preweaning period than during the postweaning period (1).

Learning of autonomic behavior has been well recognized in the study of hypertension (7,78) and forms the theoretical basis for behavioral approaches to the pathogenesis and treatment of cardiovascular illness (79,80). Cruikshank and Weinberger (8) recently reviewed the evidence for experience-dependent plasticity and suggested three models for such learning to occur. In these simplified, conceptual models (Fig. 1) a stimulus (tone) used in a pairing treatment influences the discharge of a postsynaptic cell. Following the pairing, a change is induced, so that presynaptic firing and postsynaptic responses are altered. In a Hebbian model (12), the tone directly influences the postsynaptic cell to develop the capacity to respond in a stereotypic manner to a given stimulus. The simple idea is that every stimulus is directly linked to one postsynaptic event. The problem is that one must then conceive of new learning as requiring new, even unique, pre- and postsynaptic pairings. Other explanations for learning are necessary, given the presence of neural systems with multiple inputs and our knowledge of its efficiency. In Figure 1, middle panel, the paired treatment results in a modulation of presynaptic neurotransmitter release, and in the interneuronal model, the pairing alters interneuronal processes that modify the connections between pre- and postsynaptic neurons. Certainly combinations of these models are possible, or possibly the use or existence of each model may be relatively different throughout growth and development. Nonetheless, these models are either implicit or explicit in many experimental paradigms that involve learning or plasticity.

One practical application of these paradigms is the study of how maternal care influences brain structure and function. Variations in maternal care promote variations in hippocampal neural growth and the development of synapses in concert with variations in spatial learning and memory in the adult animal (26,27,81). In these experiments changes resulting from high (or low) maternal licking are transduced through systems that are well known to respond to other experiential paradigms. As a result, individual differences in adult behavior can result from naturally occurring variations in maternal behavior.

A similar paradigm is found in the study of the development of the respiratory phenotype. Okubo and Mortola (15), and Ling et al. (2) present evidence that exposure to either hypoxia or hyperoxia in early life resulted in

Hebbian

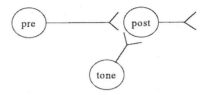

Presynaptic

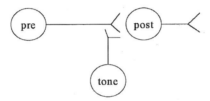

Interneuronal

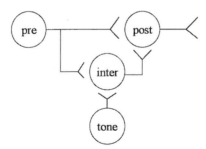

Figure 1 Three models for "conditioning" a neural circuit. Pre, presynaptic neurons or systems; post, postsynaptic neurons or systems; tone, a stimulus intervention such as an auditory tone; inter, interneuron(s).

a blunting of the respiratory response to hypoxia in the adult animal. In our studies (13,17,82), we use somatosensory stimuli and hypoxia in neonatal life to produce respiratory pauses during sleep in the adult animal. As will be discussed, white noise, a common counter-conditioning stimulus used to disrupt learned behavior, reduces the number of respiratory pauses in neonatally conditioned rats (17). Thus, learning may occur in early life with regard to ventilatory behavior.

In summary, research in animals has identified a neonatal period of rapid growth, development, and potential modification of postsynaptic networks responsible for both nonrespiratory and ventilatory behavior in the adult animal. In this period brain cellular events and system responses can be strongly influenced by environmental perturbations.

V. Active Sleep and Neural System Behavior

Active sleep may be a critical part of the mechanism by which these neonatal interventions produce changes in neural structure and function that, in turn, result in physiological alterations in adult respiratory behavior. Stimuli including hyperoxia, hypoxia, petting, or noise fit into a paradigm of (1) interruption or modification in the amount of AS, and/or (2) state-dependent conditioning. These sensory experiences direct developmental events along different pathways and result in an alteration from the norm (2,13,52,66).

In association learning paradigms, both endogenous and exogenous sensory input produced by environmental perturbations occurring in temporal proximity with sleep act as part of the conditioning paradigm (83). As such, interruption of sleep becomes or acts as a secondary conditioning stimulus that is able to provoke an autonomic response that affects breathing.

This concept leads to a new interpretation of studies (2,15) that examine the effects of various respiratory challenges during the neonatal period and their effects on respiratory activity in the adult animal in the absence of the original provoking stimulus. For example, Okubo and Mortola showed the long-term effects of hypoxia and hypercapnia presented to neonates on subsequent respiratory behavior in the adult rat (15,16). Active sleep was one component of their environmental challenge, although it was a variable that was not under direct measurement or manipulation.

In summary, studies have indicated a high degree of plasticity for nonrespiratory neural networks as a direct result of specific chemical and behavioral interventions in the first days of life in the rat. We propose that as in other physiological systems, the developing respiratory control system will be characterized by (1) plasticity for structural and biochemical differentiation, (2) configuration or reconfiguration of respiratory neuronal networks which are experience dependent and modifiable, and (3) a dependence on the predominance of AS during the first week of life for the acquisition of normal behavior.

VI. Neonatal Perturbations and the Adult Ventilatory Phenotype

Our original studies (82) were predicated on the idea that we might be able to alter breathing by conditioning (paired learning) in the neonatal period. For these studies, we used Sprague Dawley rats and raised pups from pregnant dams purchased from a single vendor (Charles River, Wilmington, MA). From pup age 3 to 28 PN days, pups and their mothers were exposed three times a week to one of three conditions: usual care, animals kept in their cage within the laboratory, or exposure in chambers to one of two different perturbations. Perturbations were presented during a 2-hr period when mother and pups would appear to be asleep. One perturbation group was exposed to either 5 min of hypoxia at a flow rate of 7 L/min for 30 sec and then 1 L/min for 5 min and presented with two conditioning stimuli, one auditory (a clicking noise) and one tactile (petting). In a second perturbation group, air was blown into the chamber at the same rate for the same length of time as was the hypoxic gas mixture for the first perturbation group, and animals were also presented with the noise and petting stimuli. One investigator presented all of the perturbations. After 28 days, pups were separated from their mothers and all animals were returned to the Animal Resource Center for usual care until 13–15 weeks of age, at which time individual animals were observed for breathing patterns.

A complete description of the results is presented by Thomas et al. (17). To summarize, there were no differences among groups in the number of pauses preceded by a sigh. However, the number of spontaneous pauses increased in both conditioned groups. The group with all three stimuli (noise, petting, and hypoxia) exhibited a greater number of spontaneous pauses than any other group ($p < 0.001$). The number of events for animals conditioned in air was significantly different from any other group. Adult animals (the mothers) that also experienced these interruptions did not exhibit an increased number of pauses or post-sigh events during behavioral sleep.

We have also observed that neonatally conditioned respiratory behavior is exhibited during sleep. To show this, five conditioned rats and three controls had chronic implantation of sleep staging electrodes. Six days after the procedure, animals were placed in a plethysmograph chamber in which ventilation could be continuously monitored. This chamber was, in turn, placed inside of a soundproof, lighted, temperature-regulated environment box, designed with a one-way glass to allow behavioral monitoring. Ventilation was constantly recorded. The rat was left undisturbed for a 2-hr sleep period, during the light phase. Records were independently scored for wakefulness, nonslow wave sleep (nSWS), SWS, and AS by standard criteria and calculations made of the number and distribution of pauses, not occurring as a result of a sigh, by state.

The absolute number of pauses (not preceded by a sigh) over a 2-hr period was 19 $+/-$ 8 (Standard Deviation [SD]) for control animals and 58 $+/-$ 16 for the conditioned animals ($P < 0.01$). There was a preferential redistribution of pauses to sleep. Figure 2 provides information on the relative distribution of respiratory pauses according to state, wakefulness, and the different stages of electroencephalogram (EEG)-defined sleep in the rat. There were no significant differences in the amount of wakefulness or sleep between the two groups (data not shown).

The results showing pauses occurring in sleep in the adult rat have been demonstrated by others (84) (see Chap. 10, this volume), but the demonstration that neonatal conditioning can increase the absolute as well as relative number of pauses during sleep is new.

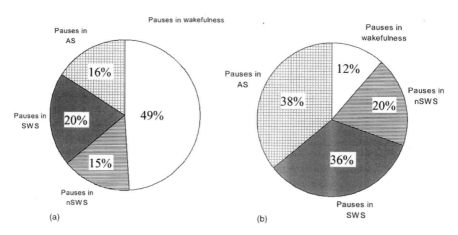

Figure 2 The pie charts show the relative distribution of pauses (apneas) during sleep in rats raised under usual-care conditions (a) or after neonatal exposures to intermitted touching, hypoxia, and auditory stimuli (b). Not only was there an absolute increase in the overall number of events, but there was redistribution from wakefulness into sleep.

VII. Respiratory Pauses During Sleep Can Be Modified in the Adult Animal

We have reported on the effect of white noise and, on a separate occasion, the effect of Equithesin (a pentobarbital-based anesthetic used in small animal surgery) on the number of respiratory and post-sigh pauses during sleep. Figure 3 displays a condensed summary of data from Thomas et al. (17). The effect of an auditory stimulus (white noise: 50 Hz, 30 db) presented for periods of 20 min on and 20 min off during behaviorally defined sleep resulted in a reduction of respiratory pauses by approximately 80%, but had no effect on the number of pauses preceded by a sigh. White noise did not alter tidal volume and respiratory frequency.

The effect of barbiturate anesthesia was to abolish all pauses. Anesthesia also resulted in a small, but insignificant reduction in tidal volume without a change in respiratory frequency.

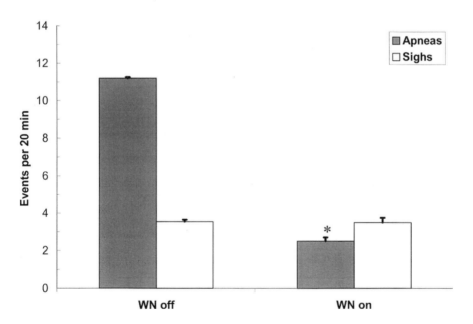

Figure 3 The bar graph describes the number of spontaneous pauses (apnea) or pauses following sighs (sighs), calculated as events/20 min, during periods with exposure to white noise (WN on) or without white noise (WN off). Bars represent the mean and standard error of the mean. The symbol (*) represents a significant difference ($p < 0.01$) in the number of apneas between the two conditions.

VIII. Effects of Suppression of Active Sleep

We also have evidence that neurotransmitter systems change as a result of neonatal exposure to drugs that suppress AS (85), and have preliminary evidence to suggest that the same is true for conditioning with noise, petting, and hypoxia. In this experimental design, Sprague Dawley pups were born, randomized among four mothers on the first day of life, and assigned to one of four groups. On days 1–7 pups received usual care, scopolamine (0.8 mg/kg in 0.3 mL of sweet milk twice a day), clonidine (100 ng/kg in 0.3 mL of sweet milk twice a day), or conditioning with hypoxia. We used oral administration to avoid potential confounding effects of behavioral and sleep responses to peritoneal injections. At day 19, animals were sacrificed and the brain was rapidly frozen. Transverse sections were made of the whole brain, and regions of the hypothalamus, prefrontal area, and hippocampus were identified (105), punched out, and prepared for high-performance liquid chromatography (HPLC) analysis of 5-hydroxytryptamine (5-HT) and norepinephrine (NE) (26,148). Results (expressed as nanograms per milligram of protein) are presented in Figure 4.

These results show that any of the three interventions result in a similar reduction in neurotransmitter levels in the hypothalamus. These could result from a decrease in production or an increase in metabolism or both. The changes are not the immediate result of the drug intervention because the time after the last dose of medication (12 days) is 10–30 half lives too long for the drug to still be attached to the receptor; in addition, the direction of change is similar to that observed with a behavioral intervention. The similarity in responses suggests, but does not prove, that the three interventions (two drugs acting on entirely different receptors and one behavioral intervention) operate through a similar function. We believe this function is sleep state and that the results support the idea that interruptions of sleep in the neonatal period have a lasting effect on biochemical functions.

The reduction in 5-HT levels in the prefrontal cortex seen with scopolamine is consistent with previous observations on the effect of neonatal AS suppression (86). The direction of change is different for NE than for 5-HT, indicating that in this region of the brain scopolamine has discordant effects on neurotransmitter systems. The finding that alpha-adrenergic receptors can be downregulated by neonatal exposure to clonidine is consistent to some extent with previous observations in a rat model (87). We are intrigue by the differences among the hypothalamus, cortex, and hippocampus following each intervention.

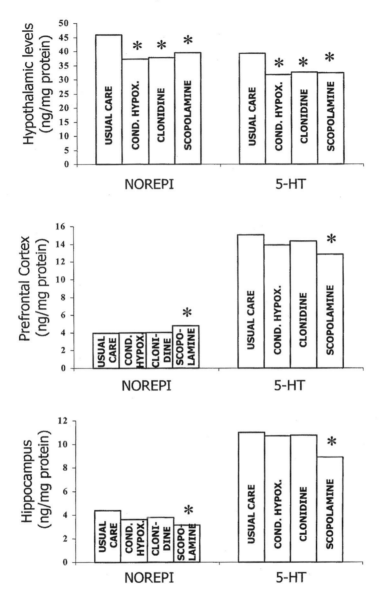

Figure 4   The bar graphs represent values (mean and standard error of the mean) of neurotransmitters, expressed as namograms per milligram of protein, for the four conditions discussed in the text. The separate graphs indicate values from three different brain regions. NOREPI, norepinephrine levels; 5-HT, 5-hydroxytryptamine. The symbol (*) represents a significant difference ($p < 0.05$).

IX. Adult Ventilatory Consequences of Neonatal Interventions

The following addresses the feasibility and the potential outcome of the experiments that are designed to address the adult consequences of neonatal interventions. The protocols described above are directly derived from the following observations. These results were collected over a 90-day period (ordering of animals to compilation of results), indicating the feasibility of a complicated protocol.

Table 1 lists the physiological variables collected at PN 19 days of the Sprague Dawley rat. Animals were born to four mothers. There were three interventions in the first 7 days of life—oral administration of clonidine (100 µg/kg); oral administration of scopolamine (0.8 mg/kg); and conditioning with hypoxia, petting, and noise—and all three interventions are compared to usual care conditions. More detailed methods are found in Thomas et al. (85).

We interpret the data in the following manner. Animals given scopolamine weighed significantly less and were shorter than the other animals. This effect was observed after 3 days of administration of scopolamine, so that at 10 days of age (3 days after the last dose of drug), animals given scopolamine weighed 20% less than those in other groups and at 19 days, they weighed 15% less. However, the Lee index, a measure of body mass, was similar among groups.

Although body temperature at the time of testing was similar, metabolic measures appeared to vary among groups at 19 days. Animals given scopolamine had slightly lower oxygen consumption, and animals conditioned with intermittent petting and hypoxia appeared to have a reduction in both oxygen consumption and carbon dioxide production.

At 19 days of life, respiratory frequency was about 20% higher in the clonidine-treated group than in the other groups. This difference was not observed at 10 days of age; in fact, at 10 days PN, respiratory rate was about 10% lower in the clonidine-treated group than in the other groups. However, it appears that the clonidine-treated group did not exhibit a decrease in respiratory frequency from PN 10 days (frequency = 165) to PN 19 days (frequency = 163), whereas the other groups exhibited a decrease in respiratory rate from an average of 183 to 135 over the same time period. To our knowledge, this is the first demonstration of this effect.

At PN 19 days, tidal volume was lower in both groups of drug-treated animals, compared to those under customary care or conditioned hypoxic animals. From PN 10 to PN 19 days, all groups exhibited an increase in tidal volume, with greater changes in usual-care and conditioned-hypoxic groups (data not shown). Therefore, at day 19, 12 days after the last dose of drug, the pattern of breathing varied with drug treatment, with the most prominent effect being a higher frequency/lower tidal volume in the clonidine-treated animals.

Minute ventilation varied among groups. The clonidine-treated animals had minute ventilation, both unadjusted and adjusted for body weight or carbon dioxide production, that was similar to that in controls. This suggests that the pattern of breathing is altered independently of metabolic load or changes in gas exchange. Although we have no measures of respiratory mechanics, at autopsy there were no discernable differences in the stiffness of the chest wall or the lung. All of these observations suggest the conclusion that the respiratory pattern generator (and not the controlled system) has changed in the clonidine-treated group.

Table 1 Ventilatory Behavior and Metabolism: Findings at Postnatal Day 19

Mean (SD)	Customary care (5, 5)[a]	Clonidine (7, 3)[a]	Scopolamine (5, 5)[a]	Conditioned hypoxic (5, 3)[a]
Weight (g)	49.8 (3.5)	46.5 (4.1)	39.6 (7)	49.1 (2)
Length (cm)	12.1 (0.5)	11.3 (0.5)	10.8 (0.4)	11.8 (0.4)
Lee index (112)	0.30 (0.01)	0.31 (0.02)	0.31 (0.2)	0.30 (0.03)
Body temperature[b]	37.7 (0.3)	37.8 (0.4)	38.15 (0.7)	37.8 (0.5)
Oxygen consumption	2.42 (0.35)	2.49 (0.22)	**2.20 (0.27)**	**2.38 (0.33)**
Carbon dioxide production	1.78 (0.16)	1.52 (0.23)	1.37 (0.24)	**1.16 (0.25)**
Respiratory quotient	**0.73 (0.05)**	0.61 (0.05)	0.62 (0.04)	0.63 (0.04)
Respiratory frequency	136 (11)	**163 (20)**	135 (18)	134 (13)
Tidal volume	0.10 (0.01)	0.08 (0.01)	0.08 (0.01)	0.09 (0.01)
Minute ventilation	13.2 (2.5)	13.2 (2.5)	**10.9 (2.0)**	**11.5 (1.5)**
Minute ventilation/gr	0.26	0.28	0.27	**0.23**
Minute ventilation/CO_2	7.4	8.6	7.9	**9.9**

[a] (n, n) = (number of males, number of females).
[b] At the time of testing for respiratory variables.
Text in bold represents findings that are emphasized in the discussion of these preliminary data.
Differences are not dependent upon the sex or maternal origin of the animal.

In contrast to the usual-care and clonidine-treated groups, there was a reduction in minute ventilation in scopolamine-treated and conditioned hypoxic groups. In the former group, the reduction in minute volume was proportionate to body weight and carbon dioxide production, whereas in the latter group there was a significant reduction in ventilation for weight or carbon dioxide production. This latter observation suggests that hypoxic-conditioned animals might exhibit differences in the controlled system. The higher values of ventilation and carbon dioxide production are an indication of a change in respiratory dead space (a controlled element)

Sleep was determined noninvasively and behaviorally by inspection of the animals (17). Figure 5 shows the data (mean and SD) collected during 2 hr of observations of each animal. These data demonstrate a significant ($p < 0.05$) decrease in frequency and in minute ventilation only in the usual-care group. The values in the scopolamine group did not reach statistical significance. Such changes did not occur in the clonidine-treated group. Indeed, respiratory frequency and minute ventilation were independent of state in these animals. These findings of a lack of reduction in minute ventilation with the onset of sleep persisted to 55 days of age in the drug-exposed animals, as compared to customary-care animals, in which there occurred a 38% decrease in metabolism with sleep onset.

We speculate that three possible scenarios may occur. First, there could be an uncoupling of respiratory behavior from sleep. Further observations in animals in which we directly measure EEG activity are needed to address this issue. Second, an inhibitory function of sleep on respiration has been lost. Again, direct measurements of sleep are necessary; nevertheless, this observation is inconsistent with the notion that respiratory changes with sleep result from the loss of a "wakefulness effect" (88). Third, the metabolic pathways have been altered so that the metabolic effects of sleep are uncoupled from sleep onset and therefore from respiratory drive.

We present these data to indicate the experimental design and power of studies in the rat to address issues of development and the influence of perturbations in the neonatal period on ventilatory behavior. Certainly, these studies need to be confirmed by us and by others; the use of more precise measures of respiratory control and mechanics should be included.

X.   Models to Incorporate Neonatal Experience into Adult Ventilatory Phenotypes

If one can accept the concept of sleep, a state that predominates the neonatal period, being a factor in any conditioning paradigm, then it is possible to create Hebbian and non-Hebbian models of how sleep alters

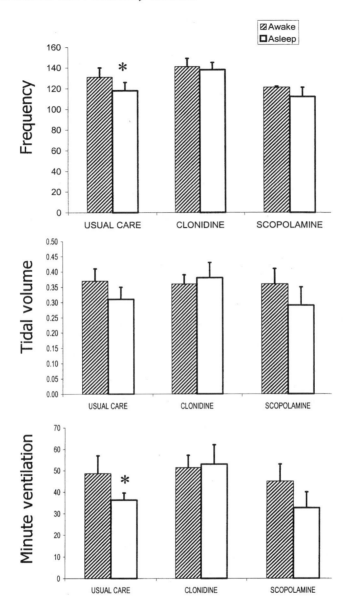

Figure 5 Bars represent the mean and standard deviation of values/group in respiratory frequency, tidal volume, and minute ventilation. Hatched bars represent the group mean values during behaviorally defined wakefulness; open bars represent the group mean values during behaviorally defined sleep. The symbol (*) represents a significant difference ($p < 0.01$) in the number of apneas between the two conditions.

respiratory drive. We currently think along the conceptual framework presented in simplified form in Figure 6. The receptive field in our models is that of control of respiratory behavior, in particular tidal volume and frequency. Currently, the location of postsynaptic events is not known. Because likely candidates are widely distributed in the brain (88), the reader should suspend anatomical assumptions to allow this model to make sense. Interactions among somatosensory input and sleep in the neonate could

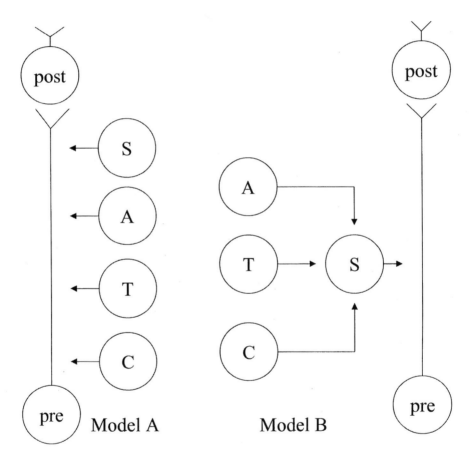

Figure 6 Two conceptual models are presented for discussion about beginning an experimental strategy to dissect mechanisms that operate in the neonatal acquisition of ventilatory behavior. Pre, presynaptic neurons or systems; post, postsynaptic neurons or systems; C, chemosensory input; T, touching or handling of animals; A, auditory stimuli; S, sleep neurons or systems regulating state.

take place with the different stimuli (auditory, hypoxia, or petting) either acting in parallel with the effect of state (model A) or acting through the state itself (model B). Our studies in the rat suggest that the three stumuli are not distinct with regard to special effects on hypothalamic transmitters, when compared to pharmacologic inhibition of AS, possibly favoring model B. However, as discussed in the opening sections of this chapter, in the neonate there is evidence for modal and amodal processing of stimuli, so that the specificity of the conditioning stimulus may not be as much of an issue as in the adult animal. This being the case, both models could be simplified even further in the neonate. In any event, future studies can be designed to address the combined and separate aspects of internal and external factors that can drive neural development and direct its functioning.

XI. Conclusions

Pathophysiologically and therapeutically, it is less constraining to consider breathing and sleep as behaviors rather than as innate programs. Evidence supports the need for more rigorous studies to demonstrate the extent to which adult sleep and respiratory control systems are modifiable by early experience and dependent in part upon uninterrupted sleep during the first week of life.

Firm demonstration of a critical period for the acquisition of autonomic cardiorespiratory behavior permits refinement in design, methods, and clinical application. Models used to describe other sensory adaptations to conditioning and/or maturation (51,76,89,90) will be applicable to understanding the behaviors of sleep and breathing (86). A need exists for future research to reconfirm observations that show these apparently robust effects of perinatal drug exposure, to examine dose-response characteristics, and to utilize emerging genomic and protenomic methods to determine molecular pathways responsible for these behaviors. Studies could examine animals for respiratory events, metabolism, and sleep state, as well as for circadian rhythms in temperature and locomotor behavior.

Critical periods of development, once identified, could lead to prospective studies of sudden infant death syndrome, and behavioral prevention and treatment of childhood sleep disorders (91,92), or to an understanding of the variance in sleep–wake behavior in the population (29,93–99).

Acknowledgments

The author would like to thank Agnes Thomas, Dong Liu, Bernadette Erokwu, Paul Ernsberger, and Bryan Yamamoto for their help in developing the concepts and approaches to this area of recent interest in the laboratory. This work was supported in part by the Department of Veterans Affairs, the National Institutes of Health (HL25830, HL58844, HL07193), and by a Sleep Academic Award (HL03650).

References

1. Alberts, J., Early learning and ontogenetic adaptation. In: Krasnegor, N., Blass, E., Hofer, M., and Smotherman, W., eds. Perinatal Development: A Psychobiological Perspective. Orlando, FL: Academic Press, 1987; 11–37.
2. Ling, L., Olson, E. J., Vidruik, E., and Mitchell, G. Attenuation of the hypoxic ventilatory response in adult rats following one month of perinatal hyperoxia. J Physiol (Lond) 1996; 495:561–571.
3. Mortola, J. Invited editorial on "Modification of conditioned apneas in rats: evidence for cortical involvement." J Appl Physiol 1995; 78(4):1213–1214.
4. Real, L. How to think about behavior: an introduction. In: Real, L. A., ed. Behavioral Mechanisms in Evolutionary Ecology. Chicago: University of Chicago Press, 1994; 1–8.
5. Rio, J., Montero, D., and DeCeballos, M. Long-lasting changes after perinatal exposure to antidepressants. Brain Res 1988; 73:173–187.
6. Stanton, H. Factors to consider when selecting animal models for postnatal teratology studies. J Environ Pathol Toxicol 1978; 2(1):201–210.
7. Dworkin, B. Learning and Physiological Organization. Chicago: University of Chicago Press, 1993.
8. Cruikshank, S. and Weinberger, N. Evidence for the Hebbian hypothesis in experience-dependent physiological plasticity of neocortex: a critical review. Brain Res Rev 1996; 22:191–228.
9. Folkow, B. Physiological organization of neurohormonal responses to psychosocial stimuli: implications for health and disease. Ann Behav Med 1993; 15(4):236–244.
10. Reppert, S. and Schwartz, W. Maternal coordination of the fetal biological clock in utero. Science 1983; 27:969–971.
11. Reppert S. Pre-natal development of a hypothalamic biological clock. Prog Brain Res 1992; 93:119–132.
12. Hebb, D. The Organization of Behavior. New York: Wiley Press, 1949.
13. Strohl, K. and Thomas, A. Neonatal conditioning for adult respiratory behavior. Respir Physiol 1997; 110:269–275.
14. Erzurumlu, R. and Guido, W. Cellular mechanisms underlying the formation of orderly connections in developing sensory pathways. Prog Brain Res 1996; 108:287–301.

15. Okubo, S. and Mortola, J. Long-term respiratory effects of neonatal hypoxia in the rat. J Appl Physiol 1986; 64:952–958.
16. Okubo, S. and Mortola, J. Control of ventilation in adult rats hypoxic in the neonatal period. Am J Physiol 1990; 259:r836–r841.
17. Thomas, A., Friedman, L., MacKenzie, C., and Strohl, K. P. Modification of conditioned apneas in rats: evidence for cortical involvement. J Appl Physiol 1995; 78(4):1215–1218.
18. Strohl, K., Thomas, A., St. Jean, P., Schlenker, E., Koletsky, R., and Schork, N. Ventilation and metabolism among rat strains. J Appl Physiol 1997; 82(1):317–323.
19. Tankersley, C. G., DiSilvestre, D. A., Jedlicka, A. E., Wilkins, H. M., and Zhang, L. Differential inspiratory timing is genetically linked to mouse chromosome 3. J Appl Physiol 1998; 85:360–365.
20. Tankersley, C. G., Elston, R. C., and Schnell, A. H. Genetic determinants of acute hypoxic ventilation: patterns of inheritance in mice. J Appl Physiol 2000; 88:2310–2318.
21. Mickley, G. A., Schaldach, M. A., Snyder, K. J., Balogh, S. A., Len, T., Neimanis, K., Goulis, P., Hug, J., Sauchak, K., Remmers-Roeber D. R., Walker, C., and Yamamoto, B. K. Ketamine blocks a conditioned taste aversion (CTA) in neonatal rats. Physiol Behav 1998; 64:381–390.
22. Kehoe, P. and Bronzino, J. D. Neonatal stress alters LTP in freely moving male and female adult rats. Hippocampus 1999; 9:651–658.
23. Slawecki, C. J., Thomas, J. D., Riley, E. P., and Ehlers, C. L. Neonatal nicotine exposure alters hippocampal EEG and event-related potentials (ERPs) in rats. Pharmacol Biochem Behav 2000; 65:711–718.
24. Ling, L., Olson, E. B. Jr., Vidruk, E. H., and Mitchell, G. S. Slow recovery of impaired phrenic responses to hypoxia following perinatal hyperoxia in rats. J Physiol (Lond) 1998; 511:599–603.
25. Hermann, P. M. and Bulloch, A. G. Developmental plasticity of respiratory behavior in Lymnaea. Behav Neurosci 1998; 112:656–667.
26. Liu, D., Diorio, J., Day, J. C., Francis, D. D., and Meaney, M. J. Maternal care, hippocampal synaptogenesis and cognitive development in rats. Nat Neurosci 2000; 3:799–806.
27. Liu, D., Diorio, J., Tannenbaum, B., Caldji, C., Francis, D., Freedman, A., Sharma, S., Pearson, D., Plotsky, P. M., and Meaney, M. J. Maternal care, hippocampal glucocorticoid receptors, and hypothalamic-pituitary-adrenal responses to stress [see comments]. Science 1997; 277:1659–1662.
28. Ludington-Hoe, S., Thompson, C., Swinth, J, Hadeed, A., and Anderson, G. Kangaroo care: research results, and practice implications and guidelines. Neonatal Network 1994; 13(1):19–26.
29. Whitelaw, A. Skin-to-skin contact for very low birth weight infants and their mothers: a randomized trial of kangaroo care. Arch Dis Child 1988; 63:1377–1382.

30. Li, Y., Liu, J., Liu, F., Guo, G., Anme, T., and Ushijima, H. Maternal child-rearing behaviors and correlates in rural minority areas of Yunnan, China. J Dev Behav Pediatr 2000; 21:114–122.

31. Gazzolo, D., Masetti, P., and Meli, M. Kangaroo care improves post-extubation cardiorespiratory parameters in infants after open heart surgery [in process citation]. Acta Paediatr 2000; 89:728–729.

32. De Leeuw, R., Colin, E. M., Dunnebier, E. A., and Mirmiran, M. Physiological effects of kangaroo care in very small preterm infants. Biol Neonate 1991; 59:149–155.

33. Jaselskis, C. A., Cook, E. H. J., Fletcher, K. E., and Leventhal, B. L. Clonidine treatment of hyperactive and impulsive children with autistic disorder. J Clin Psychopharmacol 1992; 12:322–327.

34. American Thoracic Society. Finding genetic mechanisms in syndromes of sleep disordered breathing. www.thoracic.org, 1999.

35. Boer, G., Feenstra, M., Mirmiran, M., Swaab, D., and Haaren, F. Biochemical basis of functional neuroteratology permanent effects of chemicals on the developing brain. Prog Brain Res 1988; 73:189–204.

36. Cusick, C. Extensive cortical reorganization following sciatic nerve injury in adult rats versus restricted reorganization after neonatal injury: implications for spatial and temporal limits on somatosensory plasticity. Prog Brain Res 1996; 108:379–390.

37. Scher, M., Steppe, D., Banks, D., Guthrie, R., and Sclabassi, R. Maturational trends of EEG-sleep measures in the healthy preterm neonate. Pediatr Neurol 1995; 12(4):314–322.

38. Oksenberg, A., Sjaffery, J., Marks, G., Speciale S., Mihailoff, G., and Roffwarg, H. Rapid eye movement sleep deprivation in kittens amplifies LGN cell-size disparity induced by monocular deprivation. Dev Brain Res 1996; 97:51–61.

39. Leon, M., Coopersmith, R., Lee, S., Sullivan, R., Wilson, D., and Woo, C. Neural and behavioral plasticity induced by early olfactory learning. In: Krasnegor, N., Blass, E., Hofe, R. M., and Smotherton, W., eds. Perinatal Development: A Psychological Perspective. Orlando, FL: Academic Press, 1987:145–168.

40. Weinberger, N. Learning-induced changes of auditory receptive fields. Curr Opin Neurobiol 1993; 3:570–577.

41. Yew, D. T., Chan, W. Y., Luo, C. B., Zheng, D. R., and Yu, M. C. Neurotransmitters and neuropeptides in the developing human central nervous system. A review. Biol Signals Recept 1999; 8:149–159.

42. Penn, A. A., and Shatz, C. J. Brain waves and brain wiring: the role of endogenous and sensory-driven neural activity in development. Pediatr Res 1999; 45:447–458.

43. Spear, N. and Molina, J. The role of sensory modality in the ontogeny of stimulus selection. In: Krasnegor, N., Blass, E., Hofer, M., and Smotherman, W., eds. Perinatal Development: A Psychobiologic Perspective. Orlando, FL: Academic Press, 1987:83–110.

44. Johnston, M., Barks, J., Greenamayr, T., and Silverstein, F. Use of neurotoxins to disrupt neurotransmitter circuitry in the developing brain. Prog Brain Res 1995; 73:425–446.

45. Ambrish, J. and Lewis, P. Brain cell acquisition and neurotropic drugs with special reference to functional teratogenesis. In: Boer, G., Finestra, M., Mirmiran, M., Swaab, D., and Van Haaren, F., eds. Prog Brain Res 1988; 73:389–403.

46. Mirmiran, M., Scholtens, J., Van De Poll, N., Uylings, B., Van der Gugten, J., and Boer, G. Effects of experimental suppression of active (REM) sleep during early development upon adult brain and behavior in the rat. Dev Brain Res 1983; 7:277–286.

47. Mirmiran, M., Matthijs, G., Dijcks, F., Nico, P., and Haaren, F. Functional deprivation of noradrenaline neurotransmission: effects of clonidine on brain development. Brain Res 1988; 73:159–172.

48. Ioffe, S., Jansen, A., and Chernick, V. Fetal respiratory neuronal activity during REM and NREM sleep. J Appl Physiol 1993; 75(1):191–197.

49. Funk, G. and Feldman, J. Generation of respiratory rhythm and pattern in mammals: insights from developmental studies. Curr Opin Neurobiol 1995; 5:778–785.

50. Mirmiran, M., Swaab, D., Kok, J., Hofman, M., Witting, W., and Van Gool, W. Circadian rhythms and the suprachiasmatic nucleus in perinatal development, aging and Alzheimer's disease. Prog Brain Res 1992; 93:151–163.

51. Frias, J. and Thomas, I. Teratogens and teratogenesis: general principles of clinical teratology. Ann Clin Lab Sci 1988; 18(2):174–179.

52. Drucker-Colin, R. The function of sleep is to regulate brain excitability in order to satisfy the requirements imposed by waking. Behav Brain Res 1995; 69:117–124.

53. Hennevin, E., Hars, B., Maho, C., and Bloch, V. Processing of learned information in paradoxical sleep: relevance for memory. Behav Brain Res 1995; 69:125–135.

54. Marks, G. A., Shaffery, J.P., Oksenberg, A., Speciale, S. G., and Roffwarg, H. P. A functional role for REM sleep in brain maturation. Behav Brain Res 1995; 69:1–11.

55. Thai, L., Galluzzo, J., McCook, E., Seidler, F., and Slotkin, T. Atypical regulation of hepatic adenylyl cyclase and adrenergic receptors during a critical developmental period: agonists evoke supersensitivity accompanied by failure of receptor down-regulation. Pediatr Res 1996; 39(4 pt 1):697–707.

56. Jouvet-Mounier, D., Astic, L., and Lacote, D. Ontogenesis of the states of sleep in rat, cat, and guinea pig during the first postnatal month. Dev Psychobiol 1970; 2(4):216–239.

57. Anders, T. and Eiben, L. Pediatric sleep disorders: a review of the past 10 years. J Am Acad Child Adolesc Psychiatry 1997; 36(1):9–20.

58. Frank, M. G. and Heller, H. C. Development of REM and slow wave sleep in the rat. Am J Physiol 1997; 272:R1792–R1799.

59. Mirmiran, M. The function of fetal/neonatal rapid eye movement sleep. Behav Brain Res 1995; 69:13–22.
60. Krueger, J., Obal, F. J., Kapas, L., and Fang, J. Brain organization and sleep function. Behav Brain Res 1995; 69:177–185.
61. Smith, C. Sleep states and memory processes. Behav Brain Res 1995; 69:137–145.
62. Mitchison, G. and Crick, F. REM sleep and neural nets. Behav Brain Res 1995; 69:147–155.
63. Salzarulo, P. and Fagioli, I. Sleep for development or development for waking?—some speculations from a human perspective. Behav Brain Res 1995; 69:23–27.
64. Benington, J. and Heller, H. Does the function of REM sleep concern non-REM sleep or waking? Prog Neurobiol 1994; 44(5):433–449.
65. Parmeggiani, P. Interaction between sleep and thermoregulation. Waking Sleeping 1997; 1:123–132.
66. Vogel, G., Neill, D., Kors, D., and Hagler, M. REM sleep abnormalities in a new animal model of endogenous depression. Neurosci Biobehav Rev 1990; 14:77–83.
67. Vogel, G. and Hagler, M. Effects of neonatally administered iprindole on adult behaviors of rats. Pharmacol Biochem Behav 1996; 55:157–161.
68. Huisjes, H., Hadders-Algra, M., and Torwen, B. Is clonidine a behavioural teratogen in the human. Early Hum Dev 1986; 14:43–48.
69. Owens, J. A., Maxim, R., Nobile, C., McGuinn, M., and Msall, M. Parental and self-report of sleep in children with attention-deficit/hyperactivity disorder. Arch Pediatr Adolesc Med 2000; 154:549–555.
70. Gruber, R., Sadeh, A., and Raviv, A. Instability of sleep patterns in children with attention-deficit/hyperactivity disorder. J Am Acad Child Adolesc Psychiatry 2000; 39:495–501.
71. Corkum, P., Moldofsky, H., Hogg-Johnson, S., Humphries, T., and Tannock, R. Sleep problems in children with attention-deficit/hyperactivity disorder: impact of subtype, comorbidity, and stimulant medication. J Am Acad Child Adolesc Psychiatry 1999; 38:1285–1293.
72. Kujala, T., Alho, K., and Naatanen, R. Cross-modal reorganization of human cortical functions. Trends Neurosci 2000; 23:115–120.
73. Ford, B., Holmes, C., Mainville, L., and Jones, B. GABAergic neurons in the rat pontomesencephalic tegmentum: codistribution with cholinergic and other tegmental neurons projecting to the posterior lateral hypothalamus. Comp Neurol 1995; 363(2):177–196.
74. Greenough, W. Experience effects on the developing and mature brain: dendritic branching and synaptogenesis. In: Krasnegor, N., Blass, E., Hofer, M., and Smotherman, W. eds. Perinatal Development: A Psychobiological Perspective. Orlando, FL: Academic Press, 1987:195–220.
75. Kaczmarek, L., Kossut, M., and Skangiel-Kramska, J. Glutamate receptors in cortical plasticity: molecular and cellular biology. Am Physiol Soc 1997; 77(1):217–255.

76. Miller, J. and Friedhoff, A. Prenatal neurotransmitter programming of postnatal receptor function. Prog Brain Res 1988; 73:509–522.
77. Wu, G.-Y., Malinow, R., and Cline, H. Maturation of a central glutamatergic synapse. Science 1996; 274:972–975.
78. Miller, N. Behavioral medicine: symbiosis between laboratory and clinic. Annu Rev Psychol 1983; 34:1–31.
79. Strumwasser, F. The relations between neuroscience and human behavioral science. J Exp Anal Behav 1994; 61(2):307–317.
80. Fokkema, D. S. The psychobiology of strained breathing and its cardiovascular implications: a functional system review. Psychophysiology 1999; 36:164–175.
81. Meaney, M. J., Mitchell, J. B., Aitken, D. H., Bhatnagar, S., Bodnoff, S. R., Iny, L. J., and Sarrieau, A. The effects of neonatal handling on the development of the adrenocortical response to stress: implications for neuropathology and cognitive deficits in later life. Psychoneuroendocrinology 1991; 16:85–103.
82. Thomas, A., Austin, W., Friedman, L., and Strohl, K. A Model of ventilatory instability induced in the unrestrained rat. J Appl Physiol 1992; 73(4):1530–1536.
83. Cohen, D. Development of a vertebrate experimental model for cellular neurophysiologic studies of learning. Conditional Reflex 1969; 4(2):61–80.
84. Mendelson, W. B., Martin, J. V., Perlis, M., Giesen, H., Wagner, R., and Rapoport, S. I. Periodic cessation of respiratory effort during sleep in adult rats. Physiol Behav 1988; 43:229–234.
85. Thomas, A. J., Erokwu, B. O., Yamamoto, B. K., Ernsberger, P., Bishara, O., and Strohl, K. P. Alterations in respiratory behavior, brain neurochemistry and receptor density induced by pharmacologic suppression of sleep in the neonatal period. Brain Res Dev Brain Res 2000; 120:181–189.
86. Kattwinkel, J. Neonatal apnea: pathogenesis and therapy. J Pediatr 1977; 90:342–352.
87. Cella, S., Mennini, T., Miari, A., Cavanus, S., Arce, V., and Muüller, E. Down-regulation of alpha 2-adrenoceptors involved in growth hormone control in the hypothalamus of infant rats receiving short-term clonidine administration. Dev Brain Res 1990; 53:151–156.
88. Strohl, K., Dick, T., and Haxhiu, M. Respiratory control. Comprehensive Textbook of Pulmonary Medicine, 1997.
89. Harper, R. The cerebral regulation of cardiovascular and respiratory functions. Semin Pediatr Neurol 1996; 3(1):13–22.
90. Lauder, J. Neurotransmitters as morphogens. In: Boer, G., Finestra, M., Mirmiran, M., Swaab, D., and van Haaren eds. Prog Brain Res 1988; 73:365–387.
91. Korner, A., Guilleminault, C., Van den Hoed, J., and Baldwin, R. Reduction of sleep apnea and bradycardia in pre-term infants on oscillating waterbeds: a controlled polygraphic study. Pediatrics 1978; 61:528–533.
92. Redline, S., Tishler, P. V., Schluchter, M., Aylor, J., Clark, K., and Graham, G. Risk factors for sleep-disordered breathing in children. Associations with

obesity, race, and respiratory problems. Am J Respir Crit Care Med 1999; 159:1527–1532.

93. Glotzbach, S., Ariagno, R., and Harper, R. Sleep and the sudden infant death syndrome. In: Ferber, R. and Kryger, M., eds. Principles and Practice of Sleep Medicine in the Child. Philadephia: W.B. Saunders, 1995:231–244.

94. Fleming, P. J., Blair, P. S., Bacon, C., Bensley, D., Smith, I., Taylor, E., Berry, J., Golding, J., and Tripp, J. Environment of infants during sleep and risk of the sudden infant death syndrome: results of 1993–95 case-control study for confidential inquiry into stillbirths and deaths in infancy. Br Med J 1996; 313:7051:191–195.

95. McKenna, J. and Mosko, S. Evolution and the sudden infant death syndrome (SIDS). Part III: infant arousal and parent-infant co-sleeping. Hum Nat 1990; 1:291–330.

96. O'Kusky, J. and Norman, M. Sudden infant death syndrome: increased number of synapses in the hypoglossal nucleus. J Neuropathol Exp Neurol 1995; 54(5):627–634.

97. Seaver, L. and Hoyme, H. Teratology in pediatric practice. Pediatr Clin North Am 1992; 39(1):111–134.

98. Van Someren, E., Mirmiran, M., and Swaab, D. Non-pharmacological treatment of sleep and wake disturbances in aging and Alzheimer's disease: chronobiological perspectives. Behav Brain Res 1993; 57:235–253.

99. Yogman, M. and Zeisel, S. Nutrients, neurotransmitters and infant behavior. Am J Clin Nutr 1985; 42:352–360.

10

The Laboratory Rat as a Model of Sleep-Related Breathing Disorders

MIODRAG RADULOVACKI and DAVID W. CARLEY

University of Illinois
Chicago, Illinois, U.S.A.

I. Introduction

An important challenge to the field today is to determine the neural bases for sleep-related changes in control of respiration. Animal models are essential in this endeavor and recent advances have been made in the studies of breathing disorders in marine mammals, preterm lambs, English bulldogs, and neonatal and mature rats. Our group has illustrated this strategy, by characterizing the respiratory instability and its neural mechanisms in the rat model of sleep apnea. In addition, our studies have indicated pharmacologic avenues for the treatment of central apneas in the rat, central/obstructive apneas in other animal species, and the potential management of human sleep apnea syndrome.

II. Rat Model of Sleep Apnea

The occurrence of centrally generated apneic events has been reported during all stages of sleep in unrestrained Fischer-344 (1), Wistar-Kyoto

265

(WKY) (2–5), Sprague Dawley (1,6–22), spontaneously hypertensive (SHR) (3–5,23), and Zucker lean and Zucker obese (24) rats. These respiratory pauses described in rats and related to sleep have been considered as models for determining the basis of sleep-related breathing disorders (SRBDs). Mendelson et al. (1) and Thomas et al. (6) have classified these events according to the presence or absence of a preceding sigh and have divided them into two types: those preceded by a large inspiration ("sighs") and those which occurred without apparent antecedent alteration in respiratory pattern. The latter, which appear to be most analogous to human apneas of clinical interest, at least in adults, varied in duration from 2.0 to 6.1 sec. We have defined both postsigh and spontaneous sleep apneas in rats as cessation of respiratory effort for at least 2.5 sec (Fig. 1). The duration requirement of 2.5 sec represents at least two "missed" breaths, and is therefore roughly analogous to a 10-sec apnea duration in humans, which also reflects two to three missed breaths. These apneas represent central apneas because loss of inspiratory effort has been documented plethysmographically (8,9) and electromyographically (2).

One may well question the relevance of the rat model of sleep apnea to the mechanisms and management of human sleep apnea syndromes. It is our view that both central and obstructive apnea reflect, at least in part, dysregulation of central neural motor output patterning to the respiratory

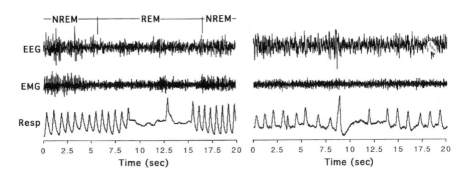

Figure 1 Typical polygraphic presentation of sleep apnea in rats. Left panel depicts a spontaneous apnea; right panel presents a postsigh apnea. Electroencephalogram and EMG activity is employed to determine sleep state. Each peak on the respiration (Resp) channel represents a single inspiration. Note the cessation of respiration, or apnea, in the center of each panel. The postsigh apnea (right) is preceded by a clearly augmented breath, or sigh. The spontaneous apnea (left) is not. These events are transient, but reflect two to three "missed" breaths. This corresponds to 10 to 15-sec apneas in man.

system. In humans with upper airways predisposed to collapse by anatomic, mechanical, or muscular factors, this dysregulation may be manifest primarily by obstructive apneas. In humans or rats with mechanically stable upper airways, dysregulation of respiratory motor output patterning may be expressed primarily by central apneas or hypopneas.

Indirect support for our view comes from several lines of investigation. Most patients with sleep apnea syndrome exhibit a combination of central, mixed, and obstructive apneas in a single sleep period, leading to the suggestion that any factor that destabilizes respiratory drive during sleep promotes apnea genesis. Önal and Lopata (25) demonstrated that patients with sleep apnea exhibited obstructive apneas when breathing through their own upper airways, but central apneas when breathing through a tracheostomy. These investigators concluded that obstructive apnea reflects unstable central respiratory drive in patients with upper airways predisposed to collapse by anatomic or neuromuscular defects. Furthermore, in some cases, continuous positive airway pressure converts obstructive apneas to central apneas, again supporting the conclusion that unstable central respiratory motor patterning contributes to the pathogenesis of obstructive apnea syndrome.

If apnea reflects unstable respiratory patterning, interventions stabilizing respiratory drive during sleep may reduce or eliminate apnea. Indeed, inspired carbon dioxide, used to elevate respiratory drive, reduced the expression of both central (26,27) and obstructive (26,28) apnea in man. Conversely, supplemental inspired oxygen that raises mean arterial oxygen saturation is often associated with longer or more frequent apneas in humans (28). The above-described human findings suggest that central and obstructive apnea during sleep share common central neural pathogenic mechanisms.

In testing the validity of the normal rat model of sleep-disordered breathing, we have demonstrated that central apneas in rats are expressed in similar patterns and are influenced by interventions in a fashion similar to human central and obstructive apnea. In patients, both central and obstructive apnea are most severe during rapid eye movement (REM) sleep (29). In the rat, central apnea is 2–10 times more frequent during REM than during non-REM (NREM) sleep (4,11,18,19). In both humans and rats, inspired hypercapnia decreases, whereas hyperoxia increases, the severity of apnea (11). Essential hypertension appears to increase the risk for sleep apnea syndrome (30), and effective treatment of hypertension can ameliorate sleep apnea (31). Genetic hypertension in rats is associated with a two- to five-fold increase in apnea, and pharmacologic treatment significantly reduces apnea expression (4). Thus, the above-described evidence depicts similar patterns of expression and responses to intervention for central and obstructive apnea in humans and central apnea in rats. In view of this similitude, we have begun to examine the factors that control apnea expression in the rat model.

III. Impact of Cranial Nerve Afferent Activity on Apnea

A. Effects of Altering Vagus Nerve Activity

Stimulation of the Vagus Nerves Produces Apnea

The vagus nerves carry both sensory and motor fibers to a wide array of visceral structures including the heart and lungs. Stimulation of vagus nerve sensory fibers by electrical, mechanical, or chemical means has a potent ability to evoke immediate apnea (loss of respiratory effort) in anesthetized animals of various species. The pathway for this reflex is shown in Figure 2.

If sensory nerve fibers of the vagus nerve are activated, their cell bodies in the nodose ganglia are stimulated to fire. This excitation is transmitted to the primary visceral sensory integrating area of the brainstem, the solitary tract nucleus. The solitary tract nucleus, in turn, suppresses (via pathways that remain to be determined) respiratory pattern generating and motor output centers, producing apnea. Serotonin (5-hydroxytryptamine [5-HT]), an important signaling molecule in the nervous system, can act at each site along this reflex arc. The actions of serotonin on reflex apnea are complex, however. At least 14 different serotonin receptor subtypes have now been identified. The receptor subtypes expressed and their net effects vary significantly at different sites within the reflex arc.

Of particular relevance is the fact that serotonin injection into the veins, hearts, or arteries of anesthetized animals produces dose-dependent

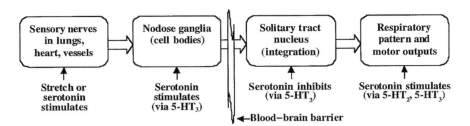

Figure 2 Pathway of vagus nerve-induced reflex apnea. The vagus nerves carry both sensory and motor fibers to a wide array of visceral structures including the heart and lungs. Stimulation of vagus nerve sensory fibers by electrical, mechanical, or chemical means has a potent ability to evoke immediate apnea (loss of respiratory effort) in anesthetized animals of various species.

reflex apnea (32–35). Yoshioka et al. (34) demonstrated that serotonin-induced reflex apnea results from activation of type 3 (5-HT$_3$) receptors in or on the cell bodies (located in the nodose ganglia) of vagus sensory fibers. Activation of 5-HT$_3$ receptors causes nodose ganglion cells to depolarize; they respond more easily and vigorously to stimulation. The ability of vagus nerve activity to provoke apnea, together with the ability of serotonin to make vagal afferent fibers more excitable, prompted our recent investigations into the role of serotonin receptors in *sleep* apnea genesis in the rat (18–20).

Serotonin Exacerbates Sleep Apneas in Rats

We demonstrated that serotonin injection into the intraperitoneal space did not produce immediate reflex apnea in sleeping rats. Instead, as depicted by Figure 3, such injections dramatically increased the intermittent, spontaneous expression of central apnea, an effect that was most prominent during REM sleep (19). Increased apnea expression resulted from stimulation of serotonin receptors in the peripheral nervous system, because serotonin does not cross the blood–brain barrier. Furthermore, the apneagenic effect of serotonin was completely blocked by pretreatment with ondansetron (GR38032F), a 5-HT$_3$ receptor antagonist, at a dose (0.1 mg/kg) that had

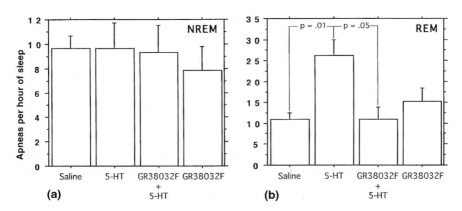

Figure 3 Effects of 5-HT (0.79 mg/kg), GR38032F (0.1 mg/kg) plus 5-HT (0.79 mg/kg), and GR38032F (0.1 mg/kg) on spontaneous apneas in NREM and REM sleep. (a) Spontaneous apneas per hour in NREM sleep were not affected by any drug treatment ($p = 0.97$). (b) Following 5-HT treatment, spontaneous apnea expression increased in REM sleep (>250% increase; $p = 0.01$), but the increase was abolished by pretreatment with GR38032F. GR38032F had no effect on spontaneous apneas ($p = 0.51$).

no independent effect on sleep, pulmonary ventilation, or apnea expression (Fig. 3) (19). At a higher dose (1.0 mg/kg), ondansetron completely suppressed apnea expression during REM sleep for several hours (Fig. 4), but had little or no impact on apneas during NREM sleep (18). In accordance, using English bulldog as an animal model of obstructive sleep apnea, Veasey et al. (36) showed that oral administration of 2.0 mg/kg ondansetron significantly reduced apneas during REM sleep but had no effect on NREM sleep apneas. This is of interest because it demonstrates the importance of the peripheral vagal 5-HT$_3$ mechanism in the pathogenesis of obstructive sleep apneas. Together, these results show that endogenous serotonergic tone at receptors within the peripheral nervous system acts to destabilize respiration during sleep—especially REM sleep.

We have now confirmed the apnea-suppressing action of serotonin antagonists using two additional compounds, mirtazapine (20) and zacopride (22). We administered mirtazapine (labeled as Remeron), an antidepressant with 5-HT$_1$ agonist as well as 5-HT$_2$ and 5-HT$_3$ antagonist properties, intraperitoneally to nine rats in three doses. At all three doses the drug reduced the apnea index (AI) during NREM sleep by more than 50% ($p < 0.0001$) and reduced the AI during REM sleep by 60% ($p < 0.0001$) for at least 6 hr (Fig. 5a). In association with this apnea suppression, normalized

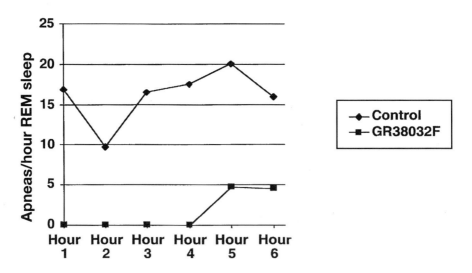

Figure 4   Effect of GR38032F (1.0 mg/kg) on the rate of apneas per hour of REM sleep. There was a significant suppressant effect of the drug on REM sleep apneas throughout the 6-hr recording period ($p = 0.01$).

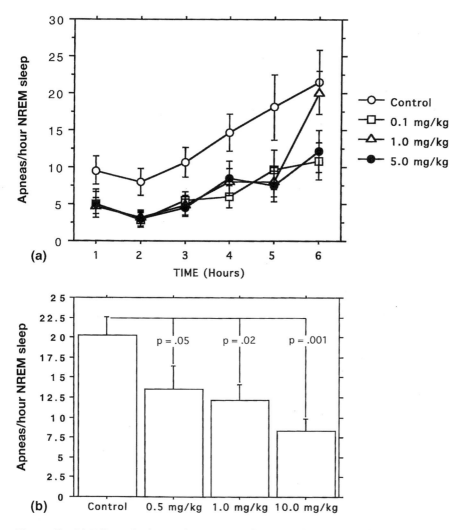

Figure 5 (a) Effect of mirtazapine on apnea index during NREM sleep. Each dose of mirtazapine significantly reduced apnea index with respect to control ($p < 0.0001$ for each). (b) Effects of (R)-zacopride on apnea expression in NREM sleep during the first 2 hr after injection. NREM sleep apnea index was significantly reduced by all three doses of (R)-zacopride. There were no statistically significant differences on NREM apnea index during the first 2 hr among the three doses of (R)-zacopride tested.

inspiratory minute ventilation increased during all wake–sleep states ($p < 0.0001$ for each state). The duration of NREM sleep was unaffected by any dose of mirtazapine, but NREM electroencephalogram (EEG) delta power was increased by more than 30% at all doses ($p = 0.04$), indicating improved NREM sleep consolidation after mirtazapine injection. We concluded that mirtazapine, over a 50-fold dose range, significantly reduced central apnea expression during NREM and REM sleep in the rat. We suggested that the efficacy of mirtazapine to suppress apnea in all sleep stages most probably arises from its mixed agonist–antagonist profile at serotonin receptors.

We also administered (R)-zacopride, a benzamide with potent 5-HT_3 receptor antagonist and weak 5-HT_4 receptor agonist properties, intraperitoneally to 10 Sprague Dawley rats. Our data showed that (R)-zacopride (0.5, 1.0, and 10.0 mg/kg) suppressed spontaneous apneas during NREM sleep by 50% and suppressed spontaneous apneas during REM sleep by 80% at all doses tested (Fig. 5b). Thus, we concluded that (R)-zacopride, over a 20-fold dose range, significantly reduced central apnea expression during NREM and REM sleep in the rat. We ascribed the efficacy of zacopride to suppress central apneas to its antagonist actions at 5-HT_3 receptors or from its mixed agonist–antagonist profile at $5\text{-HT}_4/5\text{-HT}_3$ receptors.

Taken together, these key observations demonstrated that endogenous tone is present at 5-HT_3 receptors in the peripheral nervous system and this predisposes the respiratory control system to experience apnea during sleep. The observations also illustrated the therapeutic potential of serotonergic drugs, especially 5-HT_3 receptor antagonists, for treatment of SRBDs.

B. Effects of Altering Glossopharyngeal Activity

Chemoreceptor Stimulation Reduces Sleep Apnea

Inspired hypoxia, hypercapnia, and hyperoxia are well known to affect the frequency and severity of apnea in humans (37–40). In rats, Thomas et al. (6) showed that apneic events in adult rats were affected by intermittent peripheral chemoreceptor perturbations during their postnatal development. Intermittent hypoxia led to markedly increased expression of spontaneous but not postsigh apnea in adulthood (6). Our studies in rats showed that apnea incidence is strongly modulated by manipulations of inspired gas (Fig. 6) (11). Increasing chemoreceptor stimulation by either hypoxia or hypercapnia significantly reduced AI, i.e., number of apneas per hour, whereas conversely, decreasing peripheral chemoreceptor drive by hyperoxia increased AI (Fig. 6). None of these effects was associated with gross changes in sleep architecture.

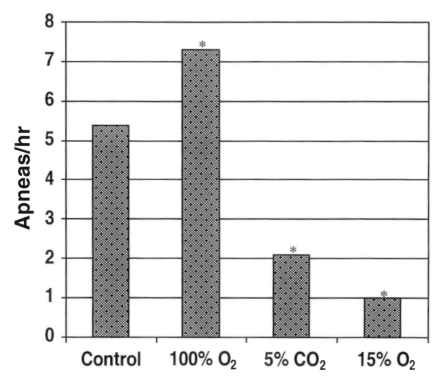

Figure 6 Effects of inspired gas on apneas per hour. Apneas per hour were significantly higher during 100% O_2 and significantly lower during 15% O_2 and 5% CO_2 compared with room air. $*p < 0.05$ for each.

Data from our studies did not allow us to discriminate the relative contributions of mechanoreceptor versus chemoreceptor feedback to postsigh apnea genesis. Activation of pulmonary stretch receptors inhibits inspiration and can potentiate expiration via the Hering-Breuer reflex (41,42). Thus, a sigh may activate this reflex, precipitating a central apnea under otherwise permissive conditions. Postsigh apnea has also been observed in humans and dogs during sleep (43), and the characteristics of the apnea have been used as a measure of the Hering-Breuer reflex. Issa and Porostocky (43) reported that 83% of spontaneously occurring sighs were followed by apnea during wakefulness and sleep in anesthetized dogs. Chow et al. (44) employed brief airway occlusion to induce brief hyperpnea in sleeping dogs. Their findings demonstrated a volume threshold for reflex apnea during sleep; apnea did not occur unless tidal volumes at least three times the eupneic levels were achieved during the hyperpnea (44). In contrast, our studies showed that postsigh apnea often occurred during sleep in the rat when tidal volume was augmented by as little as 25%. Less than 20% of the postsigh apneas measured in our studies were preceded by tidal breaths >300% of baseline. This percentage was not significantly affected by manipulations of inspired gas, and the effects of inspired gas on postsigh apneas were similar for larger (>300% baseline) and smaller (<300%) sighs. These observations argued that a significant volume threshold for postsigh apnea genesis was not present in the rat under the experimental conditions employed. The disparity of results may have also reflected species differences as well as differential effects of spontaneous sighs versus occlusion-induced augmented breaths.

The significance of our studies on the effects of inspired gas on sleep-related apneas in rats is that we demonstrated for the first time that the sleep AI was higher during 100% O_2 compared with room air, and was lower during 15% O_2 and 5% CO_2 compared with room air. Thus, we concluded that stimulation of chemoreceptors acts to oppose apnea in the rat.

Adenosine Agonists Suppress Apnea

It is generally recognized that adenosine administration to the peripheral nervous system has a stimulant effect on respiration. Indeed, intra-arterial infusion of adenosine to humans and animals stimulated respiration (45–49) and potentiated chemoreflexes (48,49). Isolated perfusion of carotid bodies with adenosine agonists augmented ventilation and chemoreflexes in rats (50). These lines of evidence suggest that adenosinergic respiratory stimulation is mediated by the peripheral nervous system. In contrast, intracerebroventricular administration of adenosine agonists to anesthetized rats and cats depressed ventilation (51,52). In addition, injection of the adenosine agonist adenosine 5′-N-ethylcarmoxamide into the nucleus tractus solitarius of anesthetized rats depressed respiration (53). Thus, the central action of adenosine on respiration follows the pattern of adenosine's general inhibitory role in the central nervous system (CNS) (54).

We tested the hypothesis that peripheral stimulation of adenosine receptors by adenosine or adenosine analogs, in accordance with their stimulant effects on breathing, may suppress apnea during sleep. We administered adenosine receptor agonists intraperitoneally to rats and observed clear dose-dependent suppression of apnea during NREM sleep, using either the A_1 receptor agonist phenylisopropyl-adenosine (L-PIA) or A_2 receptor agonist 2-p-(2-carboxyethyl)phenethylamino-5′-N-ethylcarbox-amido-adenosine hydrochloride (CGS 21680) (8).

Because L-PIA and CGS 21680 cross the blood–brain barrier, we were interested in ascertaining whether the apnea suppression can be produced by peripherally selective adenosine agonists and whether the effects is receptor mediated. For that purpose we intraperitoneally administered to rats, singly and in combination, N^6 (p-sulfophenyl)adenosine, a selective A_1 adenosine receptor agonist, and 8-(p-sulfophenyl)theophylline (p-SPT), a peripherally selective (55) adenosine receptor antagonist (56). Our results showed that p-SPA, like L-PIA and CGS 21680, suppressed apneas in NREM sleep and that this effect was blocked by pretreatment with an equimolar dose of p-SPT (Fig. 7) (21), indicating that p-SPA suppression of apneas was receptor mediated in the peripheral nervous system. Administration of p-SPT alone to rats had no effect on apneas, sleep, or blood pressure (BP) (21). The lack of p-SPT effect on sleep apneas argued against a physiological role for endogenous adenosine in the peripheral nervous system as a modulator of sleep apnea expression under baseline conditions.

These studies were limited because although hypotension and hypothermia are well-known effects of systemically administered adenosine agonists, BP and core temperature were not measured. We then tested another A_1 receptor agonist, N-[(1S, *trans*)-2-hydroxycyclopentyl]adenosine (GR79236), on apnea expression in rats, and measured BP and core temperature to determine whether this agonist would suppress apnea at doses not associated with significant hypotension or hypothermia. Our data showed that GR79236 administration was associated with significant respiratory stimulation and significant dose-dependent suppression of

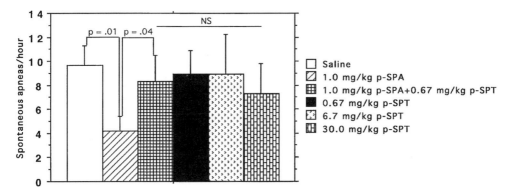

Figure 7   The effect of p-SPA (1.0 mg/kg), p-SPA (1.0 mg/kg) plus p-SPT (0.67 mg/ kg), and p-SPT (0.67, 6.7, and 30.0 mg/kg) on spontaneous apneas in NREM sleep. Apnea expression decreased following p-SPA treatment (50% decrease), but the decrease was abolished by an equimolar dose of p-SPT.

apneas. The drug was equipotent in suppressing NREM- and REM-related spontaneous apneas (Fig. 8) without effects on BP, core temperature, or sleep architecture (15).

Baroreceptor Stimulation Impacts Apnea Expression

Acute Hypotension Reduces Sleep Apnea

Increased prevalence of SRBD has been reported in patients with essential hypertension. It has been suggested that SRBD may predispose to hypertension, and also that hypertension may predispose to SRBD. With respect to the latter possibility, hypertensive patients demonstrate an increased prevalence of sleep apnea in some studies (30,57), but not in others (58). In addition, pharmacological treatment of hypertension in patients with SRBD may improve sleep-related respiratory function (59). The mechanisms underlying the connection between hypertension and SRBD remain poorly defined.

It is commonly accepted that increases in BP inhibit ventilation, whereas decreases in arterial pressure disinhibit, or stimulate, ventilation (60,61). Even small reductions of BP in awake dogs stimulate ventilation (62). We hypothesized that lowering of BP would stimulate ventilation,

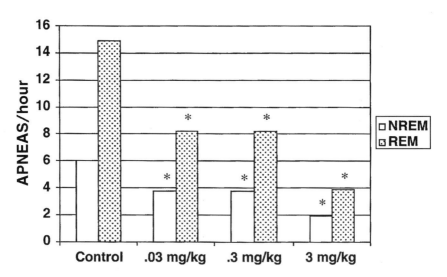

Figure 8   Effects of A_1 receptor agonist GR79236 on the rate of spontaneous apneas per hour of NREM and REM sleep. Each bar represents mean $\pm$ SE over all 6 hr of recording. $*p < 0.01$ versus control.

presumably by reducing baroreceptor activity, and would thereby reduce the expression of central apneas during sleep in rats.

We examined the effects of mild hypotension induced by hydralazine on apnea expression in Zucker lean and Zucker obese (24), Sprague Dawley (13), WKY, and SHR (4) rats because the effects of BP on respiratory control are believed to result from baroreceptor reflexes (60–62), which differ among these strains. We used two strains Zucker rats: (1) heterozygous phenotypically lean animals and (2) homozygous phenotypically obese animals. Obese Zucker rats are normotensive but have impaired baroreflexes compared to lean strain control animals (63,64). We compared the hypotension-induced changes in ventilation and apnea expression during sleep in these two groups of animals. We demonstrated a clear decrease in the rate of sleep apnea during hypotension (Fig. 9), but were unable to identify a differential effect between the lean and obese strains of Zucker rat. This finding was of interest because the reduced rate of expression was found for spontaneous as well as for postsigh apneas (Fig. 9). Finally, in addition to the apnea suppression associated with hydralazine-induced hypotension, significant respiratory stimulation was also observed, supporting the possibility that hypotension acts indirectly, via modulation of respiratory drive, to suppress apnea.

To further test the possibility that hypotension reduces sleep apneas via modulation of respiratory drive in normotensive animals, we intraperitoneally administered hydralazine to Sprague Dawley rats (13). Our study showed that transitions from wakefulness to NREM and REM sleep were associated with progressive decreases in relative minute ventilation (RVi)

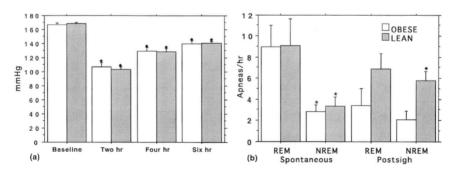

Figure 9 (a) Blood pressure in Zucker lean and Zucker obese rats for 6 hr following intraperitoneal administration of hydralazine (◆$p < 0.0001$ related to baseline). (b) Sleep state dependence of apnea expression in Zucker lean and Zucker obese rats (*$p < 0.02$ related to respective REM sleep of each animal group; ◆$p = 0.005$ related to obese NREM postsigh apneas per hour).

and increases in apnea expression (Fig. 10). The 15–25% decrease in RVi with sleep onset was associated with significant apnea expression, whereas increasing RVi by 25% via hydralazine administration was associated with near total apnea suppression. Hydralazine significantly increased respiratory rate and minute ventilation during all behavioral states in the rat (Fig. 10).

Whatever the mechanisms, changes in apnea expression during sleep and after hydralazine administration correlated with changes in integrated respiratory drive. Although hydralazine is believed to exert its primary effects on the circulatory system, some of its metabolites are known to cross the blood–brain barrier, and direct effects of these metabolites could not, therefore, be excluded. For example, hydralazine potentiates the production of nitric oxide within the vasculature, and this may have led to increased nitric oxide concentration in the brain. It is possible that increased brainstem interstitial nitric oxide concentrations contributed to the observed respiratory stimulation after hydralazine administration.

Taken together, these manipulations of chemoreceptor and baroreceptor stimulation suggest that integrated respiratory drive is an important factor that determines the likelihood of apnea expression during sleep in the rat. In this interpretation, sustained states of decreased drive render the respiratory network more vulnerable to apnea expression, whereas interventions or conditions that increase the baseline respiratory drive diminish apnea expression. These findings suggest that sleep-related apnea in normotensive rats is promoted by sustained states of decreased respiratory drive.

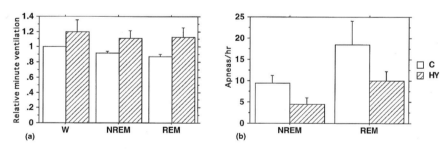

Figure 10 (a) Group mean data, obtained from final 4 hr of each recording for relative minute ventilation (RVi). RVi exhibited progressive decreases with transitions from W to NREM and from NREM to REM sleep. (b) Expression of spontaneous apneas per hour of NREM and REM sleep. In all cases, group data demonstrate a significant decrease in apnea expression after hydralazine (HY) administration ($p < 0.05$).

Chronic Hypertension Exacerbates Sleep Apnea

We have shown that genetic hypertension in rats is associated with increased apnea expression (3,4). We have used SHR, a well-characterized substrain of WKY rats, as a model of genetic hypertension and demonstrated that these animals exhibited nearly 10-fold more apneas than WKY rats (4). Moreover, when BP was acutely normalized by systemic administration of hydralazine, apnea fell to the level of normotensive WKY animals (vide supra, Ref. 4). However, our previous study did not demonstrate the effects of sustained normotension on sleep-related breathing in SHR.

Sustained normotension in SHR was achieved by Berecek et al. (65) who showed that in utero and postnatal (up to age 8 weeks) treatment of SHR rats by an angiotensin-converting enzyme inhibitor, captopril, completely blocked the development of hypertension and related cardiovascular derangements in adult animals (66).

We recorded respiration, BP, heart rate, and sleep in captopril-treated SHR (cap-SHR), SHR, and WKY rats (5). Our study showed for the first time that sleep-related respiratory abnormalities persist in genetically hypertensive but phenotypically normotensive rats. In untreated SHR, the rate of spontaneous apneas versus WKY animals was elevated 15-fold during NREM sleep and 10-fold during REM sleep. Captopril treatment, despite normalizing BP and heart period, yielded no reduction in NREM apnea expression and the REM-related spontaneous AI remained elevated by 500% (Fig. 11). Despite the significant sleep-related respiratory disorder exhibited by treated and untreated SHR, mean respiratory rate and minute ventilation were equivalent among all three animal groups in all behavioral states.

Our earlier finding, that acute normalization of BP in SHR by hydralazine (vide supra) produced a decrease in apnea expression, contrasted with the study in cap-SHR rats in which sustained control of hypertension did not correspond to a sustained reduction in apnea expression. It is possible that acute suppression of apnea in the rat by hydralazine bolus injection reflected a transient reduction in baroreceptor feedback to the brainstem. Even a slight lowering of BP can disinhibit respiratory drive, yielding significantly increased ventilation in conscious animals (62). In support of this possibility, we demonstrated that hydralazine-induced hypotension produced respiratory stimulation and suppressed apnea in Sprague Dawley (13) and Zucker (24) rats. Effects of long-term hydralazine administration on breathing have not been tested. It is possible that baroreflex resetting, alterations in receptor expression or localization, or other factors may result in a loss of apnea suppression during sustained pharmacological management of hypertension.

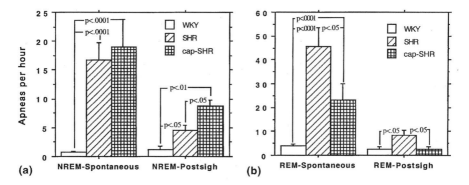

Figure 11 Ordinate shows apneas per hour of NREM or REM sleep for each animal group. (a) Both spontaneous and postsigh apneas per hour during NREM sleep were significantly elevated in SHR and cap-SHR versus WKY animals. (b) Spontaneous apneas per hour during REM sleep were significantly elevated in SHR and cap-SHR versus WKY animals, whereas postsigh apneas per hour were significantly elevated only in SHR versus WKY animals.

We suggest that differences in respiratory or cardiovascular behaviors between SHR and cap-SHR rats reflect the differences in the developmental course of the nervous system induced by administration of captopril from conception to postnatal age 8 weeks. Our study showed that untreated SHR rats demonstrated clear cardiovascular and respiratory derangements with respect to the normotensive WKY control strain. However, captopril treatment dissociated these derangements: cardiovascular parameters remained normal throughout the adult life of the animal (65,66), whereas sleep-related respiratory disorder persisted.

The results of our studies showed that phenotypically normotensive but genetically hypertensive rats exhibited striking sleep-disordered respiration, which was equivalent to untreated hypertensive animals with a mean AI of more than 20/hr. This elevation in apnea genesis occurred without alteration in sleep architecture, respiratory rate, or inspiratory minute ventilation, using normotensive WKY animals as a control. Our findings strongly suggest that sleep-disordered respiration in SHR rats is genetically determined and not secondary to hypertension or other cardiovascular derangement.

Baroreceptor Stimulation Increases Sleep Apnea

We hypothesized that the acute effects of altering BP on sleep apneas are mediated via baroreflexes that may influence the respiratory pattern generator (67,68) as well as CNS-mediated control of BP (68,69). Because baroreceptor stimulation induces ventilatory depression (70–72), we suggested that acute hypotension, which inhibits baroreflex activity, causes disinhibition of respiration, leading to fewer apneas (4,24).

We evaluated further the role of baroreflexes on sleep apnea by using protoveratrine (PV) A and B (PVA and PVB, respectively), known to exert their effect on the cardiovascular system via stimulation of baroreceptors in the carotid sinus, heart, aorta, and pulmonary vascular bed (73,74). In addition, systemic administration of PVs to cats and dogs (75) yielded respiratory suppression that was ascribed to stimulation of carotid sinus baroreceptors and pulmonary venous stretch receptors. We tested the hypothesis that baroreceptor afferent stimulation by PV inhibits respiratory drive and leads to an increased apnea expression.

Our study demonstrated that pharmacological stimulation of barore-flexes in the rat is associated with increased apnea expression. Administration of 1 mg/kg of PV increased spontaneous AI in NREM sleep almost five-fold in comparison to control (Fig. 12), whereas the postsigh AI increased almost four-fold. The fact that BP did not decrease, whereas the heart period increased, indicated the presence of compensatory increases in stroke volume, vascular resistance, or both. The absence of hypotension reduced the likelihood that the observed respiratory effects were due to nonspecific circulatory changes. These findings also suggested, therefore, that hydrala-zine-induced hypotension most probably suppressed apnea (4) by decreasing baroreceptor stimulation, rather than indirectly, as a result of hypotension per se. In addition, the strong correlation between AI and decreased Vi

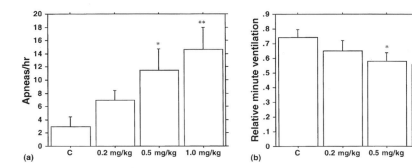

Figure 12 (a) Effect of 0.2, 0.5, and 1.0 mg/kg of protoveratrines on spontaneous apneas per hour during NREM sleep (*$p = 0.02$ and **$p = 0.001$ in relation to control). (b) Effects of 0.2, 0.5, and 1.0 mg/kg of protoveratrines on minute ventilation during NREM sleep (*$p = 0.04$ and **$p = 0.01$ in relation to control).

(Fig. 12) supported the theory that one mechanism underlying central apnea is reflex inhibition of the respiratory center (76).

In addition to their peripheral effects on cardiovascular system, PVs may have direct CNS effects. One possibility is that they may affect proposed central baroreceptors similar to those of the carotid sinuses (77). Their central effect on respiration could be either stimulatory, possibly through medullary areas, or inhibitory, through another intracranial area, possibly meningeal (73). Regardless of their action, central or peripheral, it is known that PVs stimulate baroreceptor nerve endings. There is also indication of direct involvement of baroreceptor afferent firing in reflex apnea genesis in anesthetized rats (78). In accordance, our study provided evidence that the PVs have a potent sleep apnea-promoting action, indicating that pharmacological stimulation of baroreflexes can indeed promote apnea expression in the sleeping rat.

IV. Central Nervous System Influences on Sleep Apnea
A. REM Sleep and Apnea

As first recognized by Aserinsky and Kleitman (79), REM sleep is uniquely characterized by two major phenomena: (1) atonia of postural muscles resulting from active inhibition of motor neurons, and (2) transient (or "phasic") events that are widespread in the brain and are typified by the REMs, for which REM sleep was named. It is important to recognize that there exist many other peripherally observable correlates of these central events. Phasic perturbations of respiratory pattern and motor outputs, sympathetic outflow, heart rate, BP, and coronary blood flow are all characteristic of REM sleep (80).

REM sleep leads to substantial changes in respiratory control. With respect to wakefulness, ventilation is consistently decreased during REM sleep, whereas changes in respiratory frequency are more variable (81,82). Although respiration during NREM sleep is determined primarily by the homeostatic control mechanisms, during REM sleep it is clear that there are phasic influences arising outside the homeostatic controllers that dramatically affect ventilation. The intermittent and variable presentation of these phasic events within and between REM periods underlies the fact that the greatest change in ventilation during REM sleep is increased breath-to-breath variability (83).

Changes in respiratory control associated with REM phasic events are relevant to the occurrence of apnea, hypopnea, and upper airway flow limitation. The English bulldog, with significant upper airway abnormalities, exhibits obstructive apneas during REM sleep (84,85). In this animal model, tonic reductions in motor output are insufficient to produce apnea; rather, apneas occur in association with further phasic decrements in muscle activities coincident with eye movements.

In the rat, eye movements are associated with irregular activation of the diaphragm and upper airway muscles, and with central apnea (86). In addition, the rate of apneas is highest during REM sleep in the rat (1,3,12), as in man (29). Similar eye movement-related changes have been noted in man, including (1) reductions in the motor outputs to upper airway muscles (87), (2) increased upper airway resistance (88), (3) decreased minute ventilation (89), and (4) apnea (90). Thus, understanding the neural basis for these phasic respiratory phenomena is both intrinsically interesting and of great clinical relevance.

B. Brainstem Phasic Events and Apnea

An understanding of the phasic respiratory behaviors characteristic of REM sleep should naturally be built upon our current knowledge of its intrinsic phasic phenomena, such as ponto-geniculo-occipital (PGO) waves. PGO waves are large-amplitude field potentials, which can be recorded from the pons, lateral geniculate, and occipital cortex of cats. They are very sensitive markers for the phasic events of REM sleep. Basically, PGO wave generation has been linked to two groups of cholinergic cells in the rostral pons, the laterodorsal tegmental nucleus (LDT) and the pedunculopontine tegmental (PPT) nucleus. Lesions out of both LDT and PPT caused a reduction of PGO waves and eye movements, which was correlated to the number of cholinergic cells destroyed (91). At least two types of bursting cells have been identified in the caudal PPT, which fire just prior to PGO waves and eye movements (92). Virtually all of this work investigating the neural basis of PGO wave generation has been performed in cats.

Field potentials fulfilling all criteria for PGO waves can also be recorded from the region of the locus coeruleus in rats (93). In fact, the pontine distribution of sites at which PGO waves can be recorded is similar in the cat and the rat (94). Although geniculate PGO waves have not been demonstrated in the rat, single-unit recordings in the dorsal lateral geniculate nucleus of rats demonstrated that discharge rates in 70% of these cells exhibit a temporal relationship with hindbrain PGO waves (95). This finding supports the existence of a phasic event system in the rat.

Our research has provided the first evidence relating PGO waves to the occurrence of apnea and hypopnea (Figs. 13 and 14). We instrumented a group of 3-month-old Sprague Dawley rats with electrodes for recording cortical EEG, nuchal muscle electromyogram (EMG), and pontine PGO waves using bilateral electrodes stereotaxically targeted to the region of the locus coeruleus. Figure 13 represents a 10-sec epoch of REM sleep extracted from the middle of a 4-min REM period. The upper tracing in this and Figure 14 is the biparietal cortical EEG, obtained using skull screws. The next tracing is nuchal muscle EMG, followed by respiration obtained by single-chamber plethysmography. The bottom tracing is PGO activity recorded by bilateral stainless steel electrodes in the region of the locus coeruleus. Figure 13 depicts the pattern of rapid, shallow, and irregular respiration typically associated with human and rat REM sleep. Notice that the beginning of this record is characterized by regular tidal breathing and an absence of PGO waves. Coincident with the onset of PGO waves, respiration becomes highly erratic, suggesting that the PGO-related phasic events of REM sleep may be the primary source of respiratory instability. This observation is consistent with the relationships between eye movements and respiration observed during human sleep.

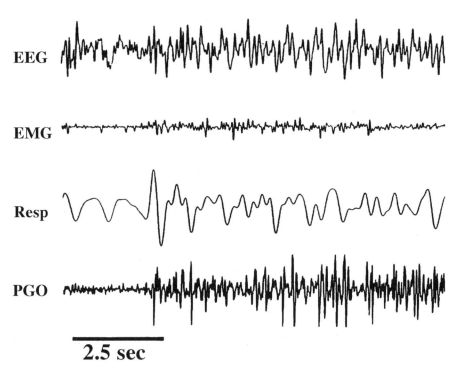

EEG

EMG

Resp

PGO

2.5 sec

Figure 13   Represents a 10-sec epoch of REM sleep. The pattern of rapid, shallow, and irregular respiration is typically associated with human and rat REM sleep.

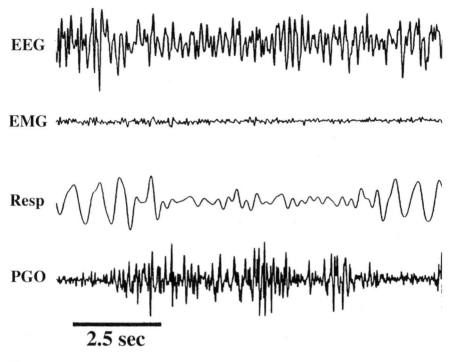

2.5 sec

Figure 14 Represents a 10-sec epoch of REM sleep. An apnea of 6 sec duration is shown coincident with the appearance of a PGO cluster wave.

Strong circumstantial evidence links the incidence of brainstem phasic events, typified by PGO waves, to the occurrence of apnea and hypopnea, but we know virtually nothing of the mechanisms that mediate this connection. Our group has characterized the respiratory instability during sleep in the rat and has demonstrated the association of spontaneous phasic events to respiratory instability. Future work must capitalize on this and related animal models to determine the neural mechanisms of sleep state-dependent respiratory control.

C. Sleep Deprivation Increases Apnea

Acute sleep deprivation precipitates numerous changes in sleep homeostatic mechanisms and autonomic function. Twenty-four-hour sleep deprivation leads to acute diathesis of sleep apnea in man (96) and sleep-disordered respiration in a canine model of experimental airway obstruction (97). Forty-eight-hour REM sleep deprivation in humans increased the frequency of breaths in which ventilation was reduced below the range for tonic REM sleep. These events were associated with longer REM periods and an increase in total phasic activity during REM sleep (98). In cats, acute sleep deprivation resulted in an increase in REM sleep-associated phasic alterations in diaphragm activity during recovery REM sleep (99). Sleep deprivation also caused an increased percentage of diaphragm bursts with decreased slope and an increased number of diaphragm fractionations. Collectively, these results demonstrate that respiratory control mechanisms during REM sleep are sensitive to prior sleep deprivation.

We examined the effects of 48 hr of REM sleep deprivation on apneas in Sprague Dawley, WKY, and SHR rats (3,12,16). Recovery sleep exhibited equivalent increases in REM sleep in all strains. Proportional increases in REM-related apnea occurred in both normotensive strains, but SHR rats demonstrated a stronger, disproportionate increase in REM apneas during recovery sleep. These observations support the hypothesis that states of low respiratory drive (e.g., hypertension) promote respiratory instability and apnea.

It appears that REM sleep deprivation, by its concomitant increase in REM pressure, may have intensified the unsteadiness of both respiration and BP, which was then reflected in elevation of apneas in the SHR rats. It seems likely that decreased tonic and phasic activity of reticular formation and respiratory neurons during REM sleep may be accountable for the occurrence of central apneas in that sleep state (100,101).

D. Benzodiazepines and Apnea

In view of the conflicting reports on the depressant, null, or stimulant respiratory effects exerted by benzodiazepines, it remains controversial whether benzodiazepines could be or should be prescribed to sleep apnea patients. The matter is further complicated by the fact that distinction should be made between central and obstructive apnea as well as between short- and long-acting benzodiazepines.

Although the conventional approach is that benzodiazepines, particularly long-acting ones, should not be given to patients with obstructive apnea (102), reports from the literature appear to support the use of short-acting benzodiazepines in the management of patients with central apnea (103,104). This is largely because of findings that short-acting benzodiazepines either produce no respiratory depression (105) or respiratory stimulation (106). Even though diazepam, one of the most widely prescribed sedatives–hypnotics, is a long-acting benzodiazepine, Rao et al. (107) believed that respiratory depression associated with its use was comparable to the changes occurring during physiologic sleep.

We tested the effects of subhypnotic and hypnotic does of diazepam on respiration, spontaneous and postsigh apneas, and sleep in the rat model of central sleep apnea (17). Our study directly supported the findings of three clinical studies where administration of short- or medium-acting benzodiazepines to central apnea patients (103,108) and normal subjects with altitude-associated central apneas (109) improved respiration and reduced central sleep apneas. We observed similar results in rats that were administered diazepam (Fig. 15), which despite having a long plasma half-life in humans, shows a relatively brief duration of central action because of redistribution out of the brain. In addition, the plasma half-life of diazepam in rats was expected to be much shorter than in humans because of the high metabolism of these animals.

As in a clinical study of triazolam in which the drug reduced apneas in sleep stage 1 with less impact on stage 2 apneas and without effect on apneas in REM sleep (103), our data showed that in rats diazepam also decreased apneas in NREM (Fig. 15) but not in REM sleep. It is of interest that triazolam at two dose levels decreased central apneas by about 50%, whereas in our study both doses of diazepam reduced spontaneous and postsigh apneas to about half of their baseline value.

The functional site and mechanism of diazepam's action on apnea expression could not be directly determined from our study. Although respiratory stimulation and apnea suppression were clearly associated during NREM sleep, that association did not persist during REM sleep. Thus, apnea suppression may not have resulted simply from respiratory stimulation.

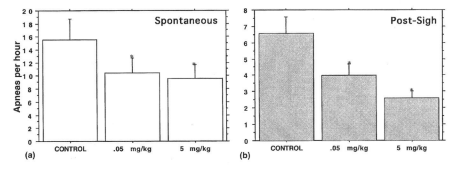

Figure 15 Effects of 0.05 and 5.0 mg/kg of diazepam on spontaneous and postsigh apneas per hour during NREM sleep. Both doses of diazepam reduced spontaneous and postsigh apneas to about half of their baseline value.

We concluded from our study that administration of diazepam to rats induced respiratory stimulation even at doses insufficient to augment NREM sleep, and that this stimulation was associated with suppression of NREM apneas. However, despite equivalent augmentation of minute ventilation by high-dose diazepam during NREM and REM sleep, REM apneas were not affected. The discordance of apnea-suppressing effects caused by diazepam during NREM versus REM sleep in rats, coupled with the identical phenomena produced by another benzodiazepine, triazolam, in humans (103), suggested different mechanisms of apnea genesis during these sleep states, a hypothesis that we had previously advanced (12).

V. Conclusions

Animal models are essential in understanding the neural bases for sleep-related changes in control of respiration. In this chapter, we characterized the respiratory instability and its neural mechanisms in the rat model of sleep apnea. Our research has determined: (1) similar patterns of expression and responses to intervention for central and obstructive apnea in humans and central apnea in the rat; (2) similar increases in apnea frequency from deep slow wave sleep to light NREM sleep to REM sleep in the rat model as is the case in humans; (3) similar effects on respiration produced by stimulation of peripheral adenosinergic system in the rat as is the case in humans; (4) a possible physiological role for endogenous 5-HT in the peripheral nervous system in producing or modulating sleep apnea expression under baseline conditions; and (5) a similarity in the reduction of central apneas in rats and obstructive apneas in English bulldogs during sleep by serotonergic antagonists.

These findings indicate pharmacological avenues for the treatment of central or obstructive apneas and the potential management of human sleep apnea syndrome.

References

1. Mendelson, W. B., Martin, J. A., Perlis, M., Giesen, H., Wagner, R., and Rapoport, S. I. Periodic cessation of respiratory effort during sleep in adult rats. Physiol Behav 1988; 43:229–234.
2. Sato, T., Saito, H., Seto, K., and Takatsuji, H. Sleep apneas and cardiac arrhythmias in freely moving rats. Am J Physiol 1990; 259:R282–R287.
3. Carley, D. W., Trbovic, S., and Radulovacki, M. Sleep apnea in normal and REM sleep deprived normotensive Wistar-Kyoto and spontaneously hypertensive (SHR) rats. Physiol Behav 1996; 59:827–831.

4. Carley, D. W., Trbovic, S. M., and Radulovacki, M. Hydralazine reduces elevated sleep apnea index in spontaneously hypertensive (SHR) rats to equivalence with normotensive Wistar-Kyoto rats. Sleep 1996; 19:363–366.
5. Carley, D. W., Berecek, K., Videnovic, A., and Radulovacki, M. Sleep-disordered respiration in phenotypically normotensive, genetically hypertensive rats. Am J Respir Crit Care Med 2000; 162:1474–1479.
6. Thomas, A. J., Austin, W., Friedman, L., and Strohl, K. P. A model of ventilatory instability induced in the unrestrained rat. J Appl Physiol 1992; 73:1530–1536.
7. Thomas, A. J., Friedman, L., MacKenzie, C. N., and Strohl, K. P. Modification of conditioned apneas in rats: evidence for cortical involvement. J Appl Physiol 1995; 78:215–218.
8. Monti, D., Carley, D. W., and Radulovacki, M. Adenosine analogs modulate the incidence of sleep apneas in rats. Pharm Biochem Behav 1995; 51:125–131.
9. Carley, D. W., Trbovic, S. M., Monti, D., and Radulovacki, M. Effects of sleep fragmentation and clonidine administration on apnea in the rat. Res Commun Biol Physiol Behav 1995; 59:827–831.
10. Monti, D., Carley, D. W., and Radulovacki, M. p-SPA, a peripheral adenosine A$_1$ analog reduces sleep apneas in rats. Pharm Biochem Behav 1996; 53:341–345.
11. Christon, J., Carley, D. W., Monti, D., and Radulovacki, M. Effects of inspired gas on sleep-related apnea in the rat. J Appl Physiol 1996; 80:2102–2107.
12. Carley, D. W., Trbovic, S., and Radulovacki, M. Effect of REM sleep deprivation on sleep apneas in rats. Exp Neurology 1996; 137:291–293.
13. Carley, D. W., Trbovic, S. M., Bozanich, A., and Radulovacki, M. Cardiopulmonary control in sleeping Sprague-Dawley rats treated with hydralazine. J Appl Physiol 1997; 83:1954–1960.
14. Trbovic, S. M., Radulovacki, M., and Carley, D. W. Protoveratrines A and B increase sleep apnea index in Sprague-Dawley rats. J Appl Physiol 1997; 83:1602–1606.
15. Carley, D. W., Hagan, R. M., Trbovic, S. M., Thai, T., and Radulovacki, M. Adenosine A$_1$ receptor agonist GR 79236 suppresses apnea during all sleep stages in the rat. Sleep 1997; 20:1093–1098.
16. Radulovacki, M., Trbovic, S. M., and Carley, D. W. Cardiopulmonary interactions following REM sleep deprivation in Sprague-Dawley rats. Exp Neurol 1997; 145:371–375.
17. Carley, D. W., Trbovic, S. M., and Radulovacki, M. Diazepam suppresses sleep apnea in rats. Am J Resp Crit Care Med 1998; 157:917–920.
18. Radulovacki, M., Trbovic, S. M., and Carley, D. W. Serotonin 5-HT$_3$ receptor antagonist GR38032F suppresses sleep apneas in rats. Sleep 1998; 21:131–136.
19. Carley, D. W. and Radulovacki, M. Role of peripheral serotonin in the regulation of central sleep apneas in rats. Chest 1999; 115:1397–1401.

20. Carley, D. W. and Radulovacki, M. Mirtazapine, a mixed-profile serotonin agonist/antagonist, suppresses sleep apnea in the rat. Am J Resp Crit Care Med 1999; 160:1824–1829.

21. Carley, D. W. and Radulovacki, M. Role of peripheral adenosine A_1 receptors in the regulation of sleep apneas in rats. Exp Neurol 1999; 159:545–550.

22. Carley, D. W. and Radulovacki, M. R-zacopride, a 5-HT$_3$ antagonist/5-HT$_4$ agonist, reduces sleep apneas in rats. Pharm Biochem Behav 2001; 69:283–289.

23. Carley, D. W., Trbovic, S. M., and Radulovacki, M. Losartan, an angiotensin AT_1 receptor antagonist, modulates sleep apnea expression in spontaneously hypertensive (SHR) rats. Sleep Res Online 2001; 4:7–12.

24. Radulovacki, M., Trbovic, S. M., and Carley, D. W. Acute hypotension reduces sleep apneas in Zucker lean and Zucker obese rats. Sleep 1996; 19:767–773.

25. Önal, E. and Lopata, M. Periodic breathing and pathogenesis of occlusive sleep apneas. Am Rev Respir Dis 1982; 126:676–680.

26. Badr, M., Grossman, J., and Weber, S. Treatment of refractory sleep apnea with supplemental carbon dioxide. Am J Respir Crit Care Med 1994; 150:561–564.

27. Steens, R., Millar, T., Su, W., Biberdorf, D., Backle, P., Ahmed, M., and Kryger, M. Effect of inhaled 3% CO_2 on Cheyne-Stokes respiration in congestive heart failure. Sleep 1994; 17:61–68.

28. Hudgel, D., Hendricks, C., and Dadley, A. Alteration in obstructive apnea pattern induced by changes in oxygen and carbondioxide concentrations. Am Rev Respir Dis 1988; 138:16–19.

29. Lugaresi, E., Coccagna, G., and Mantovani, M. Hypersomnia with periodic apneas. In: Weitzman, E., ed. Advances in Sleep Research. New York: Spectrum, 1987:68–70.

30. Lavie, P., Ben-Yousef, R., and Rubin, A. Prevalence of sleep apnea syndrome among patients with essential hypertension. Am Heart J 1984; 108:373–376.

31. Meyer, J., Weichler, U., Herres, M. B., Schneider, H., Marx, U., and Peter, J. H. Influence of metoprolol and cilazapril on blood pressure and on sleep apnea activity. J Cardiovasc Pharmacol 1990; 16:952–961.

32. Jacobs, L. and Comroe, J. H. Reflex apnea, bradycardia, and hypotension produced by serotonin in cats. Circ Res 1971; 29:145–155.

33. Szereda-Przestaszevska, M. and Wypych, B. Effects of vagal and laryngeal efferents on apnoeic response to serotonin in cats. Respir Physiol 1995; 101:231–237.

34. Yoshioka, M., Goda, Y., and Togashi, H. Pharmacological characterization of 5-hydroxytryptamine-induced apnea in the rat. J Pharmacol Exp Ther 1992; 260:917–924.

35. Zucker, I. and Cormish, K. Reflex cardiovascular and respiratory effects of serotonin in conscious and anesthetized dogs. Circ Res 1980; 47:509–515.

36. Veasey, S. C., Chachkes, J., Fenik, P., and Hendricks, J. C. The effects of ondansetron on sleep-disordered breathing in the English bulldog. Sleep 2001; 24:155–160.

37. Fletcher, E. C. and Munafo, D. A. The role of nocturnal oxygen therapy in obstructive apnea. When should it be used? Chest 1990; 98:1497–1504.

38. Martin, R. J., Sanders, M. H., Gray, B. A., and Pennock, B. E. Acute and long-term ventilatory effects of hyperoxia in the adult sleep apnea syndrome. Am Rev Respir Dis 1982; 125:175–180.

39. McNicholas, W. T., Carter, J. L., Rutherford, R., Zamel, N., and Phillipson, E. A. Beneficial effects of oxygen in primary alveolar hypoventilation with central sleep apnea. Am Rev Respir Dis 1982; 125:773–775.

40. Smith, P. L., Haponik, E. F., and Bleecker, E. R. The effects of oxygen in patients with sleep apnea. Am Rev Respir Dis 1984; 130:959–963.

41. Berger, A. J., Mitchell, R. A., and Severinghaus, J. W. Regulation of respiration (pt 1–3). N Engl J Med 1977; 297:92–97, 138–143, 194–201.

42. Phillipson, E. A. Control of breathing during sleep. Am Rev Respir Dis 1978; 118:909–939.

43. Issa, F. and Porostocky, S. Effect of sleep on changes in breathing pattern accompanying sigh breaths. Respir Physiol 1993; 93:175–187.

44. Chow, C. M., Xi, L., Smith, C. A., Saupe, K. W., and Dempsey, J. A. A volume-dependent apneic threshold during NREM sleep in the dog. J Appl Physiol 1994; 76:2315–2325.

45. Biaggioni, I., Olafson, B., Robertson, R., Hallister, A. S., and Robertson, D. Cardiovascular and respiratory effects of adenosine in conscious man: evidence of thermoreceptor activation. Circ Res 1987; 6:779–788.

46. Gleeson, K. and Zwilich, C. W. Adenosine stimulation, ventilation, and arousal from sleep. Am Rev Respir Dis 1992; 145:453–457.

47. Jonzon, B., Sylven, C., Beerman, B., and Brant, R. Adenosine receptor mediated stimulation of ventilation in man. Eur J Clin Invest 1089; 19:65–71.

48. Maxwell, D. L., Fuller, R. W., Nolop, K. B., Dixon, C. M. S., and Hughes, J. M. B. Effects of adenosine on ventilatory responses to hypoxia and hypercapnia in humans. J Appl Physiol 1986; 61:1762–1766.

49. McQueen, D. S. and Ribeiro, J. A. Effect of adenosine on carotid chemoreceptor activity in the cat. Br J Pharmacol 1981; 74:129–136.

50. Monteiro, E. C. and Ribeiro, J. A. Ventilatory effects of adenosine mediated by carotid body chemoreceptors in the rat. Naunyn Schmiedebergs Arch Pharmacol 1987; 335:143–148.

51. Eldridge, F. L., Millhorn, D. E., and Kiley, J. P. Respiratory effects of a long acting analog of adenosine. Brain Res 1984; 301:273–280.

52. Hedner, T., Hedner, J., Wessberg, P., and Jonason, J., Regulation of breathing in the rat: indication for a role of central adenosine mechanisms. Neurosci Lett 1982; 33:147–151.

53. Barraco, R., Janusz, C. A., Schoener, E. P., and Simpson, L. L. Cardiorespiratory function is altered by picomole injections of 5′-N-ethyl-carboxamidoadenosine into the nucleus solitarius of rats. Brain Res 1990; 507:234–246.

54. Phillis, J. W. and Wu, P. H. The role of adenosine and its nucleotides in central synaptic transmission. Prog Neurobiol 1981; 16:187–239.

55. Finlayson, K., Butcher, S. P., Sharkey, J., and Olverman, H. J. Detection of adenosine receptor antagonists in rat brain using a modified radioreceptor assay. J Neurosci Methods 1997; 77:135–142.

56. Shamim, M. T., Ukena, D., Padgett, W. L., and Daly, J. W. Effects of 8-phenyl and 8-cycloalkyl substituents on the activity of mono-, di-, and trisubstituted alkylxanthines with substitution at the 1-, 3-, and 7- positions. J Appl Physiol 1983; 55:813–822.

57. Fletcher, E., DeBehnke, R., Lovoi, M., and Gorin, A. B. Undiagnosed sleep apnea in patients with essential hypertension. Ann Intern Med 1985; 103:190–195.

58. Warley, A., Mitchell, J., and Stradling, J. Prevalence of nocturnal hypoxaemia amongst men with mild to moderate hypertension. Q J Med 1988; 256:637–644.

59. Weichler, U., Herres, M. B., Mayer, J., Weber, K., Hoffmann, R., and Peter, J. H. Influence of antihypertensive drug therapy on sleep pattern and sleep apnea activity. Cardiology 1991; 78:124–130.

60. Sant' Ambrogio, G. and Remmers, J. E. Reflex influences acting on the respiratory muscles of the chest wall. In: Roussos, C., Macklem, P. T., eds. The Thorax (Lung Biol Health Dis series). New York: Marcel Dekker, 1985:531–594.

61. Widdicombe, J. G. Respiratory reflexes. In: Handbook of Physiology. Respiration. Washington, DC: American Physiological Society, 1964:585–630.

62. Ohtake, P. J. and Jennings, D. B. Ventilation is stimulated by small reductions in arterial pressure in the awake dog. J Appl Physiol 1992; 73:1549–1557.

63. Barringer, D. L. and Bunag, R. D. Uneven blunting of chronotropic baroreflexes in obese Zucker rats. Am J Physiol 1989; 256:H417–H421.

64. Bunag, R. D. and Barringer, D. L. Obese rats, though still normotensive, already have impaired chronotropic baroreflexes. Clin Exper Theory Prac 1988; A10(suppl 1):257–262.

65. Cheng, S., Swords, B., Kirk, K., and Berecek, K. Baroreflex function in lifetime captopril-treated spontaneously hypertensive rats. Hypertension 1989; 13:63–69.

66. Lee, R., Berecek, K., Tsoporis, J., McKenzie, R., and Triggle, C. Prevention of hypertension and vascular changes by captopril treatment. Hypertension 1991; 17:141–150.

67. Aviado, D. M., Cerletti, A., Li, T. H., and Schmidt, C. F. The activation of carotid sinus pressoreceptors and intracranial receptors by veratridine and potassium. J Pharmacol Exp Ther 1955; 115:329–338.

68. Schmidt, R. F. and Thews, G. The control of respiration. In: Schmidt, R. F. and Thews, G. eds. Human Physiology. Berlin: Springer-Verlag, 1983:479–486.

69. Aviado, D. M. and Schmidt, C. F. Reflexes from stretch receptors in blood vessels, heart, and lungs. Physiol Rev 1955; 35:247–300.

70. Bishop, B. Carotid baroreceptor modulation of diaphragm and abdominal muscle activity in the cat. J Appl Physiol 1974; 34:12–19.

71. Grunstein, M. M., Derenne, J. P., and Milic-Emili, J. Control of depth and frequency of breathing during baroreceptor stimulation in cats. J Appl Physiol 1975; 39:395–404.
72. Heistad, D. D., Abboud, F. M., Mark, A. L., and Schmid, P. G. Effect of baroreceptor activity on ventilatory response to chemoreceptor stimulation. J Appl Physiol 1975; 39:411–416.
73. Krayer, O. and Meilman, E. Veratrum alkaloids with antihypertensive activity. In: Gross, F. ed. Handbook of Experimental Pharmacology. Antihypertensive Agents. Berlin: Springer-Verlag, 1977:547–570.
74. Benforado, J. M. The veratrum alkaloids. In: Root, W. S. and Hoffmann, F. G. eds. Physiological Pharmacology. The Nervous System. New York: Academic Press, 1967:331–398.
75. Wang, S. C., Ngai, S. H., and Grossman, R. G. Mechanism of vasomotor action of veratrum alkaloids: extra vagal sites of action of veriloid, protoreactrine, germitrine, neogermitrine, germerine, veratridine and vera-tramine. J Pharmacol Exp Ther 1955; 113:100–114.
76. Bradley, T. D., McNicholas, W. T., Rutherford, J., Popkin, J., Zamel, N., and Phillipson, E. A. Clinical and physiologic heterogeneity of central sleep apnea syndrome. Am Rev Respir Dis 1986; 134:217–221.
77. Rodbard, S. and Saiki, H. Mechanism of the pressor response to increased intracranial pressure. Am J Physiol 1952; 168:234–244.
78. Sapru, H. N., Gonzalez, E., and Krieger, A. J. Aortic nerve stimulation in the rat: cardiovascular and respiratory responses. Brain Res Bull 1981; 6:393–398.
79. Aserinsky, E. and Kleitman, N. Regularly occurring periods of eye motility, and concomitant phenomena during sleep. Science 1953; 118:273–274.
80. Verrier, R. L., Muller, J. E., and Hobson, J. A. Sleep, dreams and sudden death: the case for sleep as an autonomic stress test for the heart. Cardiovasc Res 1996; 31:181–211.
81. Dempsey, R. J., Smith, C. A., Harma, C. A., Chow, C., and Saupe, K. W. Sleep-induced breathing instability. Sleep 1996; 19:236–247.
82. Stradling, J. R. and Phillipson, E. A. Breathing disorders during sleep. Q J Med 1986; 225:3–18.
83. Pack, A. I. Changes in respiratory motor activity during rapid eye movement sleep. In: Regulation of Breathing, 2nd ed., Dempsey, J. A. and Pack, A. I. eds. New York: Marcel Dekker, 1995; 983–1010.
84. Hendricks, J. C., Kline, L. R., Kovalski, R. J., O'Brien, J. A., Morrison, A. R., and Pack, A. I. The English bulldog: a natural model of sleep-disordered breathing. J Appl Physiol 1987; 63:1344–1350.
85. Hendricks, J. C., Kovalski, R. J., and Kline, L. R. Phasic respiratory muscle patterns and sleep-disordered breathing during rapid eye movement sleep in the English bulldog. Am Rev Respir Dis 1991; 144:1112–1120.
86. Sherrey, J. H. and Megirian, D. Respiratory EMG activity of the posterior cricoarytenoid, cricothyroid and diaphragm muscles during sleep. Respir Physiol 1980; 39:355–365.

87. Wiegand, L., Zwillich, C. W., Wiegand, D., and White, D. P. Changes in upper airway muscle activation and ventilation during phasic REM sleep in normal men. J Appl Physiol 1991; 71:488–497.

88. Gaultier, C. Upper airway muscles and physiopathology of obstructive sleep apnea syndrome. Neurophysiol Clin 1994; 24:195–206.

89. Gould, G. A., Gugger, M., Molloy, J., Tsara, V., Shapiro, C. M., and Douglas, N. J. Breathing pattern and eye movement density during REM sleep in humans. Am Rev Respir Dis 1988; 138:874–877.

90. Hanly, P. J. Mechanisms and management of central sleep apnea. Lung 1992; 170:1–17.

91. Webster, H. H. and Jones, B. E. Nerotoxic lesions of the dorsolateral pontomesencephalic tegmentum-cholinergic cell area in the cat. II. Effects upon sleep-waking states. Brain Res 1988; 458:285–302.

92. Datta, S. Neuronal activity in the peribrachial area: relationship to behavioral state control. Neurosci Biobehav Rev 1995; 19:67–84.

93. Farber, J., Marks, G. A., and Roffwarg, H. P. Rapid eye movement sleep PGO-type waves are present in the dorsal pons of the albino rat. Science 1980; 209:615–617.

94. Marks, G. A., Farber, J., and Roffwarg, H. P. Metencephalic localization of ponto-geniculo-occipital waves in the albino rat. Exper Neurol 1980; 69:667–677.

95. Marks, G. A., Farber, J., and Roffwarg, H. P. Phasic influences during REM sleep upon dorsal lateral geniculate nucleus unit activity in the rat. Brain Res 1981; 22:388–394.

96. Persson, H. E. and Svanborg, E. Sleep deprivation worsens obstructive sleep apnea. Comparison between diurnal and nocturnal polysomnography. Chest 1996; 109:645–650.

97. O'Donnell, C. P., King, E. D., Schwartz, A. R., Smith, P. L., and Robotham, J. L. Effect of sleep deprivation on responses to airway obstruction in the sleeping dog. J Appl Physiol 1994; 77:1811–1818.

98. Neilly, J. B., Kribbs, N. B., Maislin, G., and Pack, A. I. Effects of selective sleep deprivation on ventilation during recovery sleep in normal humans. J Appl Physiol 1992; 72:100–109.

99. Veasey, S. C., Hendricks, J. C., Kline, L. R., and Pack, A. I. Effects of acute sleep deprivation on control of the diaphragm during REM sleep in cats. J Appl Physiol 1993; 74:2253–2260.

100. Hobson, J. A., Lydic, R., and Baghdoyan, H. A. Evolving concepts of sleep cycle generation: from brain centers to neuronal populations. Behav Brain Sci 1986; 9:371–392.

101. Lydic, R. and Biebuyck, J. F. The Clinical Physiology of Sleep. Bethesda, MD: American Physiological Society, 1988.

102. Guilleminault, C. Benzodiazepines, breathing and sleep. Am J Med 1990; 88(suppl 3A):25S–28S.

103. Bonnet, M. H., Dexter, J. R., and Arand, D. L. The effect of triazolam on arousal and respiration in central sleep apnea patients. Sleep 1990; 13:31–41.

104. Mendelson, W. B. Safety of short-acting benzodiazepine hypnotics in patients with inspired respiration. Am J Psychiatry 1991; 148:1401.
105. Cohn, M. A. Hypnotics and control of breathing: a review. Br J Clin Pharmacol 1983; 16(suppl 2):245S–259S.
106. Dodson, M. E., Yousseff, Y., Maddison, S., and Pleuvry, B. Respiratory effects of lorazepam. Br J Anaesth 1986; 48:611–612.
107. Rao, S., Sherbaniuk, R. W., Prasad, K., Lee, S. J. K., and Sprole, B. J. Cardiopulmonary effects of diazepam. Clin Pharmacol Ther 1973; 14:182–189.
108. Guilleminault, C., Crowe, C., Quera-Salva, M. A., Miles, L., and Partinen, M. Periodic leg movement, sleep fragmentation and central sleep apnea in two cases: reduction with clonazepam. Eur Respir J 1988; 1:762–765.
109. Nickolson, A., Smith, P. A., Stone, B. M., Bradwell, A. R., and Coote, J. H. Altitude insomnia: studies during an expedition to the Himalayas. Sleep 1988; 11:354–361.

11

The English Bulldog Model of Sleep-Disordered Breathing

SIGRID CARLEN VEASEY and JOAN C. HENDRICKS

University of Pennsylvania
Philadelphia, Pennsylvania, U.S.A.

I. Overview

Just more than three decades ago, obstructive sleep-disordered breathing (OSDB) was recognized as a clinical disorder (1,2). Since recognition of OSDB as a clinical entity, research has been tremendously helpful in characterizing the varying presentations of this disorder, and at the same time, has brought much insight into the pathophysiology of this disorder and provided several therapeutic options for management of this disease. Other pursuits in OSDB research have revealed significant neurobehavioral and cardiovascular consequences in some, but not all persons with OSDB. Given the complexities in not only the disease presentation, but also in therapeutic responses and in consequences of OSDB, it is clear that many different animal models of OSDB are necessary to address the vast array of questions concerning this disease. In the first part of this chapter, we characterize sleep-disordered breathing (SDB) in the English bulldog, comparing and contrasting OSDB in the bulldog and human. After describing the attributes and limitations of this animal model, the types of

297

research questions that this model is particularly suited to address are discussed. The studies performed using the English bulldog are reviewed in relation to results obtained using different animal models and human studies, and we conclude by describing the potential for this model in future studies.

II. Characterization of the English Bulldog as a Natural Model of Sleep-Disordered Breathing

The initial characterization of SDB in the English bulldog involved a study of seven bulldogs, most of which were volunteered for study by their owners (3). The dogs underwent a daytime polysomnography in which data from electroencephalogram (EEG) and electromyogram (EMG) electrodes were recorded along with nasal thermistor signals and inductive plethysmographic signals for both rib cage and abdominal movement. Sleep-disordered breathing events were qualified as $\geq 4\%$ oxyhemoglobin saturation decreases accompanied by a $>30\%$ reduction in airflow signal amplitude. The SDB index was >10 events/hr in four of the six dogs. In these dogs, the SDB index in REM sleep was >20 events/hr. Only the leanest bulldog had no desaturation events (respiratory disturbance index [RDI] < 5 events/hr). Within the group, the average SDB index was higher in rapid eye movement (REM) sleep (27 events/hr) versus non-REM (NREM) sleep (7 events/hr, $p < 0.05$). Control dogs of similar skeletal size had very few SDB events (range 0–1 event/hr) and fewer events than the bulldogs ($p < 0.05$). In the English bulldogs, the average nadir for oxyhemoglobin saturation in NREM sleep was 88%, and the average nadir in REM sleep was 73%. In contrast, the NREM and REM sleep nadirs for control dogs were 94% and 98%, respectively. Apneas occurred almost exclusively in REM sleep in bulldogs, and events, as defined in human studies (4), were a combination of obstructive, central, and mixed apneas. Bulldogs, but not control dogs, demonstrated sleep state-dependent abnormal patterns of respiratory and abdominal movements. Specifically, there were timing shifts in abdominal and respiratory movements, which at times were 180° out of phase, or paradoxical in movement. In addition to the respiratory phase changes in bulldogs, large periodic reductions in amplitudes of rib cage and abdominal inspiratory movements in REM sleep were seen in bulldogs and not in the control dogs. Sleep latencies were measured for each daytime polysomnography. The average sleep latency for bulldogs was 12 min, significantly shorter than control dogs' latencies, which were >150 min ($p < 0.0001$). Arousal indices and sleep architecture (depth of

REM sleep, sleep bout length, percent REM sleep) were not measured in this study.

One of the initial concerns about the bulldog as an animal model of SDB was that it was difficult to understand why the dogs had significant daytime hypersomnolence. The bulldogs did not arouse from REM SDB events, had very few NREM sleep events, and yet had profound hypersomnolence. Although very few nighttime studies were performed, the total sleep time for bulldogs was similar to total sleep time in control dogs. We hypothesized that hypersomnolence in this breed occurs because of respiratory-related arousals and hypopneas in NREM sleep. We have added parameters used in most clinical studies in humans, including improved airflow measures, snore signals, and higher quality EEG signals. Esophageal manometry was poorly tolerated in bulldogs; the dogs are obligate nasal breathers with extremely narrowed nasal passages.

To improve detection of respiratory-related arousals, we implanted frontoparietal skull EEG and nuchal EMG electrodes attached to a radiotransmitter placed subcutaneously over the dorsal thorax. As our placement of the electrodes has improved, many more aspects of human sleep are evident. We may now detect K complexes, spindles, delta activity, and transient arousals in the dogs (5). Currently, we are staging NREM sleep in the dogs as light NREM sleep (for what would be scored in humans as stages 1/2) and deep NREM sleep for what would be scored as human stage 3/4 sleep. Because we have not placed occipital leads, we are unable to measure alpha activity in quiet waking. Recent electroencephalographic signals in a bulldog with waveforms characteristic of human sleep are presented in Figure 1. This greater resolution in EEG activity, along with measurement of snoring, has allowed us to detect snores with arousal events and respiratory-related arousals with desaturations less than 4%. Consequently, we have expanded our definition of SDB events to include both respiratory-related arousals with desaturations $\geq 2\%$ and snores with arousals (5). In the bulldogs, approximately three-fourths of NREM SDB events are respiratory-related arousals with desaturations and snores with arousals. We believe that the fragmentation of NREM sleep by respiratory-related arousals, and perhaps the repeated mild desaturation followed by reoxygenation, explains, at least in part, the daytime hypersomnolence in bulldogs.

The improved ability of measuring sleep stages and the capacity to detect the complete spectrum of SDB events scored in human clinical trials strengthens the use of this model in pharmacotherapeutic trials. That is, this model with respiratory-related arousals, hypopneas, and apneas allows assessment of drug effectiveness for each category of SDB events, as well as

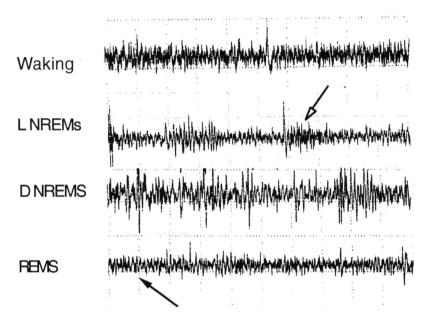

Figure 1 Frontoparietal EEG signals across behavioral states. Waking EEG signals in the dogs show characteristic high-frequency, low-amplitude waveforms. Light NREM sleep (L NREMS) in the bulldogs shows slowing relative to waking with spindles and K complexes. In contrast to humans, rolling eye movements are not seen in light NREM sleep. The open arrow highlights a K complex followed by a typical spindle in the dogs. Deep NREM sleep (D NREMS) shows at least 30% delta waveforms in a 30-sec epoch. REM sleep in the dogs frequently shows sawtooth waveforms (closed arrow), characteristic of human REM sleep.

measurement of sleep consolidation, sleep quality, and daytime hypersomnolence.

There are many similarities in SDB in humans and bulldogs. Notably, the events are primarily obstructive or mixed and occur in both NREM and REM sleep. Furthermore, events are more frequent and exhibit larger desaturations in REM sleep, as evidenced by the occurrence of apneas and lower oxyhemoglobin desaturations. Daytime hypersomnolence is present in the dogs, and sleep latency is negatively correlated with the SDB index. The polysomnographic features (EEG, EMG, snore, airflow, and respiratory signals) in the English bulldog during NREM sleep are remarkably similar, as described above, to electrographic findings in persons with upper airways resistance syndrome (6).

EEG

DIA EMG

SH EMG

GH EMG

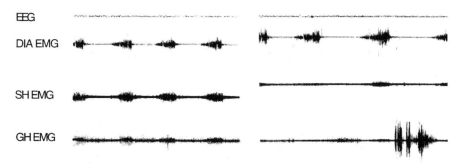

Figure 2 Polysomnographic tracings with respiratory muscle electromyographic signals. The left panel shows typical deep NREM sleep respiratory EMG activity. Upper airway dilator muscles, sternohyoid (SH EMG) and geniohyoid (GH EMG), are synchronized with the diaphragm (DIA) EMG activity and very slightly precede DIA EMG activity. The right panel shows phasic REM sleep changes in respiratory muscle activity. The diaphragm is only minimally affected with occasional fractionations. In contrast, the inspiratory activity for the SH and GH are diminished in some bursts and absent in others. In addition, DIA EMG activity precedes GH and SH activity, rendering upper airway dilator activity less efficient. These changes in timing are frequently associated with paradoxical rib cage and abdominal movements in bulldogs.

There are, however, several important differences between SDB in the bulldog and OSDB in adult humans. In contrast to the severity of disease at presentation in humans, NREM OSDB in the bulldog is, in most cases, quite mild with rare apneas and rare desaturations >4%. We have not found NREM SDB indices of >15, including snores with arousal events. That is, even in the bulldogs with frequent and severe desaturations in REM sleep, events in NREM sleep are typically snores with arousals and hypopneas with desaturations of 2–4%.

In addition to the relative infrequency of NREM apnea and hypopnea events, the bulldogs have fewer and less pronounced cardiovascular sequelae than have humans (7,8). Cardiovascular consequences of OSDB have just begun to be explored in bulldogs. Systemic arterial blood pressures have been measured in three dogs and are only slightly higher than those in control dogs. In bulldogs, transthoracic echocardiograms have not revealed obvious differences in either ventricular sizes or wall thickness. In two of the older dogs, however, dilated chambers and decreased wall motion were found. The cause of cardiomyopathy in these dogs is uncertain. Although postmortem evaluation excluded ischemic and infectious causes, vascular histology, sympathetic nerve activity, and angiotensin–renin changes have not been explored in the bulldog.

The absence of hypertension in the bulldog model is indeed intriguing. The induced OSDB dog model (Ref. 9, and Chap. 7, this volume) shows statistically significant changes in blood pressure after just 1–2 weeks of induced sleep apnea. Notably, this particular model allows each dog to serve as its own control, allows the induction of frequent NREM and REM sleep events with hypoxia, and takes advantage of a chronic indwelling cannula for measurement. With each animal serving as its own control, the induced OSDB model is a far more powerful model for cardiovascular cause and effect, and this model will be enormously valuable in determining which aspects of OSDB (arousals, hypoxia time, hypoxia arousal, etc.) contribute to hypertension. Thus, although the English bulldog is a very limited model for cardiovascular studies, a superb model exists with the induced OSDB dog model. The rat model of intermittent hypoxia is also an excellent model with which to determine the pathogenesis of hypertension related to intermittent hypoxia observed in some persons with OSDB (Ref. 10 and Chap. 6, this volume). In particular, this latter model can be extremely useful in determining which genes and proteins are altered in responses to intermittent hypoxia within the brain regions involved in vasomotor responses, carotid bodies, adrenals, kidneys, and within arterial vessels. This model also permits determination of dose effects of intermittent hypoxia on sympathetic nerve activity and vascular morbidity.

That the bulldog does not demonstrate significant hypertension is interesting and may relate in part to the minimal NREM SDB and/or the minimal fluctuations in oxygen levels in NREM sleep. Alternatively, the bulldog may be relatively resistant to either oxidative stress or the cardiovascular sequelae from oxidative stress (11). It is interesting that in humans there appears to be a differential vulnerability to hypertension from OSDB. Specifically, hypertension may develop in young persons with mild SDB, and this condition can improve with treatment of OSDB (12). Although the absence of cardiovascular morbidities in the bulldog is interesting, we believe that animal models in which microarray and proteomics can be used to identify mechanisms of disease will be far more useful than the English bulldog model.

III. Strengths and Weaknesses of the English Bulldog as a Model of OSDB

What would be the ideal animal model of OSDB? The ideal model would have OSDB as defined in humans and would also have a spectrum of severity of disease, as is seen in humans. The mechanisms involved in the pathogenesis of disease would be identical to those in the human disease process, including neurochemical control mechanisms, and risk factors for disease would parallel human risk factors. The capacity to turn on and off the disease process at any time would enable identification of genes involved in the disease process. A relatively short life span of the model would allow the progression of disease to be followed within a reasonable study period. The model should be widely available, inexpensive to house in laboratories, and readily reproducible. Littermates without the disease would also be advantageous. The ideal model would allow measurements of cardiovascular as well as sleep and respiratory parameters.

Although the English bulldog has few of the desired attributes, this dog breed has several unique strengths as a model of OSDB. Understanding which attributes the model does and does not have helps us to identify the research niches for this animal as well as areas of research in which use of other models would be more appropriate.

Perhaps the greatest strength of the English bulldog as a model of OSDB is that this animal has OSDB events, which result from a remarkably similar pathogenesis as that described in humans with the disorder (13). Other important strengths of this animal model are the chronicity and progression of disease. The English bulldog is a natural model in which the disease process is present for years. Furthermore, the clinical presentation of the disease process is within the spectrum of human OSDB presentations. OSDB is present in almost all bulldogs studied to date and in varying degrees of severity. These combined attributes make the English bulldog a potentially powerful animal model. There are, however, several features that present challenges for studying the bulldog.

The primary challenge in using this model has been the difficulty in obtaining and/or breeding enough bulldogs to maintain a large enough colony for various types of studies. Thus, the use of the English bulldogs in nonsurvival research protocols has not been possible. Although increasing colony size is not impossible, there are now other animal models more readily available to answer questions related to cardiovascular, developmental, and neurochemical state-related changes. At the same time, it is hoped that simpler models will be developed to take advantage of genetics approaches. Large-scale mutagenesis screens of mice and *Drosophila* for abnormal vulnerability to sleep loss, intermittent hypoxia, and other components of SDB, and for craniofacial abnormalities (mice) that would predispose to OSDB may provide novel models available for genetic studies. Indeed, realization of this sample size limitation and the difficulties in genetic studies with this breed has helped launch our pursuits in developing *Drosophila* (14) and murine models (15) for determining basic sleep–wake regulation and genetic factors involved in determining the individual vulnerability to consequences of sleep apnea.

We believe that the English bulldog can best be used to address questions concerning the pathogenesis of OSDB, particularly the musculature and basic neural mechanisms underlying state-dependent changes in muscle function, and that this particular model may provide insight into the progression of disease. Furthermore, this animal model should be valuable for rapidly executed, adequately powered, and inexpensive pharmacotherapeutic trials prior to study in humans.

IV. Pathogenesis of OSDB in the English Bulldog

Obstructive respiratory events occur exclusively in sleep in humans with sleep apnea and in bulldogs with OSDB. The principle mechanism resulting in upper airway collapse in humans during sleep is a relative reduction in the activity of at least one of the upper airway dilator muscles (13). As in the human with sleep apnea, respiration in quiet wakefulness in the English bulldog is normal in most bulldogs. In sleep, coincident with reductions in upper airway dilator activity, OSDB events occur.

In bulldogs and in humans, OSDB events occur intermittently. The episodic nature of events in REM sleep was difficult to attribute to changes in arousal and ventilatory thresholds. Specifically, the onsets and offsets of events did not coincide with state change. We hypothesized that intermittent phasic REM sleep influences on respiratory musculature could explain irregularly occurring REM SDB events (16). Although this could also be studied in humans, there are several advantages to performing these studies in dogs. First, transcutaneous electromyography can be performed in the dogs on multiple respiratory muscles, including the diaphragm and several upper airway dilators; the studies can be performed more rapidly, and the cost of performing sleep studies is far less in the dogs than in humans. Thus, the bulldog provides an excellent model for determining the role that phasic influences play in OSDB. Five English bulldogs were implanted with EEG, electro-oculogram (EOG), and nuchal EMG electrodes to determine sleep state and to distinguish phasic and tonic REM sleep. Transcutaneous electrodes were inserted into the diaphragm and several upper airway dilator muscles (16). Several observations were made. First, the majority (80%) of SDB events occurred during REMs, whereas the most severe SDB events occurred at the onset of REM sleep when phasic activity is very high. Another important observation helped link OSDB events in REM sleep to phasic influences on respiratory muscles. That is, rather than a tonic suppression in dilator activity, REM SDB events in the bulldogs were associated with phasic changes in muscle activity, including fractionations (17), intermittent suppressions (18), and asynchrony of respiratory muscle activity (19). Examples of the phasic influences on both timing and muscle activity are shown in Figure 2. Many events ended in resolution of phasic respiratory muscle activity without an arousal. Furthermore, events were aperiodic, and termination of events was independent of oxygen saturation (SaO$_2$) values. Notably, suppression of upper airway dilator activity was greater and of longer duration than suppression of the diaphragm.

An important conclusion can be drawn from these data. Sleep-disordered breathing in the English bulldog in REM sleep may be largely explained by phasic influences on respiratory muscle activity. Similar phasic influences have been related to SDB events in humans (20,21). This mechanism of phasic influences could not explain NREM SDB events. Indeed, the results of this study suggested that the neurochemical mechanisms underlying REM SDB must differ, at least in part, from the mechanisms underlying NREM SDB, in which episodic changes in behavioral state and ventilatory thresholds may contribute to disordered breathing.

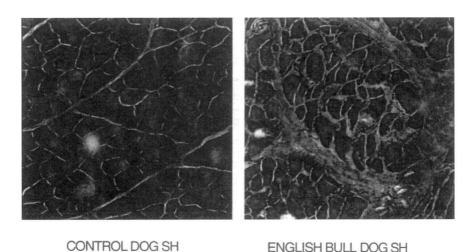

CONTROL DOG SH   ENGLISH BULL DOG SH

Figure 3 Light microscopic images of hematoxolyn- and eosin-stained cross-sectional slices in the sternohyoid (SH) muscles of a healthy control dog (beagle) and an English bulldog with a respiratory index of 11 events/hr for total sleep and 40/hr for REM sleep. Myocytes in the bulldogs were lighter, smaller, and more irregularly shaped. Copious endomysial connective tissue encases muscle fibers. These changes are consistent with a contraction–expansion injury myopathy.

The work described above identified a basic mechanism underlying SDB events in REM sleep—normal phasic influences on respiratory musculature—but at the same time, it led to a larger question. Why do phasic influences on upper airway muscle activity lead to OSDB in the bulldog and humans with sleep apnea, and not in all individuals? There were two plausible explanations for collapse of the airway and SDB events in REM sleep. Phasic activity during REM sleep could be more intense in bulldogs and in humans with sleep apnea than in normals. Alternatively, disruption of upper airway dilator activity secondary to normal phasic influences of REM sleep may have a greater impact in beings with either collapsible or narrowed upper airways.

V. Comparison of State-Dependent Changes in Upper Airway Dilator Muscle Activity in Bulldogs and Control Dogs

For phasic REM sleep influences to cause SDB events in bulldogs but not in control dogs, we hypothesized that a given level of upper airway muscle activity in the bulldogs is necessary to maintain a patent airway, and therefore, sleep-related changes in upper airway dilator activity are more profound in the bulldog. Sleep-related reductions in muscle activity in the bulldogs would help explain both REM and NREM OSDB events. As mentioned above, an alternative explanation was that phasic influences on respiratory musculature might be more pronounced in the bulldogs, and this increased disruption of respiratory activity would result in SDB in bulldogs.

To explore both hypotheses, we compared the sleep-related changes in upper airway dilator muscle activity in English bulldogs to sleep-related changes in muscle activity in dogs without SDB (22). The muscles from which activity was recorded were the sternohyoid (SH) and the diaphragm. Although in humans the genioglossus is the dilator most studied, the SH in the bulldog is the largest upper airway dilator muscle and is a dilator with typically respiratory-related activity. In contrast, the genioglossus in this prone-positioned animal only infrequently demonstrates respiratory activity. In addition, SDB events in the bulldog are associated with phasic changes in SH activity.

Several observations were made in this study of upper airway muscle activity to support one of the hypotheses. First, English bulldogs were far more likely than control dogs to have respiratory-related activity in SH recordings in NREM sleep. Second, the bulldogs demonstrated less SH activity in REM sleep than in NREM sleep. In contrast, the control dogs had either the same or increased SH activity in REM sleep as in NREM sleep. The most important finding in REM sleep was that the overall SH activity was indistinguishable between bulldogs and control dogs. Specifically, the level of activity and the frequency of phasic influences on respiratory musculature were similar in the two groups. The larger differences in SH activity between bulldogs and control dogs were present in NREM sleep. Together, these findings further support the concept that SDB in the bulldogs occurs in REM sleep largely because of normal phasic influences on respiratory musculature, and the findings suggest that the bulldogs rely upon increased upper airway dilator muscle activity to maintain airway patency in NREM sleep. Although phasic changes in upper airway dilator muscle activity in control dogs are of little consequence, these phasic influences on respiratory musculature in the English bulldog result in SDB.

VI. Age-Related Changes in SDB and Upper Airway Muscle Function in the English Bulldog

In the English bulldog, as in the human, OSDB is a chronic disease process, and one that may progress over years. In individual bulldogs observed in the colony over several years, the SDB indices have increased with time in most of the dogs. Four of the older bulldogs demonstrated a progression to chronic hypoventilation. This significant deterioration in respiration occurs over 2–3 years. OSDB appears to be acquired in bulldog puppies within the first few weeks of life. Specifically, we have found that neonatal pups (<2 weeks of age) show no SDB events ($n = 3$); slightly older pups, 6–12 weeks of age, exhibit disordered breathing events in waking and in both NREM and REM sleep. By 16 weeks, the adult pattern of SDB is established with no waking events, rare NREM sleep events, and a predominance of REM SDB events. Typically, from 12 weeks to 4 years, the SDB indices are relatively stable. Beyond 4 years, it appears that many, but not all bulldogs begin to decompensate. The dogs demonstrate exercise intolerance or syncope when stressed. By age 6–7 years, oxyhemoglobin saturations in NREM sleep are reduced from 92–95% to 87–90%. Four older dogs developed hypercapnia (resting partial pressure of CO_2, arterial [$PaCO_2$] 50–60 mmHg). These older dogs with hypoventilation occasionally demonstrate snoring, paradoxical respiration, and rarely stridor in waking. Therefore, the bulldog is an excellent model in which to study determinants of progression of disease. We hypothesized that the decompensation over time might be related, in part, to upper airway muscle damage from increased use.

To look for evidence of damage of dilator muscles in the bulldogs, Petrof et al. compared myosin content in bulldogs and the histology of upper airway dilator muscles, SH, and geniohyoid (GH) to a nonrespiratory muscle (anterior tibialis), and contrasted the finding in bulldogs to the findings in control dogs (beagles) (23). Overall, the findings were consistent with an overuse injury to upper airway muscles in the older bulldogs. There was an increase in myosin type II fibers in the SH, which is consistent with resistive load training of this dilator muscle. There were no differences in myosin type in the anterior tibialis muscles of bulldogs and control dogs. Both dilator muscles in the bulldog showed morphologically abnormal muscle fibers and fibrosis (Fig. 3). These findings may occur as a result of repetitive concentric contractions from OSDB events. These findings may explain, at least in part, a decompensation of respiration in the English bulldog with age.

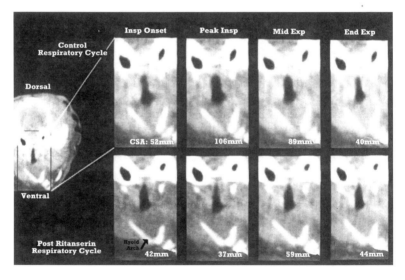

Figure 4   Effects of a broad-spectrum serotonin (5-HT) antagonist (ritanserin) on the respiratory dynamics of the upper airway. Shown here are cinematic computerized tomographic images (3-mm cuts) within the hypopharyngeal region of the bulldog. The upper four panels show waking dynamics of the airway (central black area) in the bulldog, with a stenting open of the airway during inspiration ($106 \, mm^2$). At end-expiration, with no muscle activity present, the airway collapses. In contrast, after systemic ritanserin, the upper airway muscle activity is lost, and then during inspiration, there is a significant collapse of the upper airway ($37 \, mm^2$). In contrast, end-expiration with little muscle activity at baseline is largely unaffected.

The extent of upper airway muscle damage in the bulldogs was examined by Schotland et al. in our laboratory and magnetic resonance imaging (MRI) of the upper airway dilators in English bulldogs showed increases in T_2 relaxation times in five dilator muscles, but not in four postural muscles (24). The lack of injury in postural muscles supports the concept that upper airway muscle damage is not a diffuse muscle injury related to hypoxia, other aspects of OSDB, or a bulldog's natural state, but rather is related to increased demands placed on the upper airway muscles. Furthermore the T_2 value for the SH (more so than for other muscles) correlates powerfully with the SDB index in the bulldogs. The overall higher T_2 values for dilators are consistent with overuse of dilator muscles with resultant edema (25–27). The correlation between severity of SDB and the magnitude of T_2 changes is consistent with either decompensation resulting from overuse or increased muscle use in dogs with more severe disease, or more severely compromised upper airway. Muscle injury in the bulldog is an important finding and may in part explain decompensation with time. A similar T_2 change with MRI is seen in the upper airway musculature in humans with OSDB (28). We believe that increased compliance of the upper airway soft tissue structures may also contribute to decompensation.

VII. Neural Mechanisms Underlying OSDB in the Bulldog

Although we now understand that sleep state-dependent neural mechanisms underlie the pathogenesis of SDB in both the English bulldog and the human with OSDB, the precise neurochemical changes remain unclear. State-dependent influences on respiration may occur at many respiratory-related sites within the brain. Ultimately, however, all state-dependent changes in upper airway dilator muscle activity must result in changes in neurochemical inputs to the upper airway motoneurons. This provides a good starting point for determining the neural basis of motonueronal suppression in both NREM and REM sleep (for a review, see Ref. 29). The neurochemical mechanisms underlying postural muscle atonia of REM sleep are well characterized (30–32). In contrast, it is less clear how much of a role these postsynaptic inhibitory mechanisms at upper airway motoneurons contribute to REM sleep-dependent effects on upper airway musculature.

In the carbachol model of REM sleep, postsynaptic inhibition of hypoglossal motoneurons (which are responsible for protrusion of the tongue) occurs, but appears to play a minimal role in motoneuronal suppression (33). The same has been shown in natural REM sleep in cats for trigeminal motoneurons; gamma-aminobutyric acid (GABA) and glycine inhibition of trigeminal motoneurons contribute only in part to REM sleep-related suppression of these brainstem motoneurons (34,35). An alternative explanation for suppression of brainstem motoneurons in REM sleep is disfacilitation of (withdrawal of excitatory influences from) these motoneurons. The excitatory influences on brainstem motoneurons include glutamate, acetylcholine, serotonin (5-hydroxytryptamine [5-HT]), and norepinephrine (29). Serotonergic and noradrenergic neurons have reduced activity in NREM sleep and many of these neurons are quiescent in REM sleep (36). Kubin et al. hypothesized that a likely etiology of brainstem motoneuronal suppression in sleep is withdrawal of 5-HT delivery from brainstem motoneurons (37). Using the pontine carbachol model of REM sleep with microdialysis probes in the hypoglossal nuclei, Kubin et al. found reduced levels of 5-HT in the hypoglossal nuclei after pontine carbachol injections (38). The reduced 5-HT extracellular levels coincided with the onset of phasic phenomena of REM sleep. Thus, 5-HT levels may be reduced to upper airway motoneurons in natural REM sleep. Whether the other excitatory neurochemicals have decreased levels at motoneurons in sleep is unknown. Horner et al. developed a rat model in which a microdialysis probe, and electroencephalographic and electromyographic electrodes are chronically implanted into one of the hypoglossal nuclei in a freely moving rat (39). His group showed that serotonin injected into the hypoglossal nucleus can completely prevent genioglossus muscle suppression in NREM sleep, and partially prevents genioglossal suppression in REM sleep. This work suggests that serotonergics may be effective in preventing NREM OSDB, and that additional neural mechanisms may be involved in REM sleep events (39).

The English bulldog is one model in which we can test the importance of 5-HT in the maintenance of patent upper airways. With this model, it is not possible currently to test the hypothesis directly with application of 5-HT antagonists at upper airway motoneurons, rather the overall importance of 5-HT can be tested with intravenous administration of 5-HT antagonists. To evaluate the importance of 5-HT in the maintenance of patent upper airways in the bulldog, we determined the effects of two broad-spectrum 5-HT antagonists administered systemically on upper airway muscle activity, upper airway caliber, and oxyhemoglobin saturations (40). Upper airway caliber was measured using cinematic computerized tomography of the upper airway. Sternohyoid and GH muscle activity were measured coincident with airway area. Both antagonists produced a dose-dependent reduction in SH and GH inspiratory muscle activity. Suppression of upper airway dilator muscle activity was greater than suppression of diaphragmatic activity. Concurrent with reductions in upper airway muscle activity were reductions in the oxyhemoglobin saturation and significant reductions in the upper airway cross-sectional area at its narrowest region, within the hypopharynx. Not only was the airway caliber reduced, but the dynamics of the airway were altered with inspiratory collapse after administration of 5-HT antagonists (Fig. 4). This collection of studies demonstrates the importance of 5-HT for maintenance of the upper airway in wakefulness in the English bulldog. The site of action could not, however, be determined in this work. This work led us to hypothesize that 5-HT is important for the maintenance of patent airways in the English bulldog, and that serotonergic drugs may have therapeutic potential in the bulldog and in humans with SDB.

Serotonergics have been tested in humans with SDB previously without demonstration of clear benefit (41–43). In general, the results are inconclusive (44). Trials were either not adequately powered to detect a difference or used relatively weak serotonergics. Selection of the optimal drug for these studies is quite difficult. Serotonin does not cross the blood–brain barrier, and there are 14 different 5-HT receptor subtypes involved in both activation and inhibition of neurons (for a review, see Ref. 45). Serotonin reuptake inhibitors may not provide enough 5-HT at motoneurons in sleep to counteract sleep state-dependent changes (42,43). One advantage of the bulldog model is that drugs not approved for human use can be tested in dogs, and the studies can be designed with multiple trials per dog to allow better detection of an ideal dose and to test dose responsiveness. In the bulldog we studied the effects of L-tryptophan (a precursor of 5-HT that increases 5-HT production and release) and trazodone (5). Trazodone is a weak 5-HT reuptake drug, but has an active metabolite that is a 5-HT agonist at $5\text{-}HT_{2A,2C}$ receptors. Earlier studies suggested that brainstem motoneurons are excited through $5\text{-}HT_{2A \text{ and/or } 2C}$ receptors in several mammalian species (46–49). Five English bulldogs were implanted with skull EEG, neck EMG, and SH EMG electrodes connected to a radiotransmitter. Each dog underwent 16 separate sleep studies, 4 studies each for placebo, a low-dose, middle-dose, and high-dose of trazodone and L-tryptophan. The 16 studies were performed in a random order. This study design allowed us adequate power in five dogs to detect a 20% reduction in SDB event frequency and provided insight into the optimal dose for effect. Each bulldog demonstrated reductions in the SDB index for the two higher doses for both NREM sleep and REM sleep events. There was no measurable drug effect, however, on the REM sleep entry SDB events, which occur with highly phasic activity of respiratory musculature. Improvements were seen, not only in the overall SDB indices, but in sleep efficiency and slow-wave sleep time. REM sleep time was unaffected.

This study suggests a tremendous potential for serotonergics in treating OSDB. The combination of L-tryptophan and trazodone at comparable doses, however, may not be safe in humans (50). We believe that the next step is to determine the serotonin receptor subtypes that contribute to excitation of upper airway dilators. To rapidly screen for all potential excitatory serotonin receptor subtypes, we have incorporated methods of single-cell, real-time polymerase chain reaction (PCR) with laser capture of single hypoglossal motoneurons. With this novel assay, we have determined that the serotonin receptor subtype mRNA present in hypoglossal motoneurons are $5\text{-HT}_{2A \text{ and } 2C}$ (51). This work provides information on the most likely serotonin receptor subtypes, but functional studies are necessary to determine which of these two receptors is active at hypoglossal motoneurons.

Once we have determined the serotonin subtypes responsible for excitation of dilator motoneurons, we may try selective serotonin agonists, targeting the active subtypes, in the English bulldog. Thus, we believe that the bulldog will be most helpful as a preliminary test model for drug effectiveness, prior to initiating human trails.

We have been asked whether serotonergics might increase muscle damage and result in earlier decompensation of OSDB. It is important to note that the muscle injury is not related to increased tonic activity, but is from contraction excitation (52) resulting from closure of the airway and a massive excitation of muscles required to suddenly open the airway against very negative intraluminal pressures. We believe that a drug effective in exciting upper airway motoneurons would maintain a patent airway and prevent the need to massively excite dilator muscles under conditions of extremely negative intraluminal pressures.

The serotonin and respiration literature is filled with many seemingly contradictory findings, and the English bulldog model has been somewhat helpful in resolving some of these conflicting reports. In addition to the direct excitatory effects of serotonin at upper airway motoneurons, serotonin might also inhibit respiratory drive through peripheral mechanisms (53,54). We have shown that two serotonin antagonists with activity at receptor subtypes $5\text{-HT}_{1,2,6, \text{ and } 7}$ cause reductions in upper airway muscle activity and cause obstructive breathing events. In contrast, a selective 5-HT_3 antagonist in this model reduces OSDB events, particularly in REM sleep (55). This work highlights the importance of determining the receptor subtypes that contribute to respiratory drive at each of the regions involved in respiratory drive to upper airway muscles.

VIII. Conclusions

All models of SDB described to date have helped advance our understanding of the pathogenesis of SDB and its cardiovascular consequences. We would consider the most important findings with the English bulldog model to be that (1) REM SDB events occur because of normal phasic influences on upper airway dilator muscles; (2) this disorder is associated with injury to the upper airway dilator muscles, and decompensation over time; and (3) serotonin is important for the maintenance of patent airways in the bulldog, and serotonergics can largely improve SDB in this model. We believe that the future for this model will be to facilitate the identification of pharmacotherapeutics for OSDB for both humans and English bulldogs.

References

1. Gastault, H., Tassinari, C., and Duron, B. Etude polygraphique des manifestations épisodiques (hypniques et respiratoires) du syndrome de Pickwick. Rev Neurol 1965; 112:568–579.
2. Jung, R. and Kuhlo, W. Neurophysiological studies of abnormal night sleep and the pickwickian syndrome. Prog Brain Res 1965; 18:140–159.
3. Hendricks, J. C., Kline, L. R., Kovalski, J. A., O'Brien, J. A., Morrison, A. R., and Pack, A. I. The English bulldog: a natural model of sleep-disordered breathing. J Appl Physiol 1987; 63:1344–1350.
4. Phillipson, E. A. and Remmers, J. E. (Chairmen). American Thoracic Society Consensus Conference on Indications and Standards for Cardiopulmonary Sleep Studies. Am Rev Respir Dis 1989; 139:559–568.
5. Veasey, S. C., Fenik, P., Panckeri, K., Pack, A. I., and Hendricks, J. C. The effects of trazodone and L-tryptophan on sleep-disordered breathing in the English bulldog. Am J Respir Crit Care Med 1999; 160:1659–1667.
6. Loube, D. I., Andrada, T., and Howard, R. S. Accuracy of respiratory inductive plethysmography for the diagnosis of upper airway resistance syndrome. Chest 1999; 115:1519–1524.
7. Peppard, P. E., Young, T., Palta, M., and Skatrud, J. Prospective study of the association between sleep-disordered breathing and hypertension. N Engl J Med 2000; 342:1378–1384.
8. Shahar, E., Whitney, C. W., Redline, S., Lee, E. T., Newman, A. B., Nieto, F. J., O'Connor, G. T., Boland, L. L., Schwartz, J. E., and Samet, J. M. Sleep-disordered breathing and cardiovascular disease. Am J Respir Crit Care Med 2001; 163:19–25.
9. Brooks, D., Horner, R., Kozar, L. F., Render-Teixeira, C. L., and Phillipson, E. A. Obstructive sleep apnea as a cause of systemic hypertension: evidence from a canine model. J Clin Invest 1997; 99:106–109.

10. Fletcher, E. C. Effect of episodic hypoxia on sympathetic activity and blood pressure. Respir Physiol 2000; 119:189–197.

11. Matsuoka, H. Endothelial dysfunction associated with oxidative stress in human. Diabetes Res Clin Pract 2001; 54:S65–S72.

12. Guilleminault, C., Stoohs, R., Shiomi, T., Kushida, C., and Schnittger, I. Upper airway resistance syndrome, nocturnal blood pressure monitoring, and borderline hypertension. Chest 1996; 109:901–908.

13. Remmers, J. E., deGroot, W. J., Sauerland, E. K., and Anch, A. M. Pathogenesis of upper airway occlusion during sleep. J Appl Physiol 1978; 44:931–938.

14. Hendricks, J. C., Finn, S. C., Panckeri, K. A., Chavkin, J., Williams, J. A., Sehgal, A., and Pack, A. I. Rest in *Drosophila* is a sleep-like state. Neuron 2000; 25:129–138.

15. Veasey, S. C., Valladares, O., Fenik, P., Kapfhammer, D., Sanford, L., Benington, J., and Bucan, M. An automated system for recording and analysis of sleep in mice. Sleep 2000; 23:1–16.

16. Hendricks, J. C., Kovalski, R. J., and Kline, L. R. Phasic respiratory muscle patterns and sleep-disordered breathing during rapid eye movement sleep in the English bulldog. Am Rev Respir Dis 1991; 144:1112–1120.

17. Orem, J. Neuronal mechanisms of respiration in REM sleep. Sleep 1980; 3:251–267.

18. Kline, L. R., Hendricks, J. C., Davies, R. O., and Pack, A. I. Control of the diaphragm in rapid-eye-movement sleep. J Appl Physiol 1986; 61:1293–1300.

19. Hendricks, J. C. and Kline, L. R. Differential activation within costal diaphragm during rapid-eye-movement sleep in cats. J Appl Physiol 1991; 70:1194–1200.

20. Millman, R. P., Knight, H., Kline, L. R., Shore, E. T., Chung, D. C., and Pack, A. I. Changes in compartmental ventilation in association with eye movements during REM sleep. J Appl Physiol 1988; 65:1196–1202.

21. Neilly, J. B., Gaipa, E. A., Maislin, G., and Pack, A. I. Ventilation during early and late rapid-eye-movement sleep in normal humans. J Appl Physiol 1992; 72:100–109.

22. Hendricks, J. C., Petrof, B. J., Panckeri, K., and Pack, A. I. Upper airway muscle hyperactivity during non-rapid eye movement sleep in English bulldogs. Am Rev Respir Dis 1993; 148:185–194.

23. Petrof, B. J., Pack, A. I., Kelly, A. M., and Hendricks, J. C. Pharyngeal myopathy of loaded upper airway in dogs with sleep apnea. J Appl Physiol 1994; 76:1746–1752.

24. Schotland, H. M., Insko, E. K., Panckeri, K. A., Leigh, J. S., Pack, A. I., and Hendricks, J. C. Quantitative magnetic resonance imaging of upper airway musculature in an animal model of sleep apnea. J Appl Physiol 1996; 81:1339–1346.

25. Prince, F. P., Hikida, R. S., and Hagerman, F. C. Human muscle fiber types in power lifters, distance runners and untrained subjects. Pflugers Arch 1977; 370:227–232.

26. Larsson, S. E., Bengtsson, L., Bodegard, L., Henrikson, K. G., and Larsson, J. Muscle changes in work-related chronic myalgia. Acta Orthop Scand 1988; 59:552–556.

27. Dennett, X. and Fry, H. J. H. Overuse syndrome: a muscle biopsy study. Lancet 1988; 2:905–908.

28. Schotland, H. M., Insko, E. K., and Schwab, R. J. Quantitative magnetic resonance imaging demonstrates alterations of the lingual musculature in obstructive sleep apnea. Sleep 1999; 22:605–613.

29. Horner, R. L. Impact of brainstem mechanisms on pharyngeal motor control. Respir Physiol 2000; 119:113–121.

30. Morales, F. R., Engelhardt, J. K., Soja, P. J., Pereda, A. E., and Chase, M. H. Motoneuron properties during motor inhibition produced by microinjection of carbachol into the pontine reticular formation of the decerebrate cat. J Neurophysiol 1987; 57:1118–1129.

31. Morales, F. R., Boxer, P., and Chase, M. H. Behavioral state-specific inhibitory postsynaptic potentials impinge on the cat lumbar motoneurons during active sleep. Exp Neurol 1987; 98:418–435.

32. Morales, F. R. and Chase, M. H. Postsynaptic control of lumbar motoneuron excitability during active sleep in the chronic cat. Brain Res 1981; 225:279–295.

33. Kubin, L., Kimura, H., Tojima, H., Davies, R. O., and Pack, A. I. Suppression of hypoglossal motoneurons during carbachol-induced atonia of REM sleep is not caused by fast synaptic inhibition. Brain Res 1993; 611:300–312.

34. Soja, P. J., Finch, D. M., and Chase, M. H. Effect of inhibitory amino acids antagonists on masseteric reflex suppression during active sleep. Exp Neurol 1987; 96:178–193.

35. Yamuy, J., Fung, S. J., Xi, M., Morales, F. R., and Chase, M. H. Hypoglossal motoneurons are postsynaptically inhibited during carbachol-induced rapid-eye-movement sleep. Neuroscience 1999; 94:11–15.

36. Heym, J., Steinfels, G. F., and Jacobs, B. L. Activity of serotonin-containing neurons in the nucleus raphe pallidus of freely moving cats. Brain Res 1982; 251:259–276.

37. Kubin, L., Tojima, H., Davies, R. O., and Pack, A. I. Serotonergic excitatory drive to hypoglossal motoneurons in the decerebrate cat. Neurosci Lett 1992; 139:243–248.

38. Kubin, L., Reignier, C., Tojima, H., Taguchi, O., Pack, A. I., and Davies, R. O. Changes in serotonin level in the hypoglossal nucleus region during carbachol-induced atonia. Brain Res 1994; 645:291–302.

39. Jelev, A., Sood, S., Liu, H., Nolan, P., and Horner, R. L. Microdialysis perfusion of 5-HT into hypoglossal motor nucleus differentially modulates genioglossus activity across natural sleep-wake states in rats. J Physiol 2001; 532:467–481.

40. Veasey, S. C., Panckeri, K. A., Hoffman, E. A., Pack, A. I., and Hendricks, J. C. The effects of serotonin antagonists in an animal model of sleep-disordered breathing. Am J Respir Crit Care Med 1996; 153:776–778.

41. Schmidt, H. S. L-tryptophan in the treatment of impaired respiration in sleep. Bull Eur Physiopathol Respir 1983; 19:625–629.
42. Hanzel, D. A., Proia, N. G., and Hudgel, D. W. Response of obstructive sleep apnea to fluoxetine and protriptyline. Chest 1991; 100:416–421.
43. Kraiczi, H., Hedner, J., Dahlof, P., Ejnell, H., and Carlson, J. Effect of serotonin uptake inhibition on breathing during sleep and daytime symptoms in obstructive sleep apnea. Sleep 1999; 22:61–67.
44. Veasey, S. C. Pharmacotherapies for obstructive sleep apnea: how close are we? Curr Opin Pulm Med 2001; 7:399–403.
45. Barnes, N. M. and Sharp, T. A review of central 5-HT receptors and their function. Neuropharmacology 1999; 38:1083–1152.
46. Larkman, P. M. and Kelly, J. S. Ionic mechanisms mediating 5-hydroxy-tryptamine- and noradrenaline-evoked depolarization of adult rat facial motoneurones. J Physiol 1992; 456:473–490.
47. Ribeiro-do Valle, L. E., Metzler, C. W., and Jacobs, B. L. Facilitation of masseter EMG and masseteric (jaw-closure) reflex by serotonin in behaving cats. Brain Res 1991; 550:197–204.
48. McCall, R. B. and Aghajanian, G. K. Pharmacological characterization of serotonin receptors in the facial motor nucleus: a microiontophoretic study. Eur J Pharm 1980; 65:175–183.
49. Berger, A. J., Bayliss, D. A., and Viana, F. Modulation of neonatal rat hypoglossal motoneuron excitability by serotonin. Neurosci Lett 1992; 143:164–168.
50. Tazelaar, H. D., Myers, J. L., Drage, C. W., King, T. E. Jr., Aguayo, S., and Colby, T. V. Pulmonary disease associated with L-tryptophan-induced eosinophilic myalgia syndrome. Clinical and pathologic features. Chest 1990; 97:1032–1036.
51. Zhan, G., Shaheen, F., Mackiewicz, M., Fenik, P., and Veasey, S. C. Single cell laser dissection with molecular beacon polymerase chain reaction identifies 2A as the predominant serotonin receptor subtype in hypoglossal motoneurons. Neuroscience 2002; 113:145–154.
52. Ploutz-Snyder, L. L., Tesch, P. A., and Dudley, G. A. Increased vulnerability to eccentric exercise-induced dysfunction and muscle injury after concentric training. Arch Phys Med Rehabil 1998; 79:58–61.
53. Carley, D. W. and Radulovacki, M. Role of peripheral serotonin in the regulation of central sleep apneas in rats. Chest 1999; 115:1397–1401.
54. Carley, D. W. and Radulovacki, M. Mirtazapine, a mixed-profile serotonin agonist/antagonist, suppresses sleep apnea in the rat. Am J Respir Crit Care Med 1999; 160:1824–1829.
55. Veasey, S. C., Chachkes, J., Fenik, P., and Hendricks, J. C. The effects of ondansetron on sleep-disordered breathing in the English bulldog. Sleep 2000; 24:155–160.

12

Sleep in Aquatic Mammals

MICHAEL A. CASTELLINI

Institute of Marine Sciences
University of Alaska Fairbanks
Fairbanks, Alaska, U.S.A.

I. Introduction

Of all the mammals, the group classified as "marine" (whales, seals, sea lions, and sirenians) may have the most unusual aspects of sleep-associated physiological patterns. Because these mammals have evolved to sleep in a marine environment, the physiological control mechanisms associated with diving, apnea, and environmental monitoring have become intermixed with the controls for sleep state. In practical terms, a seal asleep at 400 m underwater does not want to take an involuntary breath. These control mechanisms have overlapped so much that true seals (phocids) go into extended breath-holds even while sleeping dry on land. By contrast, the whales have evolved to sleep only in the water, mostly while resting at the surface. However, in this case, there is strong evidence that these animals demonstrate unihemispheric slow-wave sleep (SWS), presumably to maintain vigilance with some neural centers. Furthermore, it is possible that cetaceans may not enter REM stages of sleep.

This review covers two aspects of sleep in marine mammals: sleep-associated apnea and asymmetric or unihemispheric sleep. It is critical to understand that these conditions are not associated with any pathology or disease state. Rather, they are evolved adaptations that allow the animal to better exploit its marine environment. Whereas sleep apnea in humans is a condition associated with negative health implications, in seals it is the normal and healthy state. The phenomenon of sleep apnea in marine mammals offers the ability for us to study nonpathological, long duration, repetitive apnea. It allows us to work with mammals, both young and old, that routinely hold their breath while sleeping, yet show no pathology or sudden infant death syndrome (SIDS)-like events. The interesting apparent lack of REM sleep in whales, coupled with unihemispheric sleep state, may be unique among the mammals and offers insights into the metabolic requirements and control mechanisms for sleep. Unlike the whales, the true seals demonstrate symmetrical electroencephalogram (EEG) patterns during sleep, whereas the sea lions seem to show asymmetry. Why would both whales and sea lions show this unusual pattern, but not the seals? What evolutionary pressures have fixed these distinct patterns?

II. The Marine Mammals

The three classes of marine mammals include the cetaceans (whales and dolphins), the pinnipeds (seals, sea lions, and walrus), and the sirenians (manatees and dugongs). As might be expected, our knowledge of sleep physiology is greatest with the pinnipeds and least with the manatees and whales. The pinnipeds are much more amenable to the laboratory studies necessary to examine sleep patterns, whereas the large whales are virtually impossible to study. However, the smaller cetaceans (dolphins and porpoises) that can be held in highly controlled laboratory conditions have been critical to the study of sleep in marine mammals. The pinnipeds are amphibious and have both land or ice phases along with periods spent entirely at sea. The whales and sirenians are totally aquatic. Thus, models of sleep in pinnipeds must contrast the land and sea phases, whereas sleep studies for the cetaceans and sirenians examine only sleep while the animal is in the water.

The habits of these animals while at sea or on land are essential to our general understanding of their sleep. Observations of apparent sleep or resting states have been made for years in all groups. It is vital to note that throughout this review, the term *apparent sleep* will be used when discussing observations of animals that seem, by behavioral criteria, to be sleeping. This is distinct from quantitative measurements of sleep state made by electrophysiological recording. The number of studies discussing behavioral sleep in marine mammals far exceed those that use physiological recordings.

There are at least three early references to behavioral sleep state in these mammals. In 1948, McBride and Hebb (1) reported "sleep periods" in captive dolphins (*Tursiops truncatus*), and in the mid 1950s, Bartholomew (2) observed that northern elephant seals (*Mirounga angustirostris*) went into long apnea periods (up to 15 min) while apparently sleeping on beaches. In 1964, Lilly (3) published an anecdotal remark about captive dolphins sleeping with one eye open. This single comment created a long-standing discussion about dolphins sleeping with only half of their brain. One of the interesting aspects of sleep apnea in seals is how this pattern is explained in public aquaria: at the National Zoo in Washington, DC, there are signs explaining to the public that the seals in the large rock pools are not dead, they are just sleeping under ledges and on the bottom of the tank.

Long-duration apnea associated with apparent sleep has been observed in only the true seals (phocids). True seals are the fusiform-shaped species that are more aquatic than the otariidae, or sea lions, that can walk on land. Thus, the "seals" in circus and zoo acts are actually members of the land-mobile sea lion family. Sleep in sea lions has not been studied as well as in phocids, but observations indicate that the otariids do not show sleep-associated apnea either on land or in water (4). Fur seals have been observed apparently sleeping while floating at the surface of the sea (5). On land, otariids appear to sleep in a manner similar to that of terrestrial mammals, with routine and regular respiration (personal observation). There is evidence of unihemispheric sleep in the otariids, which will be discussed later in this chapter.

The cetaceans and sirenians are the most aquatic of all these groups. Whales have been observed apparently sleeping both floating at the surface and suspended, motionless, at depth. The most interesting aspect of sleep in this group is the appearance of unihemispheric SWS EEG patterns, which suggest that the animals sleep with only "half a brain" at any given time (6). Perhaps this relates to a need for constant vigilance while resting at the surface or to their highly developed acoustic communication system. Thus, this pattern would not seem to be related to the marine environment per se. However, if whales also sleep while drifting underwater, then there would be a strong drive to control sleep state and respiration state by similar mechanisms as those proposed in the true seals. Furthermore, no REM sleep has ever been recorded in cetaceans. Sleep in sirenians also appears to exhibit the interhemispheric asynchrony of the SWS EEG (7).

III. Sleep-Associated Apnea

A. Diving Physiology

To facilitate a better understanding of sleep-associated apnea in marine mammals, it is first necessary to discuss a few issues about overall apnea tolerance in this group. In general, marine mammals can dive for extended periods by both increasing their oxygen stores compared to terrestrial mammals and by controlling blood flow and oxygen utilization patterns throughout the body. Dive-associated apneas can extend for up to 2 hr in seals, though normal diving times are usually much less. However, even routine "short" dives for some species, such as elephant seals and Weddell seals (*Leptonychotes weddellii*) can average 10–15 min. During these apneic periods, there is extensive bradycardia, peripheral restriction of blood flow, and significant hematological changes. For example, the hematocrit (Hct) can vary from about 35% in a breathing, awake, resting Weddell seal to more than 70% during the dive. The extra pool of red blood cells (RBCs) are thought to be stored in the large spleen and are mobilized through splenic contraction during diving bouts, presumably to maximize oxygen carrying capacity of the blood. In some species, after an individual dive, the Hct begins to decline, but usually the next dive occurs within a few minutes and the Hct remains elevated until an entire diving bout is finished, several hours later. In species such as elephant seals, that may be at sea for 4–5 months making nonstop dives 24 hours a day with only minimal surface times, we must assume that Hct remains elevated for months.

During diving, arterial blood oxygen partial pressure (P_aO_2) can reach values in the high teens, postdive lactate can reach more than 25 mM, and the arterial partial pressure of carbon dioxide (P_aCO_2) can reach more than 60 torr. These values are important to remember when we examine the changes that occur during sleep-associated apneas. Clearly, these species are tolerant to repeated bouts of hypoxia and hypercapnia far beyond the tolerance of most terrestrial mammals. Even more remarkable is that the animals can withstand multiple bouts of low O_2 and elevated CO_2 many times per day, and in some cases, many times per hour. Reviews of general diving physiology and biochemistry in these species can be found in Refs 8–12.

B. History of Sleep Observations

Because only the phocids appear to exhibit sleep-associated apnea, this discussion deals mainly with patterns seen in these species. No observations of long-duration apnea during apparent sleep have been seen in the otariids, and there have only been recent observations of cetaceans apparently sleeping while floating underwater in the ocean (S. Moore, personal observation).

When published reports of long-duration sleep-associated apnea in seals began appearing in the literature, there were no data to prove that the animals were truly sleeping. Outward appearance of the seals suggested that they were asleep, but this was not confirmed with EEG recordings. Early observations usually noted apnea duration and in some species, investigators were able to place their hands on the chest of the animals, count heartbeats, and note a significant reduction in average heart rate (HR) associated with the apnea (2). Apart from these field observations, however, not much work was conducted on the physiology of this behavior until the 1970s.

In 1975, Ridgway et al. (13) obtained EEG and electrocardiogram (EKG) recordings from resting gray seals (*Halichoerus grypus*) and confirmed that apnea periods were associated with various stages of sleep and with a bradycardia. Later, Pasche and Krog (14) documented the existence of bradycardia during apparent sleep apnea in harbor (*Phoca vitulina*) and hooded (*Cystophora cristata*) seals. In the mid 1980s, Huntley (15) obtained simultaneous EKG, EEG, and respiration data from sleeping, but restrained northern elephant seal pups. Starting about the same time, Castellini et al. began obtaining simultaneous EKG, instantaneous HR, EEG, respiration, and blood data from unrestrained northern elephant seals sleeping in both natural and laboratory settings (16–19). In the 1970s, Mukhametov et al. began studies of the electrophysiological characteristics of sleep in marine mammals (6). These studies dealt more with the EEG patterns than with apnea tolerance per se, therefore, their work will be described in detail in the sections dealing with asymmetric EEG patterns during sleep. Williams and Bryden (20) documented sleep apnea durations and HR patterns in apparently sleeping harbor, leopard (*Hydrurga leptonyx*), and southern elephant seals (*Mirounga leonina*), and Blackwell and Le Boeuf summarized apparent sleep-associated apnea duration patterns in northern elephant seals and discussed how those patterns change with age of the seal (21). Recently, investigators from South America have documented bradycardia and respiratory patterns during apparent sleep apnea in southern elephant seals (22).

C. Apnea Pattern

When seals sleep on land, or while resting at the water surface, they will exhibit periods of repeated apnea–eupnea bouts that can last for close to an hour before the pattern is broken and the seal awakens. In elephant seal pups, there is an apnea period of 7–10 min, followed by a eupneic period of

2–3 min, and then another apnea period follows. Figure 1 shows a bout of apnea and eupnea patterns in a 3-month-old northern elephant seal pup (16). However, there is a strong developmental component to this pattern (17,21). As the seal pup develops, the periods of apnea become longer. In adult northern elephant seals, the longest recorded sleep-associated apnea is more than 20 min. There does not seem to be an age-associated change in the eupneic duration period. There is also no evidence that the sequence pattern of an apnea–eupnea bout changes with age. That is, both seal pups and adults will go through three to four apnea–eupnea bouts before they awaken and the pattern changes.

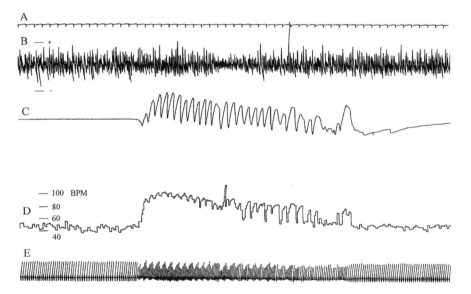

Figure 1 Electrophysiological tracings associated with an episode of eupnea during SWS under dry conditions for a 3-month-old northern elephant seal pup. The five traces, from top to bottom, show: (A) 5-sec time marks; (B) the EEG depicting continuous SWS signal range from ± 100 μV; (C) the respiratory trace at the end of an 8-min apnea followed by 2.5 min of eupnea and the beginning of another apnea; (D) the cardiotachograph depicting a low heart rate during the apnea, a ventilatory-driven tachycardia, and the appearance of the normal sinus arrhythmia, which becomes more prominent late in the eupnea, and finally the low heart rate during the ensuing apnea; (E) the ECG. (From Ref. 16.)

D. Sleep State

Before EEG data were collected on sleeping seals, it was not possible to discern if the seals had to awaken to take a breath or what stages of sleep were associated with different respiratory patterns. Figure 1 shows the EEG data from a northern elephant seal pup during bouts of apnea. The figure illustrates that the seal can remain in SWS throughout a period of apnea–eupnea–apnea cycles, and therefore, does not need to awaken to breathe. Notably, this pattern does not need to change if the seal is sleeping underwater. We obtained EEG data from elephant seal pups that were sleeping in tanks of water and documented that they could come to the surface, terminate the apnea bout, go through several minutes of eupnea, and sink to the bottom of the pool again, all while in continual SWS (16). Although gray seals seem to follow the same pattern (13), Caspian seals (*Phoca caspica*) seem to awaken each time they need to breathe (23). Thus, some species of seals appear able to swim and sleep at the same time, at least in SWS. In all species studied so far, with the exception of gray seals, apnea can be associated with either SWS or REM sleep. During REM, the general muscle atonia seemingly overrides the control mechanisms for movement and the seals do not move in this stage. In elephant seals, sleep eupnea only occurred during SWS. No instances of eupnea while in REM were ever observed in either elephant seals (16) or harp seals (24). In gray seals, however, Ridgway et al. (13) found regular respiration during REM sleep and no REM underwater. This discrepancy in the respiratory patterns during REM between gray and other seals has not yet been resolved.

Though it will be discussed in some detail later in this chapter, only bilaterally symmetric EEG patterns have been seen in sleeping phocid seals. There is no evidence of any asymmetric EEG patterns in these species. By contrast, there is evidence that the otariids may show asymmetric EEG patterns during sleep, but they do not exhibit long-duration apnea periods.

E. Characteristics of the EEG During Sleep Apnea

Beginning with the work of Ridgway et al. (13), three separate laboratories have worked extensively on the EEG patterns of sleeping phocids. Mukhametov and Lyamin focused on the characteristics of the EEG in terms of bilateral symmetry, and Castellini et al. worked on the physiological consequences of sleep state. In all three laboratories, no electrophysiological patterns have been detected that are unique to the marine mammals with respect to spike frequency, voltages, etc. Normal mammalian patterns of SWS and REM seem to be apparent. In both elephant seals (16) and harp seals (24) REM sleep was associated with muscle atonia accompanied by increased facial twitching. During SWS,

Lyamin (25) further quantified both deep and light stages. The actual patterns of transitions from various stages of sleep and respiration are more appropriately discussed below in reference to diving and sleep underwater (Sec. III.G.). However, in most cases, the animals move from awake, to quiet awake, to light SWS, to deep SWS, and then, about 50% of the time, to REM. In all species (except for the gray seal), REM was terminated by waking and respiration. No transitions from REM back into SWS were ever recorded in elephant seals (16) or harp seals (24). SWS stages can continue for hours and therefore make up the greatest percentage of time in the sleep state, whereas % REM is usually much less. In harp seal pups (25), about 9 hr/day were spent in SWS and about 2 hr in REM. In elephant seal pups, about 1.5 hr/day was spent in REM and did not change if the animal was sleeping either dry or wet (16).

In summary, the staging of the sleep cycle and the electrophysiological characteristics of the various sleep states in phocid species are typically mammalian. For these groups, it is the relationship between sleep state, respiration, and diving that is unusual.

F. Can Sleep or Apnea State Be Manipulated?

Only one study has attempted to manipulate sleep and respiratory state in marine mammals (19). In that study, northern elephant seal pups slept in large tanks where the O_2 and CO_2 of the inspired gases could be manipulated. The goal of the study was to examine how hypoxia and hypercapnia impact both sleep state and apnea state. Both hypoxic (13% O_2) and hypercapnic (6% CO_2) conditions doubled eupneic breathing rates during SWS and reduced the number of apnea bouts, although their lengths were not altered. However, if the inspired gas levels were raised further, all episodes of apnea during sleep were entirely eliminated. Moreover, as when the animals were breathing room air, breathing never occurred during REM sleep, regardless of how much respiratory drive was driven by the inspired gases. When seals were hypercapnic, the eupneic periods did not get longer, however, the breathing rate and therefore, the total number of breaths per eupneic period increased. At 7.5% inspired CO_2 and 14% O_2, the seals would drop into SWS, breath continuously, and never exhibit REM. Upon rebreathing room air, short periods of sleep occurred that consisted largely of REM sleep, which suggested a period of REM rebound after the period of REM deprivation.

These experiments demonstrated that sleep and apnea could be decoupled in these seals and thus it is possible for seals to sleep without apnea. However, at high enough levels of respiratory drive, the sleep patterns were altered by the elimination of REM. It should be noted that seals are also capable of going through periods of awake apnea, although these apneic bouts are usually short (less than 2 min). The experiments with changed respiratory gases did not alter this pattern.

The results of this study are interesting in light of later studies that examined the respiratory patterns of freely swimming elephant seals (26). In those later studies, the authors noted that juvenile elephant seals had eupneic breathing rates between free dives of about 19 ± 2 breaths/min. At the highest levels of inspired gases in the manipulative studies, the seal pups respired at about 15 ± 2 breaths/min. This suggests that the postdive respiratory drive at sea may be slightly higher than that induced by $\sim 7\%$ CO_2 inspired gas.

G. Relationships Between Sleep Apnea and Diving

As discussed above, the primary characteristics of diving apnea are bradycardia, significant changes in peripheral vasoconstriction, progressive hypoxia and hypercapnia, alterations in hematocrit, and for long dives, marked production of lactate as a result of hypoxic metabolism in the peripheral tissues such as muscle. A major interpretive complication to studying apnea in the freely diving phocids is that the seals are also exercising: they are swimming underwater while holding their breath. Thus, there is an immediate regulatory conflict between apnea tolerance, which strives to conserve oxygen, and exercise, which increases oxygen utilization. Therefore, we sought to characterize the physiology of sleep apnea to see if it could be used to study the response to diving apnea without the conflicting demands of exercise.

In experiments with Weddell seals, we were able to obtain arterial blood gas measurements and lactate values from sleeping animals (27). PaO_2 values fell to about 25 Torr after 8 min of apnea and $PaCO_2$ increased to almost 60 Torr. These values are almost identical to arterial gas levels in freely diving animals in which postdive carbon dioxide can reach 55 Torr (27) and oxygen tensions can drop to less than 20 Torr (28). Despite this level of hypoxia, lactate levels have never been seen to increase during sleep apnea in elephant seals (29) or Weddell seals (27,28). This implies that the sleep apneic periods are, on balance, aerobic in nature, much like short, aerobic dives. However, the average dive duration is longer than the average sleep apnea duration in Weddell seals (30) and in elephant seals (21).

In a series of experimental laboratory dives with Weddell seals, Elsner et al. (31) were able to show that EEG patterns in the seals did not show any response to hypoxia until arterial tensions fell below 12 Torr. Thus, the EEG patterns in sleeping seals are probably not influenced by progressive hypoxia because it is unlikely that arterial oxygen tensions fall much below about 20 Torr.

In 1980, Kooyman et al. noted that the postdive Hct levels of freely diving seals were always higher than resting values (27) and Qvist et al. (28) were able to show that the Hct started to increase soon after the dive was initiated. Castellini et al. (32) showed that Hct could remain elevated through several bouts of diving. Working with catheterized northern elephant seal pups, Castellini et al. (29) demonstrated that Hct changed in an identical manner during quiet sleep apnea bouts in elephant seals. Subsequent work now suggests that splenic contraction, initiated by neurological inputs associated with the onset of apnea, increase the circulating Hct by moving red blood cells from the spleen to the circulation (33). Clearly, the same mechanisms exist at the onset of sleep apnea as dive apnea and thus, Hct increases accordingly. However, if this is an adaptation that allows more RBCs to be loaded into the circulation to allow for rapid reoxygenation during short surface intervals, then what advantage is it to resting, sleeping seals that can acquire oxygen at any time on the surface? This adaptation may very well be a response to apnea per se and not to the diving or sleeping condition. Thus, the selection pressure may have been to increase Hct for diving apnea, but the neurological control mechanisms for apnea are not specific enough to differentiate sleep for diving apnea. As a consequence, even though there is no metabolic need for it, Hct increases during sleep apnea. Because this hematological change can occur in both diving and sleeping seals, it also implies that being underwater, wetting of the face (stimulation of trigeminal nerves), or increased hydrostatic pressure from diving to depth are not necessary to initiate the response.

Another hallmark of a diving seal is the bradycardia seen upon immersion. The significant reduction in HR in diving mammals was one of the first variables measured in studies of diving (34). Kooyman et al. (35) were able to show that the HR response in freely diving seals was graded to the length of the dive: long dives had lower HRs compared to shorter dives. Bartholomew (2) was the first to note that there was a bradycardia associated with sleep apnea in elephant seals. Subsequent studies have characterized the bradycardia seen during sleep apnea. The most salient features are that the HR declines in sleep apnea in the same manner to about the level seen in most diving species (36,37), the response is instantaneous to the onset of apnea and therefore not driven by hypoxia and hypercapnia (19), and the relationships between HR stability and apnea duration are under developmental influence (17,21,22). These findings suggest that the control of HR during apnea follows patterns similar to the control of splenic contraction; that is, it may have been selected by evolutionary pressure to maximize diving apnea duration, but is not specific enough to separate sleep-induced apnea.

Of some interest is the strong sinus arrhythmia seen in the HR during the eupneic period between apneas in the sleeping elephant seal. In these cases, the instantaneous HR during expiration falls to the same low HR seen during the apnea (16). Thus, in terms of HR control, the argument can be made that the apneic HR occurs during an extremely long expiratory pause. In fact, sleep apnea periods begin on a long expiratory pause (19). The implication is that the control of HR during diving is actually the control of HR during a long expiratory pause with the added ability of the animal to consciously decrease HR to extremely low values if necessary (36).

However it is interpreted, it is clear that the control of circulatory and respiratory adjustments seen during diving and sleep apnea have many common characteristics. Because some species of seals can spend months at sea, it is reasonable to expect that they must sleep at some time. The elephant seals can spend 5–6 months at sea and satellite tracking data show that they are always diving, 24 hours a day, with just short 2- to 3-min surface intervals between dives the entire time. When do they sleep? It must be while they are underwater. Thus, the control mechanisms of diving, sleep, and apnea have become interrelated such that it is virtually impossible to separate them in phocid seals.

H. Relationships to Human Medicine

Despite the convoluted control mechanisms, it is vital to re-emphasize that these patterns of sleep-associated apnea in seals are not respiratory disorders. They are the normal and adaptive responses to living in a marine environment. Thus, they provide evidence of the plasticity of the mammalian respiratory system and provide valuable comparative data for work with humans or other species that are not as apnea and hypoxia tolerant. For example, there is strong developmental control of the sinus arrhythmia during eupnea and the stability of the HR during the apnea. Young seal pups are relatively apnea intolerant and have very poor cardiorespiratory control, as demonstrated by a noisy HR during apnea and very poor sinus arrhythmia. As the pups mature, the eupneic sinus arrhythmia becomes more pronounced and the HR during apnea becomes more stable and deeper (17). We have explored this phenomenon in detail in relationship to SIDS and suggested that the development of a stable sinus arrhythmia is evidence of a maturing cardiorespiratory system that can more readily tolerate both long-duration apnea and, more importantly, always correctly signal the end to apnea and the need to rebreathe (37).

IV. Asymmetric EEG Patterns During Sleep

A. History of Observations

Early observations (before 1970) of sleeping patterns in dolphins were the original basis for many years of subsequent study on how these small cetaceans may sleep with only "half a brain." Today, even a quick search of an Internet site with a query about "sleep and marine mammals" will usually yield a list of sites describing how dolphins sleep with one eye open in order to maintain vigilance and that they do not exhibit REM sleep.

As discussed earlier in the section on phocid seals, there are links between sleep state and respiration in dolphins that have coevolved to allow the animal to adapt to the marine environment. As with the seals, cetaceans must swim or float to the surface in order to breathe. When do they sleep, or can they sleep while swimming near the surface in order to breathe?

Three early observations began these studies. In the first, in 1948, McBride and Hebb (1) produced an article on captive dolphin behavior that contained a discussion about sleep. They noted that sleeping dolphins would hang motionless in the water, perhaps floating at the surface, or slightly under, for 30–40 sec and then slowly swim to the surface to breathe. They wrote that "... sleep may be quite profound with only enough motion to provide for respiration and maintaining constant position." Furthermore, "... the eyelids are usually closed or almost so during sleep, but they open a few times a minute or when another animal comes near. ... The eyes during profound sleep remain closed for 15 to 30 sec on average." Notably, they did not discuss a pattern of just one eye open and, because they did not have electrodes on the animals, could not speculate about REM state.

In the second article, a review on the biology of aquatic mammals, Lilly (3) wrote that he observed captive dolphins sleeping with one eye open. Unfortunately, neither of these early papers were able to verify the sleep state. However, they did observe several important points: "sleeping" dolphins seem to be aware of other nearby animals, there are no long periods of apnea, the animals can swim while apparently sleeping, and the often open eyes suggest short sleep states and perhaps some ability to sleep with one eye shut.

In the third early observation, Shurley et al. (38) were the first to place EEG electrodes on a captive pilot whale (*Globicephala scammoni*). They observed an asynchronous and asymmetric EEG, nonconjugate eye movement, and SWS and REM sleep states. During REM, which constituted about 10% of sleep time, they noted marked loss of muscle tone.

Beginning in the 1970s, Russian scientists began a long series of investigations into sleep state that focused on determining the pattern of asymmetric EEGs in marine mammals in relation to breathing, movement, and activity level. They have documented such patterns in cetaceans, sea lions, and manatees. To date, they remain the only research group that has worked on this problem in such detail (6,39) and most of the following discussion focuses on their work.

B. EEG Symmetry Patterns in Cetaceans

Mukhametov, Lyamin, and Oleksenko have recorded EEG patterns from three species of dolphins (bottlenose dolphin, *T. truncatus*; harbor porpoise. *Phocoena phocoena*; and Amazonian dolphins, *Inia geoffrensis*). The primary characteristics of sleep in these species include strong SWS EEG asymmetry, constant motion during sleep (paddling or swimming), and the apparent complete lack of electrophysiological or behavioral evidence for REM sleep (rapid eye movement, muscle atonia, etc.) (6,39,40). By contrast, the pilot whale from the Shurley et al. study (38) showed SWS asymmetry, but a clear REM state. It is not known why the pilot whale may be different from the other three species.

An example of the asymmetric pattern in SWS in shown in Figure 2 for a harbor porpoise (6). Such unihemispheric SWS is the primary type of sleep in dolphins and can last for more than 2 hr. Notably, deep (delta) SWS has only been recorded during asymmetric stages. Detailed recordings from several sections of the brain show that the unilateral stage involves the entire hemisphere and is cortical as well as subcortical. Moreover, the absence of

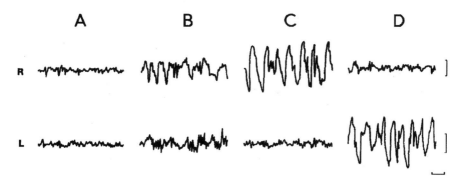

Figure 2 EEG patterns in right (R) and left (L) brain hemispheres in a harbor porpoise. (A) Bilateral desynchronization; (B) bilateral intermediate synchronization; (C and D) unilateral delta waves. Unipolar recording from roughly symmetrical areas of the parietal cortex. Time calibration, 1 sec; amplitude calibration, 200 μV. (From Ref. 6.)

sleep in one hemisphere is not compensated for by sleep in the other hemisphere. Sleep recovery occurs independently.

The evidence for marked EEG SWS asymmetry seems substantial for the species studied, but what is the adaptive need for this type of brain activity during sleep? To best discuss that question, it is necessary to examine the other two primary aspects of dolphin sleep: REM and swimming.

Electrophysiological evidence of REM state has never been recorded in any dolphin species (39) with the exception of the pilot whale (38). From the earliest references of small dolphin behavior, all authors have always noted almost constant levels of activity and swimming when the animals were apparently sleeping. In one of the latest studies of diurnal behavior of captive white-sided dolphins (*Lagenorhynchus obliquidens*), Goley (41) recorded constant swimming whether the animals were awake or behaviorally sleeping. If sleep swimming can only occur during SWS (because of the muscle atonia associated with REM) and if the animals must constantly swim to stay near the surface to breathe, then it follows that REM sleep would be extremely rare for these pelagic species. Clearly, although it is not necessary for these animals to remain motionless for them to sleep, it would be interesting to see if manipulating motion state impacted sleep state. For example, one could assess the sleep state of a small dolphin that was in a very shallow tank or perhaps in a stretcher for transport to see if REM occurred when the animal did not need to swim. Just as the hypoxia and hypercapnia experiments altered sleep state by eliminating REM in elephant seals (19), then perhaps small cetaceans would drop into REM if they did not need to swim—provided, of course, that they are capable of REM sleep under any conditions.

An intriguing aspect of the link between motion and sleep comes from recent visual observations that some of the large cetaceans (sperm whales and humpback whales), may sleep while hanging motionless underwater (S. Moore, personal observation) (42). If this is the case, then it is possible that these species may exhibit REM under those conditions of motionless apnea. To test this idea, Lyamin et al. (39) conducted behavioral sleep observations on a juvenile captive gray whale (*Eschrichtius robustus*) that had the ability to rest quietly underwater in a large enclosure. Although they could not use EEG recorders, they did look carefully for the behavioral signals of REM sleep: apparent muscle relaxation and facial twitching or body jerking. This animal could seemingly enter a sleep state by sinking to the bottom of the tank and resting on the bottom. The authors recorded eyelid movement and body twitching during these sleep periods, which could have indicated REM. Notably, both eyes could be open, but usually one or both were closed. The longest apnea periods were also recorded during this stage (up to

460 sec). The vast majority of respiratory pauses longer than 2 min occurred only in this stage of sleep as opposed to while sleeping near the surface.

Taken together, these data suggest that just as diving and sleep apnea are linked together for the seals, motion, apnea, and sleep state may be linked in the whales. If a whale needs to swim to stay near the surface to breathe, then it probably cannot enter REM. On the other hand, if it can sleep motionless underwater in an apneic state, then REM may be possible. It is not known, however, how this model would fit with the pelagic pinnipeds that also are completely aquatic for portions of their life cycles. Elephant seals exhibit REM when sleeping on land and can swim, like dolphins, during SWS. If the dolphin model suggests that swimming and REM are not compatible, does this imply that elephant seals suspend REM sleep while continually swimming at sea?

C. EEG Symmetry Patterns in Seals, Sea Lions, and Sirenians

Some of the questions involving sleep state, motion, and apnea can be approached by examining the electrophysiological sleep patterns of other species beyond cetaceans. Phocid seals seem to enter REM whether sleeping wet or dry, and have been shown to have bilaterally symmetric EEG patterns. Like phocid seals, northern fur seals have clear SWS and REM sleep stages, but can exhibit delta-stage SWS in either both or single hemispheres (4). This is similar to, but not exactly the same, as the dolphins that never showed bilateral delta-state sleep. Like dolphins, fur seals can also be completely pelagic at certain points in their life cycle. Fur seals, however, show REM whereas dolphins do not. Similar data have been recorded in the Cape fur seal (*Arctocephalus pusillus*) (43). In the wild, fur seals sleep floating at the surface and quietly paddle with one flipper to maintain orientation. The best evidence suggests that the hemisphere controlling the paddling is the awake center (44). Thus, like the dolphins, this would suggest that the motion of swimming requires an awake hemisphere.

The last animal to consider is the totally aquatic Amazonian manatee (*Trichechus inunguis*). Mukhametov et al. (7) did not record an electrophysiological REM state during sleep in this species, but did see muscle atonia, although no rapid body or facial twitching was present. Like the sea lions, this species also showed both interhemispheric asymmetry of SWS and periods of REM.

D. Why Sleep with Only One Hemisphere at a Time?

If dolphins do not enter REM sleep in order to maintain swimming ability, then do they sleep with only one hemisphere at a time in order to maintain awareness of their environment or to facilitate swimming (and breathing)? Many authors have noted that the animals seem aware of their surroundings at all times, that they watch each other (41), or that they maintain the open eye toward an area of stimulus (39). The evidence suggests that sleeping with only one hemisphere does not make up for the lack of sleep in the other (6), so this is probably not an adaptation to maximize sleep time. Oleksenko et al. (45) and Mukhametov and Lyamin (46) presented dolphins with visual stimuli when only one eye was open during apparent sleep swimming. The animals exhibited signs of behavioral arousal when the open eye could see the patterns. These data suggest that visual input from the open eye is processed by the dolphin when exhibiting unihemispheric sleep. Does this mean that the animals are capable of predator or danger awareness when sleeping? As McBride and Hebb (1) noted more than 50 years ago, sleeping dolphins were able to respond when other animals came near.

V. Conclusions

More than 50 years of study indicate that the linking of motion, sleep state, pelagic state, diving, and the option for terrestrial sleep must all be considered together when examining sleep in marine mammals. Because these animals live in the sea, the supposedly simple act of sleeping takes on new requirements. In some species, like the phocid seals, the sleep state and diving state have become so intercontrolled that it is almost impossible to tell a diving seal from a sleeping seal using most physiological or biochemical monitors. For the dolphins, there is a clear adaptation to eliminate REM and to show asymmetric SWS while they are sleep swimming. This makes sense for these pelagic species, but do the seals show the same pattern when they are totally pelagic? The sea lions show asymmetric SWS, but not sleep apnea, and the large whales may show both apnea and, perhaps, REM sleep. How does respiratory drive alter these conditions? The experiments with seal pups breathing low oxygen and high carbon dioxide were able to override REM state, but never apnea. If the large whales can sleep, motionless, at depth, then does this require a different regulation of respiratory drive and sleep than that seen at the surface?

It is clear that the adaptive pressures determining sleep state in these mammals come from many directions and that there remains much more work to do to better explain sleep in these interesting mammals. However, in all cases studied, the ties between respiration and sleep state are normal, adaptive responses to a marine lifestyle. Thus, extended-duration sleep apnea and asymmetric EEG patterns during sleep are not disorders, nor are the mammals dysfunctional. Rather, they are healthy conditions that offer a comparative window into the physiology of respiration and sleep.

References

1. McBride, A. F. and Hebb, D. O. Behavior of the captive bottlenose dolphin, *Tursiops truncatus*. J Comp Physiol Psychol 1948; 41:111–123.
2. Bartholomew, G. A. Body temperature and respiratory and heart rates in the northern elephant seal. J Mammal 1954; 35:211–218.
3. Lilly, J. C. Animals in aquatic environments: adaptations of mammals to the ocean. In: Dill, D. B., Adolph, E. F., Wilber, C. G., eds. Adaptation to the Environment. Washington, DC: American Physiological Society, 1964; 741–747.
4. Mukhametov, L. M., Lyamin, O. I., and Polyakova, I. G. Interhemisperic asynchrony of the sleep EEG in northern fur seals. Experientia 1985; 41(8):1034–1035.
5. Wynne, K. Guide to Marine Mammals of Alaska. Fairbanks, A. K.: Alaska SeaGrant, University of Alaska, Fairbanks, 1992.
6. Mukhametov, L. M. Sleep in marine mammals. In: Borbely, A., Valatx, J. L., eds. Sleep Mechanisms. Berlin: Springer-Verlag, 1984; 227–238.
7. Mukhametov, L. M., Lyamin, O. I., Chetyrbok, I. S., Vassilyev, A. A., and Diaz, R. P. Sleep in an Amazonian manatee, *Trichechus inunguis*. Experientia 1992; 48(4):417–419.
8. Castellini, M. A. The biology of diving mammals: Behavioral, physiological and biochemical limits. In: Gilles, R., ed. Advances in Comparative and Environmental Physiology. Berlin: Springer-Verlag, 1991; 105–134.
9. Castellini, M. A., Davis, R. W., and Kooyman, G. L. Diving behavior and ecology of the Weddell seal: annual cycles. Bull Scripps Inst Oceanogr 1992; 28:1–54.
10. Elsner, R. W. and Gooden, B. Diving and asphyxia: a comparative study of animals and man. Physiological Society Monograph 40. Cambridge: Cambridge University Press, 1983.
11. Kooyman, G. L. Diverse divers: physiology and behavior. Berlin: Springer-Verlag, 1989.
12. Butler, P. J. and Jones, D. R. Physiology of diving of birds and mammals. Physiol Rev 1997; 77(3):837–899.
13. Ridgway, S. H., Harrison, R. J., and Joyce, P. L. Sleep and cardiac rhythm in the gray seal. Science 1975; 187:553–555.
14. Pasche, A. and Krog, J. Heart rate in resting seals on land and in water. Comp Biochem Physiol 1980; 67A:77–83.
15. Huntley, A. C. Relationships between metabolism, respiration, heart rate, and arousal states in the northern elephant seal. Santa Cruz, CA: University of California, 1984. Ph.D. thesis.

16. Castellini, M. A., Milsom, W. K., Berger, R. J., Costa, D. P., Jones, D. R., Castellini, J. M., Rea, L. D., Bharma, S., and Harris, M. Patterns of respiration and heart rate during wakefulness and sleep in elephant seal pups. Am J Physiol 1994; 266:R863–R869.

17. Castellini, M. A., Rea, L. D., Sanders, J. L., Castellini, J. M., and Zenteno-Savin, T. Developmental changes in cardiorespiratory patterns of sleep-associated apnea in northern elephant seals. Am J Physiol 1994; 267:R1294–R1301.

18. Castellini, M. A. Apnea tolerance in the elephant seal during sleeping and diving: physiological mechanisms and correlations. In: LeBoeuf, B. J., Laws, R. M., eds. Elephant Seals. Population Ecology, Behavior and Physiology. Berkeley, Los Angeles, London: University of California Press, 1994; 343–353.

19. Milsom, W., Castellini, M., Harris, M., Castellini, J., Jones, D., Berger, R., Bahrma, S., Rea, L., and Costa, D. Effects of hypoxia and hypercapnia on patterns of sleep-associated apnea in elephant seal pups. Am J Physiol 1996; 271(40):R1017–R1024.

20. Williams, R. and Bryden, M. M. Observations of blood values, heart rate and respiratory rate of leopard seals (*Hydrurga leptonyx*). Aust J Zool 1993; 41:433–439.

21. Blackwell, S. B. and Le Boeuf, B. J. Developmental aspects of sleep apnea in northern elephant seal pups. J Zool 1993; 231:437–447.

22. Falabella, V., Lewis, M., and Campagna, C. Development of cardiorespiratory patterns associated with terrestrial apneas in free-ranging southern elephant seals. Physiol Biochem Zool 1999; 72(1):64–70.

23. Mukhametov, L. M., Supin, A. Y., and Polyakova, I. G. The sleep in Caspian seals (*Phoca caspica*). J High Nerve Activity 1984; 34:259–264.

24. Lyamin, O. I. Sleep in the harp seal (*Pagophilus groenlandica*). Comparison of sleep on land and in water. J Sleep Res 1993; 2:170–174.

25. Lyamin, O. I. Sleep in the harp seal (*Pagophilus groenlandica*). Peculiarities of sleep in pups during the first month of their lives. J Sleep Res 1993; 2:163–169.

26. Le Boeuf, B. J., Crocker, D. E., Grayson, J., Gedamke, J., Webb, P. M., and Blackwell, S. B., et al. Respiration and heart rate at the surface between dives in northern elephant seals. J Exp Biol 2000; 203(pt 21):3265–3274.

27. Kooyman, G. L., Wahrenbrock, E. A., Castellini, M. A., Davis, R. W., and Sinnett, E. E. Aerobic and anaerobic metabolism during voluntary diving in Weddell seals: evidence of preferred pathways from blood chemistry and behavior. J Comp Physiol 1980; 138:335–346.

28. Qvist, J., Hill, R. D., Schneider, R. C., Falke, K. J., Liggins, G. C., and Guppy, M., et al. Hemoglobin concentrations and blood gas tensions of free-diving Weddell seals. J Appl Physiol 1986; 61:1560–1569.

29. Castellini, M. A., Costa, D. P., and Huntley, A. C. Hematocrit variation during sleep apnea in elephant seal pups. Am J Physiol 1986; 251:R429–R431.

30. Castellini, M. A., Kooyman, G. L., and Ponganis, P. J. Metabolic rates of freely diving Weddell seals: correlations with oxygen stores, swim velocity and diving duration. J Exp Biol 1992; 165:181–194.

31. Elsner, R. W., Shurley, J. T., Hammond, D. D. and Brooks, R. E. Cerebral tolerance to hypoxemia in asphyxiated Weddell seals. Respir Physiol 1970; 9:287–297.

32. Castellini, M. A., Davis, R. W., and Kooyman, G. L. Blood chemistry regulation during repetitive diving in Weddell seals. Physiol Zool 1988; 61(5):379–386.

33. Hurford, W. E., Hochachka, P. W., Schneider, R. C., Guyton, G. P., Stanek, K. S., Zapol, D. G., Liggins, G. C., and Zapol, W. H. Splenic contraction, catecholamine release, and blood volume redistribution during diving in the Weddell seal. J Appl Physiol 1996; 80(1):298–306.

34. Irving, L., Solandt, O. M., Solandt, D. Y., and Fisher, K. C. The respiratory metabolism of the seal and its adjustments to diving. J Cell Comp Physiol 1935; 7:137–151.

35. Kooyman, G. L. and Campbell, W. B. Heart rates in freely diving Weddell seals, *Leptonychotes weddelli*. Comp Biochem Physiol 1972; 43A:31–37.

36. Andrews, R. D., Jones, D. R., Williams, J. D., Thorson, P. H., Oliver, G. W., Costa, D. P., and LeBoeuf, B. J. Heart rate of northern elephant seals diving at sea and resting on the beach. J Exp Biol 1997; 200:2083–2095.

37. Castellini, M. A. Dreaming about diving: sleep apnea in seals. News in Physiological Sciences 1996; 11:208–214.

38. Shurley, J. T., Serafetinides, E. A., Brooks, R. E., Elsner, R., and Kenney, D. W. Sleep in cetaceans: the pilot whale, *Globicephala scammoni*. Psychophysiology 1969; 6(2):230.

39. Lyamin, O. I., Manger, P. R., Mukhametov, L. M., Siegel, J. M., and Shpak, O. V. Rest and activity states in a gray whale. J Sleep Res 2000; 9(3):261–267.

40. Mukhametov, L. M. Unihemispheric slow-wave sleep in the Amazonian dolphin, *Inia geoffrensis*. Neurosci Lett 1987; 79(1–2):128–132.

41. Goley, P. D. Behavioral aspects of sleep in Pacific white-sided dolphins (*Lagenorhynchus obliquidens*, Gill 1865). Mar Mamm Sci 1999; 15(4):1054–1064.

42. Robbins, J., Mattila, D. K., Palsboll, P. J., and Berube, M. Asynchronous diving pairs of humpback whales: implications of a newly described behavior observed in North Atlantic wintering grounds. World Marine Mammals Science Conference, 1998; 20–24.

43. Lyamin, O. I. and Chetybrok, I. S. Unilateral EEG activation during sleep in the cape fur seal, *Arctocephalus pusillus*. Neurosci Lett 1992; 143:263–266.

44. Lyamin, O. I., Mukhametov, L. M., and Polyakova, I. G. Peculiarities of sleep in water in northern fur seals. J High Nerve Activity 1986; 34:1039–1044.

45. Oleksenko, A. I., Chetybrok, I. S., Polyakova, I. G., and Mukhametov, L. M. Rest and active states in Amazonian dolphins. In: Sokolov, V. E., ed. The Amazonian Dolphin. Moscow: Nauka, 1996; 257–266.

46. Mukhametov, L. M. and Lyamin, O. I. The Black Sea bottlenose dolphin: the conditions of rest and activity. In: Sokolov, V. E., Romanenko, V., eds. The Black Sea Bottlenose Dolphin. Moscow: Nauka, 1997; 650–668.

AUTHOR INDEX

Italic numbers give the page on which the complete reference is listed.

SUBJECT INDEX

A

Acetylcholine (ACh)
  dose-response curve, 194
  transporter, 76
    protein, 72
Acetylcholinesterase (AChE) inhibitor,
    59
Acoustic-induced sleep fragmentation,
    204–205
Acquired abnormalities, craniofacial
    structure, 10
Actinomycin D, 150
Active glottal closure, spontaneous
    apnea, preterm lamb, 230
Active REM/paradoxical sleep,
    cholinergic modulation, Koch's
    postulates, 60–62
Active sleep
  neural system behavior, 246–247

[Active sleep]
  perinatal period, 241–243
  suppression, 250–251
Acute blood pressure elevation
  episodic eucapnic hypoxia versus
    episodic hypocapnic hypoxia,
    187–188
Adenosine agonists, apnea, 274–276
Adenovirus EIA-associated 300 kDa
    protein, 137–138
Adrenal medulla cells, 129
Adult behavior, neonatal modulation,
    243–246
Adult ventilatory consequences,
    neonatal interventions, 252–254
Adult ventilatory phenotypes
  neonatal experience, 254–257
  neonatal perturbations,
    247–248